**Patient Care in
Pediatric Surgery**

Patient Care in Pediatric Surgery

Lucian L. Leape, M.D.
Professor of Surgery,
Division of Pediatric Surgery,
Tufts University School of Medicine;
Formerly, Chief of Pediatric Surgery,
New England Medical Center, Boston

Little, Brown and Company
Boston / Toronto

Copyright © 1987 by Lucian L. Leape

First Edition

All rights reserved. No part of this book may be reproduced in any form or by any electronic or mechanical means, including information storage and retrieval systems, without permission in writing from the publisher, except by a reviewer who may quote brief passages in a review.

Library of Congress Catalog Card No. 86-82951

ISBN 0-316-51821-2

Printed in the United States of America

MV

To Thomas M. Holder, M.D., partner, mentor, counselor, friend; role model for a generation of pediatric surgeons

Contents

Preface xiii

Surgery of the Neonate

I Care of the Neonatal Surgical Patient

1 Neonatal Surgery 5

2 Neonatal Physiology 9

3 Preparation of the Neonate for Operation 15

4 Operative Care of the Neonate 21

5 Neonatal Postoperative Care 23

6 Troubleshooting Neonatal Emergencies 27

7 Ventilatory Assistance 67

8 Neonatal Nutrition 73

9 Total Parenteral Nutrition 79

II Neonatal Surgical Diseases

10 Respiratory Distress 85

11 Airway Obstruction 89

12 Pneumothorax 93

13 Lobar Emphysema 95

14 Lung Cysts 99

15 Diaphragmatic Hernia 103

vii

16 Esophageal Atresia and Tracheoesophageal Fistula	109
17 Omphalocele and Gastroschisis	117
18 Umbilical Anomalies	123
19 Umbilical Hernia	125
20 Abdominal Masses	127
21 Neonatal Ascites	131
22 Neonatal Gastrointestinal Bleeding	133
23 Intestinal Obstruction	137
24 Duodenal Atresia and Annular Pancreas	141
25 Malrotation	145
26 Jejunoileal Atresia	149
27 Meconium Ileus	153
28 Meconium Peritonitis	157
29 Necrotizing Enterocolitis	159
30 Hirschsprung's Disease	165
31 Imperforate Anus	171
32 Gastrostomy	175
33 Colostomy and Ileostomy	179
34 Ambiguous Genitalia	181
35 Vaginal Anomalies	187
36 Conjoined Twins	191

Surgery of the Older Child

III Care of the Older Child

37 Preparation of the Child for Operation	197
38 Postoperative Care	203

IV Head and Neck

39 Neck Masses	211
40 Cystic Hygroma	219
41 Torticollis	223
42 Thyroid Nodules	227
43 Hemangioma	231
44 Tracheostomy	235

V Chest

45 Endoscopy	241
46 Foreign Bodies of the Airway	247
47 Pectus Excavatum	251
48 Breast Disease	255
49 Mediastinal Masses	257
50 Empyema	263
51 Chylothorax	267
52 Gastroesophageal Reflux	269
53 Achalasia	277
54 Caustic Ingestion	279

VI
Abdomen

55	Foreign Bodies	287
56	Chronic Abdominal Pain	291
57	Pyloric Stenosis	295
58	Gastrointestinal Bleeding	299
59	Peptic Ulcer	305
60	Meckel's Diverticulum	307
61	Gastrointestinal Duplications	311
62	Intussusception	313
63	Appendicitis	317
64	Primary Peritonitis	323
65	Crohn's Disease	325
66	Ulcerative Colitis	329
67	Colonic Polyps	335
68	Constipation	339
69	Rectal Prolapse	345
70	Anal Disorders	347
71	Mesenteric Cysts	349
72	Biliary Atresia and Choledochal Cyst	351
73	Portal Hypertension	357
74	Gallbladder Disease	363
75	Pancreatitis	367

76	Splenectomy	369
77	Inguinal Hernia	373
78	Hydrocele	379
79	Undescended Testis	381
80	Torsion of the Testis	385
81	Circumcision	389

VII Tumors

82	Tumors: General Principles	393
83	Wilms' Tumor	397
84	Neuroblastoma	401
85	Teratoma	405
86	Rhabdomyosarcoma	409
87	Hodgkin's Disease	413
88	Non-Hodgkin's Lymphoma	417
89	Liver Tumors	421
90	Ovarian Tumors	425
91	Adrenal Tumors	429

VIII Trauma

92	Trauma: General Principles	435
93	Head Injuries	439
94	Chest Injuries	443
95	Abdominal Trauma	447

96 Spleen Injuries		451
97 Liver Injuries		455
98 Pancreas Injuries		459
99 Pancreatic Pseudocyst		463
100 Intestinal Injuries		465
101 Retroperitoneal Hematoma		469
102 Urinary Tract Injuries		471
103 Kidney Injuries		475
104 Burns		479
105 Child Abuse		487
IX **Common Procedures**		
106 Vascular Access		493
107 Endotracheal Intubation		499
108 Thoracentesis and Tube Thoracostomy		501
109 Peritoneal Lavage		505
110 Bladder Aspiration		507
X **Appendixes**		
A Drug Dosages		511
B Normal Laboratory Values		514
C Trauma Checklists		515
Index		519

Preface

Patient Care in Pediatric Surgery was written for practitioners, residents, students, and nurses who have limited familiarity with pediatric surgical problems and their management. It is a "what to do" book, not a complete textbook of pediatric surgery. It is designed to provide the information needed to recognize, diagnose, and manage pediatric surgical problems under the supervision of a competent pediatric surgeon. It is intended to be a reference that will enable you to be certain that nothing critical to the optimal management of the infant or child is overlooked.

The first two parts are devoted to Surgery of the Neonate, the remainder to Surgery of the Older Child. Neonates are considered separately because they have different diseases and because of the unique physiologic requirements of newborns, particularly those who were born prematurely.

The introductory chapters should be read first since the information contained therein is not repeated in the chapters on the individual diseases. The chapter on neonatal physiology explains the rationale of therapeutic details. Individual diseases (nearly 100 in all) are presented in a standard format to facilitate rapid reference.

Surgery of infants and children differs from that of adults in several fundamental ways: Children have different diseases, they respond to surgical trauma in different ways, and the physician has responsibility for both patient and parents. Recognizing and managing these differences is the essence of both the art and the science of pediatric surgery. The peculiarities and physiologic limitations of infants demand special care. Their unique strengths make success possible. The vast majority of children undergoing surgery are cured of their affliction and can look forward to a normal life.

Care of the parent is nearly as important as care of the child. Every parent is anxious, and most parents feel guilty about the child's illness. Probably for fundamental biologic reasons, parents are much more anxious about a child's illness than about an equivalent illness in themselves, a spouse, or a parent. Individuals vary greatly in how this anxiety is expressed, but it is never absent, even when the parent seems remarkably "cool." The surgeon's kindness and understanding, as well as competence, are needed.

Little in this book is new. It is merely passed on from those from whom I have learned so much, and to whom I am forever indebted: my teachers, my colleagues, and, most of all, the pediatric and surgical residents who have taught me more than I have taught them. If they find it useful in the everyday care of the sick child, its purpose will be achieved.

L. L. L.

Notice

The indications and dosages of all drugs in this book have been recommended in the medical literature and conform to the practices of the general medical community. The medications described do not necessarily have specific approval by the Food and Drug Administration for use in the diseases and dosages for which they are recommended. Because standards for usage change, it is advisable to keep abreast of revised recommendations, particularly those concerning new drugs.

Surgery of the Neonate

I Care of the Neonatal Surgical Patient

1 Neonatal Surgery

I. **Prematurity.** "The child is not a little man." Nowhere in medicine is this more obvious than in the care of the newborn infant, especially the tiny premature.
   A. **The first few hours** after birth are a period of rapid homeostatic adjustment in which certain organs (such as the lungs) are functioning for the first time. The full-term infant makes this transition easily. The premature infant's immature homeostatic mechanisms respond less well.
   B. **Most newborn infants who require surgery are born prematurely.** Polyhydramnios is a common mechanism in premature infants with obstruction of the gastrointestinal tract.
   C. The recent impressive **reduction in postoperative mortality** of premature infants results from rapid progress in the understanding of neonatal physiology, coupled with the development of highly sophisticated methods of support, particularly nutritional and ventilatory.

II. **Physiologic limitations**
   A. **Stress** of any kind is **poorly tolerated** by premature infants. Chilling, dehydration, hypovolemia, hypoxia, or acidosis can be rapidly fatal. Prevention is the key to successful management.
   B. **Hypothermia occurs easily.** Temperature regulatory mechanisms are poorly developed. The large body surface–weight ratio and lack of insulating subcutaneous fat enhance heat loss.
   C. **Ventilatory insufficiency** may result from airway obstruction, ineffective secretion-clearing mechanisms, hypoventilation, periodic apnea, and decreased surfactant levels, as well as from the numerous diseases common in premature infants: hyaline membrane disease, aspiration, atelectasis, and bronchopulmonary dysplasia.
   D. **Acidosis,** both respiratory and metabolic, is common. Ventilatory insufficiency leads to carbon dioxide retention and hypoxia, which in turn causes tissue hypoxia and anaerobic metabolism.
   E. **Renal insufficiency** is manifested as the inability to concentrate or dilute the urine fully (i.e., lack of tolerance for extremes of solute or water load).
   F. **Hepatic insufficiency** is reflected in limited ability to conjugate or detoxify drugs, maintain blood glucose levels, synthesize coagulation factors, and excrete abnormal bilirubin loads.

III. **Assets.** The premature infant also has significant **strengths**, which help in recovery.
   A. **The cardiovascular system is remarkably resilient.** The heart is developmentally the most mature organ, and the arteries and veins have an elasticity that enables them to adapt to a wide range of vascular volume.
   B. **The brain and heart are more resistant to hypoxia** than those of the older child or adult. Full recovery is common after cardiac arrest.
   C. **Recovery from surgical trauma is much faster** than in adults if appropriate support is provided.
   D. **Wounds heal faster** and with less scar formation.

IV. Principles of management. Although premature infants tolerate most forms of stress poorly, they **tolerate surgical stress** remarkably well—as long as other forms of stress are prevented or minimized. The principles of management are the same as those applied to older children or adults: **Replace losses** and **support failing organ systems.** It is the details of their application that differ.

A. All **fluid losses** must be accurately measured or carefully estimated, including alterations caused by humidified ventilation and radiant heating.

B. **Precision in fluid replacement** is essential, for there is no margin for error.

C. **Medication doses vary,** not only because of the size of the patient, but because of the decreased ability of the immature liver and kidney to detoxify drugs and excrete the breakdown products. Doses must be accurately calculated.

D. **Failing organ systems** are supported by means of ventilatory assistance, radiant heating, parenteral nutrition, and so on.

E. **Constant monitoring** is essential to detect derangements in function so that complications can be prevented or promptly diagnosed and treated.

V. Timing of neonatal operations

A. **Immediately life-threatening conditions** (diaphragmatic hernia, airway obstruction, perforated or infarcted bowel) require immediate operation.

B. **Urgent** conditions are those that are life-threatening but in which an operation can be delayed until the patient is in optimal condition. **Resuscitation is necessary** if there is shock or acidosis from intestinal obstruction, cooling during transport, or hypoxia from inadequate ventilation.

C. **Elective operations** (hernias, asymptomatic masses) should be deferred for a week or so in premature infants.

1. **Priorities of treatment may change** after complete evaluation. For example, a serious cardiac anomaly may take precedence over a non-life-threatening intestinal atresia.

2. The infant should be metabolically **stable** and **growing.**

3. **Anesthetic risk** is greater in prematures. The risk of postanesthetic apnea necessitates careful postoperative monitoring.

VI. Ethical considerations

A. **Congenital malformations are often multiple.** The surgeon is sometimes confronted with a child who has several serious malformations, not all of which are amenable to surgical correction. The question is sometimes raised whether any treatment is appropriate.

B. **Each patient is entitled to individual consideration.** The opinions of all appropriate medical specialists should be obtained before making a recommendation to the parents. Treatment may need to be delayed until chromosome analysis is completed.

C. **Most physical malformations are correctable,** and patients often do far better than their physicians expect initially.

D. **Significant advances** have occurred in both surgical and rehabilitative treatment in the past 20 years. Many children who previously would have been consigned to a caretaking institution live useful and productive lives on their own. More will benefit in the future.

E. **At the present state of our knowledge,** therefore, surgical treatment is appropriate for most newborn infants with reparable lesions unless an uncorrectable condition is present that will result in his early demise or he has no cerebral function (e.g., anencephaly).

VII. Costs

A. Neonatal intensive care is **very expensive**—more than $1000 per day in many institutions. Tiny premature infants may require months of intensive care if they survive. While many subsequently develop normally, others are left with severe disabilities.

B. Society has yet to place this problem in perspective with other expenditures for children, such as for those who are physically sound but disadvantaged and in need of better nutrition or education.

C. On the other hand, it is impossible to know how much we can "afford" to spend on health care.

D. Although his input is critical, the physician is but one of many who should be involved in decisions about allocation of resources. The doctor's primary concern must be to do what is best for the patient, but it is sometimes difficult to know what "best" is.

2 Neonatal Physiology

I. **Prematurity**

   A. The premature infant's response to surgical trauma is significantly different from that of the normal full-term infant. It is essential that anyone who undertakes surgical care of these tiny babies be familiar with their physiologic differences and limitations.

   B. **Immaturity** of organ systems varies as a function of developmental stage. The heart, for example, serves as an effective pump from the twelfth or thirteenth week of gestation, whereas the lungs do not perform their function until birth.

   C. After **26 weeks** of gestation, all organ systems in an otherwise normal premature infant are adequate to sustain life if management is precise and complications are prevented.

   D. It is the **range** of function that is limited. The intestinal and renal systems, for example, will tolerate neither excessive fluid nor high osmotic load. As long as these limits are observed (i.e., as long as feeding or fluid administration is properly calculated and given), the infant will thrive.

II. **Body composition**

   A. One of the major intrauterine events of the last 6–8 weeks of prenatal life is the deposition of **subcutaneous fat**. Consequently, prematurely born infants are deficient in fat, and fluid volumes represent higher fractions of the body weight (see Fig. 2-1).

   B. Fat comprises only **3.5%** of the weight of a 1500-gm infant, compared to 16% in the full-term infant and 23% in an adult male.

   C. **Total body water** comprises more than 80% of the body weight in the tiny premature, compared to 55–60% in an adult.

   D. **Blood volume** represents 10% of body weight in a premature infant, compared to 7½% in a full-term newborn and 6–7% in an adult.

III. **Gestation versus size**

   A. While full-size, normal-weight babies are almost always full-term, small infants are not necessarily premature. Normal weights can be predicted by gestational age. If an infant is smaller than predicted by gestational age, growth retardation has occurred in utero. Such infants are referred to as small for gestational age (**SGA**).

   B. This difference is not merely academic. The low-birth-weight infant who is small for gestational age may have suffered from **intrauterine malnutrition** or **infection** or be afflicted with one or several **congenital anomalies**.

   C. Certain **complications** are associated with severe prematurity, while others are more characteristic of the SGA infant.

   1. **Premature**
      a. Hyaline membrane disease
      b. Hypocalcemia
      c. Poor temperature regulation

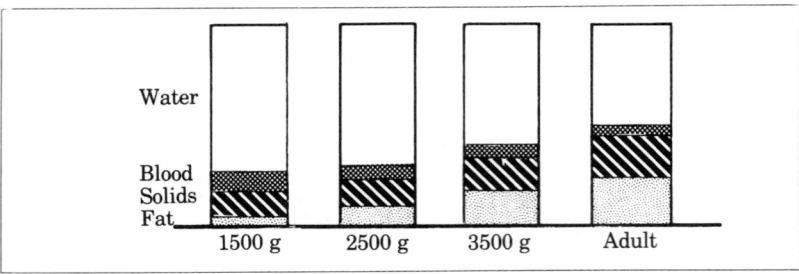

Fig. 2-1. Comparison of body composition of infants and adults.

2. **SGA**
   a. Meconium aspiration
   b. Hypoglycemia
   c. Increased metabolic rate

D. **Estimation of gestational age** is more reliably done by physical examination of the infant than by calculation of maternal dates. The degree of maturation of the skin, ear cartilage, nipples, and genitalia is most useful. The standard neonatology texts give details for such evaluations.

IV. **Temperature regulation**

A. Maintenance of normal core temperature (37.5°C rectal) requires a precise balance of heat production with heat loss. The premature infant is at a disadvantage in both processes.

B. **Heat production** is already considerably greater than that in an adult, when calculated on a body-weight basis, and cannot be readily increased in response to cold stress.

C. **Heat loss** occurs more readily than in the mature organism for several reasons: The **body surface–weight** ratio is much greater, there is much less insulating subcutaneous **fat,** the infant cannot **shiver,** and control of cutaneous blood flow is impaired because of **immaturity of the sympathetic nervous system.** (Readily observed clinically as the "blotchy" skin of the newborn when exposed to cold.) Cutaneous blood flow determines skin temperature, a major factor in heat loss.

D. When the newborn infant is placed in a cool environment, heat loss increases. To maintain body temperature, heat production must be correspondingly increased. The premature infant's ability to do this is significantly impaired.

E. The term **thermal neutrality** refers to that environmental temperature at which metabolic activity (and thus oxygen consumption) necessary to maintain body temperature is minimal, that is, metabolic activity is in the basal state.

F. Significant deviations from this thermal neutral zone overtax the infant's limited compensatory mechanisms and rapidly lead to **hypothermia** or **hyperthermia.**

G. Prolonged cooling does not decrease oxygen consumption but increases it as the metabolic activity rises to maintain body temperature. Increased metabolic work results in exhaustion of body energy stores and accumulation of metabolic breakdown products with acidosis and tissue hypoxia. This leads to **anaerobic** glycolysis, which further contributes to the metabolic acidosis.

H. **Practical considerations**
   1. The major avenue of heat loss is by **radiation** to cooler surroundings. Other mechanisms are **convection** due to cool air currents; **conduction,** if the

infant is in contact with cool equipment, or **evaporation,** if the humidity is especially low. All of these should be controlled for the tiny premature infant.

2. Maintenance of a thermally neutral environment is best accomplished by use of a servo-controlled **radiant heater** with a protective plastic shield to prevent exposure of the infant to cool air breezes. The skin temperature is maintained by a skin thermistor–activated servo-control mechanism.

3. If **ventilatory assistance** is required, the gases must be **humidified** and **heated** to prevent extensive heat loss. The heater must have a fail-safe control mechanism to prevent accidental overheating.

4. The **radiant heater** is far superior to the incubator for the sick infant who requires extensive monitoring and interventions. All procedures (e.g., venipuncture, starting IVs) are done with the unclothed baby exposed to the heater to maintain body temperature.

V. **Nutrition and fluids**

A. The newborn infant requires **100–200 cal/kg/day** for normal growth. This requirement is significantly increased by stress, cold, infection, and trauma.

B. Minimum requirements per kilogram are 3 gm of **protein,** 11–16 gm of **carbohydrate,** and small amounts of essential **fatty acids.** Although these requirements are provided by the usual formulas, the very small premature infant's gastrointestinal tract may be unable to absorb adequate amounts, and supplementation by the intravenous route may be required. If all calories are provided intravenously, adequate growth can be accomplished with fewer calories.

C. **Fluid requirements** change rapidly during the first week after birth. The very low-birth-weight infant (28–32 weeks' gestation) has an extracellular fluid (ECF) volume equal to 50% of his weight. The volume drops to 40% within the first week, catching up to that of the full-term infant.

1. Postnatal reduction in ECF is of high priority, occurring even if there is a large fluid intake. It is probably a major factor in physiologic stabilization of the very small infant during the first week.

2. **Fluid needs are increased** by 50–100 ml/kg/day by the use of **radiant heaters** or **Bililites** or by **low humidity** and decreased by covering the infant with plastic or by humidification of the environment and the inspired gases.

3. Maintenance amounts of fluids are **70 ml/kg/day** for a full-term infant in the first few days of life, increasing to **100 ml/kg/day** after that. Tiny premature infants have high transcutaneous losses and may require twice that amount, depending on the environment in which they are nursed.

4. Once the baby is receiving a full complement of calories by the enteric route, the fluid requirement is 150 ml/kg/day, which is the ratio provided in the standard formulas.

VI. **Gastrointestinal function.** By 28–30 weeks of gestation, the intestinal tract is sufficiently developed to sustain life, but there are significant limitations.

A. **Esophageal motility** is disordered and gastroesophageal reflux is usually present, but these are easily compensated for by feeding in the semiupright position.

B. **Gastric acid** is present at or shortly after birth in all infants of 30 weeks or more of gestational age. Gastric emptying is readily slowed by stress, sepsis, and virtually anything else that bothers the newborn!

C. **Intestinal absorption** of carbohydrates is adequate, but absorption is decreased for fats, partly because of a deficiency of bile salts and lipase. Medium-chain triglycerides are readily absorbed and thus are used for the fat in proprietary "preemie" formulas (Pregestimil, Portagen). Trypsin production increases rapidly in response to feeding, facilitating protein breakdown and absorption.

D. **Practical considerations**
1. Few tiny premature infants have the strength to suck adequate amounts to sustain themselves. **Gavage feedings** must be used. If these are poorly tolerated, parenteral nutrition is required.
2. Virtually any complication—diarrhea, sepsis, congestive failure, surgical stress, CNS disease—may result in disordered gastric and intestinal peristalsis and makes **parenteral nutrition** necessary.

VII. **Hepatic function**
A. The major hepatic deficiency of early and serious significance is in **glycogen storage.** Very premature infants have little energy stored in the liver as glycogen and consequently have difficulty maintaining their blood glucose level. This is particularly true if the baby's mother is diabetic or if the infant is in shock, septic, or asphyxiated at birth. Frequent monitoring and parenteral replacement are required from the first few hours of life.
B. **Conjugation of bilirubin** is impaired in prematures, a disability of particular concern because of the excessive breakdown of red cells in the neonatal period. If there is maternal-fetal red cell incompatibility, increased pigment load may result in severe jaundice. Bile excretion is decreased, as is the enterohepatic circulation of bile.
C. **Protein synthesis,** including albumin and clotting factors, prothrombin, and fibrinogen, is usually adequate even in very tiny premature infants.

VIII. **Cardiac function**
A. If there is no congenital heart disease, the premature infant's greatest physiologic asset is his cardiovascular system. A normal heart can handle intravenous fluids and blood products as necessary provided the administration is precise and appropriate. Heart failure is rare in the absence of heart disease or gross errors in fluid administration.
B. **Persistent fetal circulation (PFC)** may result from the failure of pulmonary vascular resistance to decrease after birth and lead to closure of the foramen ovale and the ductus arteriosus, separating the pulmonary and the systemic circuits.
1. **Prenatal hypoxia** and other factors predispose to PFC by causing pulmonary vascular muscular hypertrophy. If vasospasm is induced by acidosis, hypoxia, hyaline membrane disease, pneumonia, or various types of heart disease, the fetal circulatory state may be reestablished or may persist. Infants with **diaphragmatic hernia** are particularly at risk of PFC.
2. The best treatment is **prevention** of **hypoxia** and **acidosis.** Tolazoline, steroids, dopamine, and chlorpromazine (Thorazine) have been tried with mixed results. Vigorous correction of acidosis, hypoxia, and hypercapnia is more effective. Once established, PFC may be resistant to all therapy.

IX. **Pulmonary function**
A. The premature infant lives on the brink of **acidosis.** Some of it is metabolic but much is respiratory in origin.
B. The infant **airway,** although relatively large compared to body size, is still quite small. Development of even a minor degree of edema can produce a crucial amount of compromise of the tracheal lumen. Small bronchi and their divisions are easily plugged with retained secretions.
C. Because **coughing** and sneezing are absent, mobilization of secretions is also impaired.
D. **Surfactant** is deficient or absent in the extremely premature infant, readily leading to atelectasis.

E. Newborns are obligate **nasal breathers**. Nasogastric tubes thus significantly decrease the airway.

F. Neonates also breathe largely with the **diaphragm**. Anything that increases intraabdominal pressure can rapidly lead to respiratory compromise.

G. **CNS control** of breathing is deficient. Premature infants tend to breathe rapidly and irregularly. Their breathing is shallow, favoring carbon dioxide retention.

H. Decreased **alveolar surface** in proportion to body weight (about half that of an adult) results in the requirement of a higher respiratory rate to accomplish an equivalent amount of oxygen exchange.

I. The net result of these deficiencies is that the newborn premature infant tends to accumulate secretions and **hypoventilate**. He frequently develops atelectasis and much of the time he is in borderline respiratory **acidosis**.

J. More than any other vital function, ventilation must be carefully monitored and skillfully managed if these infants are to survive—even in the absence of a surgical assault. Frequent and expert pulmonary physiotherapy is essential. **Ventilatory assistance** is often required.

K. The premature newborn has a serious predisposition to **retrolental fibroplasia** and blindness caused by high oxygen concentrations. For this reason it is essential that oxygen administration and its effect be carefully monitored so that no more is given than necessary.

X. Renal function

A. Renal function in small premature infants is markedly diminished.

  1. Renal blood flow, glomerular filtration rate, and concentrating ability are decreased in the premature infant. Water excretion, however, is superior to that of adults, a key mechanism in mobilization of the extracellular fluid excess at birth.

  2. Sodium excretion is relatively fixed, so that the premature infant can neither conserve sodium when it is inadequate, nor excrete a sodium load.

  3. The infant has a poor tolerance for water deprivation or excess, salt loss, vomiting, diarrhea, or other conditions that seriously upset the fluid-salt balance.

B. If one stays within the infant's range of function in the management of fluids and solute, however, the infant kidneys will handle their task very well. Thus, fluid therapy must be precise—matching intake with losses and physiologic needs. A high fluid load can be tolerated (as in parenteral nutrition) provided there is adequate solute. It is the extremes of concentrating and diluting that must be avoided.

C. Unlike adults, the infant also has an **obligatory sodium and potassium loss** in the urine. This persists even in the face of electrolyte restriction. IV fluids must contain sodium and potassium as part of the maintenance fluid therapy or the infant will become depleted.

D. Renal function **improves markedly with postnatal age**. Within 2 weeks, the tiny premature doubles his glomerular filtration rate (GFR) and increases concentrating ability. With careful attention to details of fluid and electrolyte administration, renal function is seldom a limiting factor in postoperative care.

XI. **Hypocalcemia.** In addition to hypoglycemia, the major metabolic abnormality that must be monitored and treated is hypocalcemia. It is more commonly seen in premature infants than in SGA infants. Stress, infection, and hypothermia are causes, but it also occurs in unstressed infants. Calcium stores are probably deficient, and calcium needs are immense, if normal fetal accumulation patterns are an accurate guide to postnatal needs in premature infants. Calcium supplementation is necessary.

3 Preparation of the Neonate for Operation

Operations in the first few days of life are, with few exceptions, performed for **life-threatening** conditions. Anatomic malformations may cause early and severe symptoms (diaphragmatic hernia), initially cause no symptoms but rapidly result in serious pathophysiologic changes (imperforate anus), or be asymptomatic and yet require urgent treatment (neuroblastoma).

I. **Environment.** The proper place for optimal care of these infants is a **neonatal surgical center.** The extraordinarily high success rate of modern neonatal surgery results from the combination of professional expertise and equipment found only in such a facility.

   A. **Neonatal surgical care is a team effort** of the highest order, requiring, in addition to the pediatric surgeon, the following professionals:

   1. **Neonatologists** and other pediatric specialists
   2. Competent **residents** in both pediatrics and surgery
   3. Neonatal intensive care **nurses**
   4. Pediatric specialists in **radiology, anesthesia,** and **pathology**

   B. A modern **intensive care unit,** fully equipped with radiant warmers, ventilators, and monitors, is essential.

   C. A **laboratory** capable of performing microdeterminations must be available 24 hours a day.

II. **Transport.** Most infants are born in hospitals that do not have a neonatal surgical center. Thus they need to be moved, sometimes a considerable distance. With modern equipment and properly trained personnel, this can be accomplished expeditiously and safely.

   A. The **referring pediatrician should confer directly** with the responsible **pediatric surgeon** to plan the transfer.

   B. **Preparation for transport** depends on the specific patient problems, but some general principles apply.

   1. **Oxygen** administration is seldom wrong.
   2. **Endotracheal intubation** should be performed if there is any compromise of ventilation.
   3. **Positive pressure** ventilation should be used with great **caution,** particularly in patients with diaphragmatic hernia, pneumothorax, lung cyst, or other conditions in which a tension pneumothorax can easily develop.
   4. **Nasogastric intubation** with a **large catheter** (14F) should be performed in all patients requiring emergency transport to prevent **distention, vomiting,** and **aspiration.**
   5. **Venous access** is essential if the infant is unstable, dehydrated, or hypovolemic, in order to give fluids and drugs as necessary during transport. The umbilical vein should not be used except as a last resort because of the risk of portal thrombosis.
   6. **Arterial blood gas determination** may assist in management of respiratory insufficiency or metabolic acidosis, but it is not necessary to place an arterial catheter before transport.

7. The infant with congenital **diaphragmatic hernia is an exception.** Venous access and arterial gas determinations should be omitted in patients with diaphragmatic hernia because they delay transport and contribute little. The hypoxia and acidosis cannot be significantly improved until the hernia is surgically reduced.
8. A portable **incubator** is essential to maintain **body heat** during transport. Cooling significantly increases the mortality rate in small sick premature infants.

C. **Helicopter transport** is faster than ground ambulance in most cases, particularly in the city at rush hour or over distances greater than 25 miles. With proper equipment, it is safe for infants with respiratory compromise as well as others.

D. **The transport team** must be trained both in resuscitation and in the details of equipment use in the helicopter or ambulance.

III. **Resuscitation.** The unstable infant with respiratory decompensation, hypovolemic shock, or acidosis must be resuscitated before the operation. Although full correction of the physiological abnormalities may not be possible, every effort must be made to **restore oxygenation and tissue perfusion** before operation.

A. **Treatment takes precedence** over diagnosis and evaluation. Hypoxia or hypovolemia must be corrected as soon as possible to prevent irreversible organ damage. This may require treatment before the exact causes are known.

B. **Ventilation is the first priority.** Providing adequate air exchange and oxygenation usually requires endotracheal intubation and ventilatory assistance in the very sick infant, regardless of the disease. Arterial blood gas analysis is essential for ventilatory management. An umbilical or radial arterial catheter is inserted.

C. **Blood volume must be restored** by administration of normal saline solution (**not** 5% D/W or 1/5N saline) as well as plasma and red cells as needed.
1. Adequate **tissue perfusion** is essential for organ function and to combat acidosis. **No patient should be operated on until the blood volume is restored, however sick he is.**
2. **Large quantities of fluid may be required.** The most common error of treatment of hypovolemia is "too little, too slow."
3. **Bolus therapy** (10/ml/kg in 10 minutes) enables the physician to determine the ultimate fluid need. Repeated boluses are given until there is evidence of reexpansion of the blood volume and tissue perfusion: decreasing pulse, rising blood pressure, improved cutaneous circulation (color and warmth), and rising urine output.

D. **Acidosis is corrected** as much as possible.
1. **Respiratory acidosis** is corrected by **adequate ventilation.**
2. **Metabolic acidosis** is corrected by **reexpansion of the blood volume,** which reestablishes tissue perfusion, halting anaerobic metabolism.
3. **Bicarbonate** should also be given (1 mEq/kg/minute), but it is not a substitute for adequate tissue perfusion and ventilation and carries the hazard of producing hypernatremia.

E. **Electrolyte** imbalance and total fluid deficits cannot be fully corrected preoperatively. Restoration toward normal will decrease the anesthetic risk by improving organ function.

F. **Coagulation** abnormalities are corrected by giving fresh frozen plasma, platelets, and vitamin K (1 mg IM).

G. **Antibiotics** are indicated because tissue hypoxia greatly decreases resistance to bacterial invasion. Ampicillin, gentamicin, and clindamycin are effective against most organisms likely to cause infection.

IV. Associated anomalies

A. Prematurity commonly accompanies the devastating maladies requiring surgical treatment in the newborn. Sometimes the mechanism seems clear (e.g., polyhydramnios in high intestinal obstruction), whereas in other instances the reason is unknown.

B. Since major **anomalies are frequently multiple,** other malformations should be suspected and searched for, particularly in organs formed at the same time in embryologic development.

C. Severe associated anomalies may affect the timing of the operation or even the decision to perform it.

    1. **Decompensated congenital heart disease** may require treatment before duodenal or esophageal atresia, for example.

    2. **Operation is not indicated** in infants with hopeless cerebral damage such as anencephaly or fatal chromosomal abnormalities.

V. Assessment of operative risk.
The risk of an operation depends on the ability of the patient's homeostatic mechanisms to withstand surgical and anesthetic stress. A normal, healthy infant can tolerate a major operation without difficulty. A child with shock or severe acidosis may not even survive anesthesia. The risk of an operation in a newborn infant depends on a number of factors, only some of which are under the surgeon's control.

A. The surgical disease. Infarcted bowel from a volvulus causes profound hypovolemia, acidosis, and sepsis. But a simple cyst in the abdomen, or even a tumor, may have no physiologic effect on the baby. In many emergent neonatal surgical conditions, the pathophysiology cannot be corrected until the diseased organ is removed.

B. Associated congenital malformations. Severe prematurity and serious congenital heart disease are examples. Delay in operating may allow significant improvement.

C. The operation itself. Both the stress and the risk of technical mishap are greater with partial hepatectomy than with gastrostomy, for example.

D. Anesthesia. Although a variety of agents are now available for eliminating pain, inducing unconsciousness, and providing muscle relaxation, many are vasodilators, cardiac depressants, hepatotoxins, or bronchial irritants.

    1. Anesthetic drugs should **never** be given to a **hypovolemic** patient. Oxygen may be the only appropriate agent.

    2. Controlled **ventilation** and **oxygenation,** as well as aspiration of tracheobronchial secretions, are positive benefits of properly administered anesthesia.

VI. Timing of operations.
The scheduling of an emergency operation must take all of the preceding factors into account, recognizing that some are improved at the expense of others.

A. Resuscitation—restoration of blood volume and ventilation—is almost always essential. (Exception: congenital diaphragmatic hernia in which resuscitation may be impossible until the hernia is reduced, if then.)

B. The **major threat** to life must take **precedence.** Resection of dead or perforated bowel must precede repair of a serious congenital heart defect, but the latter may take precedence over repair of esophageal atresia.

VII. Preoperative preparation

A. The **objectives** of preoperative preparation are to minimize the risk of operation and optimize the outcome. These are best accomplished by accurate evaluation of all physiologic abnormalities and correction of as many as possible.

B. In the **emergency** patient, one must balance the need for resuscitation against the progressive effects of untreated surgical disease. One corrects what one can, but doesn't take too long doing it!
C. A number of **details** must be attended to. They vary with the urgency of the operation.
   1. **Universal** (required by all patients)
      a. History and physical examination
      b. CBC
      c. Vitamin K, 1 mg IM
      d. Blood samples (infant's and mother's) in the blood bank
   2. **Emergency** (when time is of the essence)
      a. **Diagnostic measures**
         (1) Chest x-ray
         (2) Abdominal and contrast x-rays
         (3) Electrolytes as indicated
         (4) Arterial blood gases as indicated
         (5) Coagulation studies as indicated
      b. **Therapeutic measures**
         (1) Blood volume restored
         (2) Ventilation adequate
         (3) Hematocrit restored
         (4) Beginning correction of acidosis, electrolyte imbalance, and dehydration
         (5) Antibiotics
         (6) Blood typed and cross-matching begun
         (7) Platelets and fresh frozen plasma available
   3. **Elective** (when time is of no concern)
      a. **Diagnostic measures.** Whatever studies are indicated to outline the problem completely.
      b. **Therapeutic** measures
         (1) All physiologic parameters should be restored to normal if possible.
         (2) Nutritional state should be optimal
         (3) Blood should be available if needed.
VIII. **Parents—advice and consent.** It is essential that the responsible surgeon personally explain the problem and the proposed operation to the parents. The circumstances under which this is done and the information imparted vary considerably according to whether the operation is an emergency or elective.
   A. **Emergency operations**
      1. The **circumstances** are poor: The mother is usually in another hospital and the father is distraught. They are appropriately afraid that the child may die. Most have never heard of the disease that now threatens to destroy their child. Family and friends are unable to give much support.
      2. **Consent** is almost a formality. The parents really have no choice in most cases: The child obviously requires an operation.

Ch 3. Preparation of the Neonate for Operation 19

3. Nonetheless, the parents have a right to a **clear explanation** of the problem in lay terms that they can understand, a description of the operation planned, and a discussion of the probable outcome. A detailed listing of potential complications is inappropriate.

4. Most of all, the parents want to hear that their baby will be alright. To the extent that he can honestly give them that assurance, the surgeon should do so.

5. **Repetition** of the explanations of the disease and the operation, with drawings when indicated, should take place after the infant has recovered when the parents are in a more receptive mood.

B. **Elective operations**

1. In non-life-threatening conditions, a fuller explanation of risks and complications is necessary, for the parents must weigh these against the benefits of the operation—there is a choice.

2. The prospect of an operation on their newborn infant is still a source of anxiety for parents. The surgeon must be sympathetic and freely answer all their questions.

3. The surgeon should still make a recommendation. It is unfair to put the entire burden of decision making on the parents. The final decision should be made by the parents in consultation with their pediatrician or family doctor.

4 Operative Care of the Neonate

Contrary to intuitive assumptions, neonates tolerate major surgery well, even better than older children or adults, if they are managed with appropriate regard for their physiologic limitations and needs. Operative deaths rarely occur anymore, except in babies who are in extremis at the time of the operation (e.g., infants with diaphragmatic hernia or perforated intestine).

I. Anesthesia

A. A skillful and knowledgeable anesthesiologist is essential to the safe conduct of a neonatal operation. Advances in anesthesia have all but eliminated "anesthetic risk" if the individual at the head of the table knows what to do and monitors the infant carefully.

B. **Anesthetic agents** are available to provide safely both muscle relaxation and anesthesia while maintaining oxygenation under the most difficult circumstances. **Endotracheal intubation** is almost always indicated for general anesthesia of the neonate.

C. Safe anesthetic management requires not only a high degree of knowledge and skill, but also **early detection** of any adverse physiologic response of the infant so that prompt corrective measures can be taken and disaster averted. Hypovolemia, hypoxia, myocardial depression, and other surgical-anesthetic consequences do not happen suddenly but have early warning signals that are easily recognized by the alert and knowledgeable physician.

D. **Monitoring** is the secret to successful anesthetic management. Temperature, heart rate, arterial pressure, arterial oxygen and carbon dioxide, and carbon dioxide in the exhaled gases are routinely measured continuously.

E. Proper functioning of **equipment** is also monitored by measurements of the pressure, temperature, humidity, and oxygen content of administered gases. Rates of fluid administration are controlled and monitored as well.

II. Temperature control

A. Because of the lack of insulating fat, poor circulatory control, and high surface-weight ratio, the neonate loses heat more rapidly than he can generate it. Hypothermia has profound, potentially lethal, effects on many physiologic responses to trauma and must be prevented. If possible, core temperature should be normal prior to making the incision.

B. Multiple measures are taken to **prevent hypothermia.**

1. The core (rectal) **temperature** is **monitored continuously.**
2. A **radiant heater** with skin thermistor servocontrol is used to maintain temperature during the induction of anesthesia, insertion of venous lines, and preparation and draping.
3. A **warming-cooling blanket** must be used under every patient.
4. **Room temperature** is kept high (85–90°F).
5. Inspired anesthetic **gases** are humidified and **warmed** (and monitored to ensure against accidental overwarming).
6. Intravenous **fluids,** blood, and plasma are warmed before administration.

7. **Exposed intestines** are covered with frequently changed warm, wet laparotomy pads to prevent both heat loss and cooling from evaporative water loss.

8. In an emergency, instillation of **warmed saline** into the peritoneal or pleural cavity is effective in raising the body temperature.

III. **Vascular access**

   A. **Reliable venous access** via percutaneous indwelling plastic cannulas is necessary for the instant administration of drugs, fluids, and blood during the operation. Cutdowns should be avoided if possible since they have no advantage over percutaneous catheters but permanently destroy the vein.

   B. Placement of a **central venous (right atrial) catheter** prior to the operation is usually advisable. It permits easy sampling, rapid fluid administration, and monitoring of central venous pressure. It can serve these same purposes postoperatively as well as providing a route for parenteral nutrition.

   C. **Blood replacement** is indicated when loss exceeds 10% of the estimated blood volume. In a small premature infant, therefore, replacement may be necessary when blood loss is as little as 10 ml. Plasma may be used initially if the hematocrit is high.

   D. The development of reliable **transcutaneous** monitoring devices has greatly decreased the need for percutaneous arterial catheters to monitor arterial gases.

IV. **Technical considerations**

   A. **Speed** is no longer a requirement for successful neonatal surgery, now that sophisticated and safe anesthesia is available, but neither should the surgeon dawdle. Like any other surgical procedure, an operation in a neonate should be well thought out in advance and expeditiously executed.

   B. The guiding principle of pediatric surgical technique has traditionally been **simplicity**. Minimal manipulation, single-layer anastomoses, and simple closures are best tolerated by the infant and give superior results.

   C. The need for **gentleness** in the handling of the fragile tissues of the newborn infant cannot be overemphasized. Subserosal hematoma of the bowel and subcapsular hematoma of the liver are readily produced by rough handling and can be disastrous if the coagulation mechanism is abnormal. Dilated ischemic bowel is easily ruptured, and the mesentery can be torn by excessive traction. The infant spleen is readily lacerated by a misdirected retractor. All of these complications are avoidable.

   D. More **delicate instruments** are needed for neonatal surgery, but an extensive array is not necessary. Most operations can be done with standard instruments. It is the skill in their use that counts.

   E. **Transverse incisions** are appropriate for almost every operation, giving better access, a stronger repair, a lower dehiscence rate, and a superior cosmetic result. Closure technique is a matter of the individual surgeon's preference, as a number of methods give equally satisfactory results. Single-layer closure of the abdominal wall with heavy (2-0) absorbable running suture is theoretically sound, efficient, and safe. Steristrip closure of the skin has similar advantages.

Bibliography

Betts, E. K., and Downes, J. J. Anesthesia. In K. J. Welch, et al. (eds.), *Pediatric Surgery*. Chicago: Year Book, 1986. P. 50.

Smith, R. M. Anesthesia and Monitoring. In T. M. Holder and K. W. Ashcraft (eds.), *Pediatric Surgery*. Philadelphia: Saunders, 1980, P. 45.

5

Neonatal Postoperative Care

General principles of postoperative care of the neonatal surgical patient are outlined below. (See Chap. 6 for brief synopses of the essentials of diagnosis and treatment of the common problems of critically ill neonates.)

I. **Neonatal response to surgical trauma**

  A. **Premature infants** tolerate major operations well if they are properly managed within the limits of their physiologic abilities. The endocrine response to surgical trauma in the infant is similar to that in adults, but accelerated. Surgical trauma stimulates adrenal corticoid and catecholamine excretion and the production of ADH causing fluid retention for the first 24–48 hours.

  B. **Protein catabolism** with negative nitrogen and phosphorus balance lasts for several days, followed by stabilization as ADH and adrenal steroid output decline and diuresis occurs.

  C. **Protein synthesis** begins and nitrogen balance turns positive by 5–7 days. Nutritional requirements accelerate. Normal growth and weight gain are to be expected by a week after a major operation.

II. **Intensive care.** Since most neonatal operations are for life-threatening conditions, most surgical neonates are critically ill and require intensive care. Constant care by an experienced nurse and the cooperative assistance of the neonatologist and other pediatric specialists are essential. Much of the success of modern neonatal surgery originates in the neonatal intensive care unit.

III. **Monitoring**

  A. **Vital signs.** Electronic monitoring of heart rate, blood pressure, central venous pressure, respiratory rate, and temperature must be periodically confirmed by physical measurements and recorded. Both surface and core temperature readings are relevant.

  B. **Electronic monitoring of ventilation equipment** (pressure, temperature, oxygen) **and intravenous pumps** is also necessary for prompt detection of malfunction.

  C. **Intake and output** from all sources is carefully measured, recorded, and totaled during each shift to detect changes requiring prompt corrective action.

  D. **Daily weights** are the most useful single item in global assessment of an infant's progress. Graphic display permits instant evaluation and smooths out normal daily variations. A newborn infant should gain an average of **1% of his body weight each day** if nutrition is adequate.

  E. **Clinical assessment**—whether the patient is progressing as expected and "looks right"—is the most important form of monitoring.

IV. **Respiratory care.** Immature lungs and airways are traumatized by intubation, anesthetic gases, and the stress of an operation. Depressed respiration, inability to raise secretions, and poor respiratory mechanics lead to ventilatory insufficiency. Ventilatory assistance is usually needed (see Chap. 7).

V. **Fluid therapy.** While the aim of fluid therapy, replacement of losses, is the same in the postoperative premature infant as in the older child or adult, physiologic differences and effects of other treatments significantly alter the requirements.

  A. **Babies are born with an excess of extracellular water,** which is a physiologic protective mechanism. (Breast milk is not available for the first 2 days.) In a nonoperated infant, loss of this excess fluid in the first week of life produces a decrease in weight of 10–20%.

B. **Radiant heaters and phototherapy lights** increase insensible water loss as much as 100 mg/kg/day. Tiny premature infants (<1000 gm) are most severely affected.

C. **Body water** retained postoperatively and through **"third space" edema** from the operation is not readily available to the circulation, and hormonal effects inhibit the normal postnatal fluid excretion.

D. **Fluid therapy calculations** are based on a number of variables: body weight, gestational age, insensible loss, renal water requirements, and water needs for growth. Extraordinary losses due to radiant heaters, phototherapy, and ventilatory assistance must be factored in. Age is critically important since mobilization of ECF in the first few days of life decreases the need for exogenous water.

E. **Sodium requirements** also vary with age and renal function, but 2 mEq/kg/day is a good starting point for a full-term infant, as is 4–5 mEq/kg/day in an infant of less than 32 weeks' gestation.

F. **Potassium** must be supplied, 1–2 mEq/kg/day, once urinary output is established.

G. On balance, the postoperative infant initially needs less fluid than the nonoperated one, once operative losses and "third space" fluid have been provided for. **Rough guidelines** for maintenance fluids for postoperative neonates (to which is added replacement of unusual losses) are as follows:

Weight	First 24 hr	Second 24 hr	After 48 hr
<1000 gm	100 ml/kg	100 ml/kg	140 ml/kg
>1500 gm	70 ml/kg	80 ml/kg	100 ml/kg

H. **The infusion rate is adjusted** according to response, which is gauged by continuous monitoring. Urine output (>1 ml/kg/hour) and specific gravity, pulse, peripheral perfusion, hematocrit, BUN, and serum electrolytes are followed closely—every 4–8 hours. Body weight is determined every 12 hours. Repeat physical examinations will detect dehydration or edema.

VI. **Nutrition** (see Chaps. 8 and 9).

VII. **Care of the parents.** Because neonatal surgical care frequently occurs in a hospital some distance from where the baby was born, communication with the parents in the immediate postoperative period is often difficult. An extra effort is required to help the parents understand and adjust to their baby's illness.

A. **The surgeon should talk with the family frequently** and keep them informed of the baby's progress—not just after the operation but throughout the postoperative period.

B. **There should be ready and frequent telephone communication** between the mother and the **nurse** taking care of her child. The provision of a direct-line phone number helps a great deal. Frequent progress reports are very reassuring to a mother separated from her child.

C. **The mother should be encouraged to visit the infant** as soon as she is physically able and as often as possible. Early contact is critical to mother-child bonding and is possible even in a critical care setting. **There should be no "visiting hours" for parents.** They are always welcome.

D. **Mothers usually feel responsible** for their child's defects. We often do not know the cause of a congenital anomaly, and when that is so, an effort must be made to reassure the mother that there was nothing she did, thought, ingested, overlooked, or was exposed to that caused the anomaly.

VIII. Genetic counseling

A. Most neonatal malformations are not the result of known hereditary factors, but some are. In either case, it is essential for the parents to know the facts relevant to their child.

B. The timing of counseling is important. In the first few days after the operation, the primary concern is whether the infant will survive. Once survival is established, and before the baby is discharged from the hospital, it is helpful for the parents to meet with the geneticist and have their questions answered.

Bibliography

Cartwright, G. W., and Schreiner, R. L. Major complications secondary to percutaneous radial artery catheterization in the neonate. *Pediatrics* 65:139, 1980.

Committee on Hospital Care and the Pediatric Section of the Society of Critical Care Medicine. Guideline for pediatric intensive care units. *Crit. Care Med.* 11:753, 1983.

Crone, R. K. Acute circulatory failure in children. *Pediatr. Clin. North Am.* 27:525, 1980.

Driscoll, D. J., Gillette, P. C., and McNamara, D. G. The use of dopamine in children. *J. Pediatr.* 92:309, 1978.

Driscoll, D. J., Pinsky, W. W., and Entman, M. L. How to use inotropic drugs in children. *Drug Ther.* 4:39, 1979.

Fineman, A. Emotional Considerations of the Pediatric Surgical Patient. In T. M. Holder and K. W. Ashcraft (eds.), *Pediatric Surgery*. Philadelphia: Saunders, 1980. P. 84.

Hersh, S. P. Psychological Implications of Operations in Children. In K. J. Welch, et al. (eds.), *Pediatric Surgery*. Chicago: Year Book, 1986. P. 125.

Katz, R., Pollack, M., and Weibley, R. Pulmonary artery catheterization in pediatric intensive care. *Adv. Pediatr.* 30:169, 1983.

Kosloske, A. M., and Stone, H. H. Surgical Infections. In K. J. Welch, et al. (eds.), *Pediatric Surgery*. Chicago: Year Book, 1986. P. 78.

Pasnick, M., and Lucey, J. Practical uses of continuous transcutaneous oxygen monitoring. *Pediatr. in Review* 5:5, 1983.

Rowe, M. I. Fluid and Electrolyte Management. In K. J. Welch, et al. (eds.), *Pediatric Surgery*. Chicago: Year Book, 1986. P. 22.

Rowe, M. I., and Petitt, B. J. Management of the Critically Ill Patient. In K. J. Welch, et al. (eds.), *Pediatric Surgery*. Chicago: Year Book, 1986. P. 31.

6   Troubleshooting Neonatal Emergencies

Successful care of neonates undergoing surgery is a team effort of the highest order requiring careful monitoring and competent care by surgeon, neonatologist, and intensive care nurse. Nowhere in the practice of medicine is a prompt and appropriate response to changes in the patient's condition more crucial to successful outcome than in the care of the sick premature neonate.

The purpose of this section is to provide the physician in the neonatal intensive care unit with a tool for making that response: a quick reference guide to pathologic signs, symptoms, and laboratory values. It is a guide, rather than a text. No attempt is made to explain the pathophysiology or the rationale for tests or treatment. The section is designed to help the reader consider all diagnostic possibilities and initiate treatment. The **format** is simple:

I. **Definition** of the abnormality
II. **Signs and symptoms** associated with an abnormal laboratory value
III. **Etiology**—a checklist of possible causes
IV. **Diagnosis**—a checklist of studies indicated to define the cause of the abnormality
V. **Treatment**—what to do immediately as well as later

A few **caveats** are in order first.

1. Remember that problems seldom occur in **isolation**. An abnormal value is a sign of trouble. Evaluate the whole patient and put the symptom, sign, or laboratory value in context.
2. **Repeat laboratory tests** when the results do not "fit." You are treating a patient, not a test. If a result does not make sense, it may be wrong. In most cases there is time to repeat the deviant test before treatment if the infant has no other symptoms.
3. No infant needs all of the diagnostic studies listed. Judgment must be exercised in deciding what is most likely to be rewarding. If you know what is wrong, you may not need to perform any tests.
4. No guide or checklist is a substitute for an understanding of neonatal physiology, neonatal disease, and the response of infants to trauma.

Acidosis (Metabolic)

I. **Definition.** Arterial blood pH less than 7.37, except in the first 24 hours of life, when 7.30 is normal, with PCO_2 near normal, and low HCO_3.

II. **Etiology**

 A. **Poor tissue perfusion** due to a low flow state is the most common cause of acidosis in the neonate who requires surgery. Causes include:

  1. Hemorrhage
  2. Postoperative "third space" fluid sequestration
  3. Diarrhea
  4. Low cardiac output
  5. Inadequate fluid replacement

 B. **Hypoxia**

 C. **Increased acid load**

  1. High casein formulas
  2. Urinary ascites or urocolonic fistula

 D. **Acute renal failure**

 E. **Inborn errors of metabolism**

 F. **Loss of buffering capacity**

  1. Diarrhea, intestinal fistula, cholestyramine administration
  2. Renal tubular acidosis

III. **Diagnosis**

 A. **Review intake and output, fluids,** body weight, and hemodynamic measurements for evidence of low vascular volume.

 B. **Calculate anion gap** (serum $Na - [Cl + HCO_3]$). A value less than 15 indicates loss of buffer.

IV. **Treatment**

 A. **Treat the underlying disorder.**

  1. Poor tissue perfusion must be corrected by administering fluids and improving cardiac output.
  2. Correct hypoxia.

 B. Give **sodium bicarbonate** if acidosis is severe (pH <7.30), 2–4 mEq/kg in 2–4 minutes. Repeat if necessary.

Alkalosis (Metabolic)

I. **Definition.** Arterial blood pH greater than 7.45. Most of the time alkalosis is respiratory in origin.

II. **Etiology**
   A. Contracted ECF volume
      1. Diuretics
      2. Nasogastric suction, vomiting
      3. Diarrhea
   B. Alkali administration, particularly after resuscitation
   C. Bartter's syndrome
   D. Massive transfusion
   E. Hypokalemia

III. **Diagnosis**
   A. Review intake and output, electrolytes.
   B. Measure urinary chloride. If less than 10 mEq/liter, the patient has a contracted ECF volume.

IV. **Treatment.** Correct the underlying disorder.

Apnea

I. **Definition.** Cessation of breathing for **20 seconds** or longer or a briefer episode associated with bradycardia, cyanosis, or pallor.

   A. Between **25 and 50% of premature infants** of gestational age less than 34 weeks will have one or more apneic spells. Premature infants may also have a periodic breathing pattern.

   B. **Apnea occurring at or near term is abnormal and serious.**

II. **Etiology**

   A. **Prematurity**

   B. **Hypoxemia** from any cause
      1. Hyaline membrane disease, pneumonia, pneumothorax
      2. Congenital heart disease
      3. Anemia
      4. Shock

   C. **Metabolic disorders**
      1. Hypoglycemia
      2. Hypocalcemia
      3. Metabolic acidosis
      4. Electrolyte imbalance

   D. Central nervous system causes.
      1. Seizures
      2. Intracranial hemorrhage
      3. Congenital malformations

   E. **Airway obstruction**
      1. Secretions
      2. Head flexion

   F. **Reflexive.** The apnea results from either depression of the respiratory center or from reflex laryngospasm and is triggered by stimulation of the esophagus, pharynx, or larynx.
      1. Nasogastric tube passage
      2. Gastroesophageal reflux

   G. **Drugs**—infant or maternal

   H. **Sepsis**

   I. **Hypothermia or hyperthermia**

III. **Diagnosis**

   A. **All infants of less than 34 weeks' gestation** should be continuously **monitored** for apneic spells and bradycardia until they reach 37 weeks' gestational age. All postoperative neonates should be monitored for at least 48 hours after operation.

   B. **Physical examination and history** of the events preceding the apneic spell will characterize its nature, duration, frequency, and association with other events. Apnea related to feeding, drugs, airway obstruction, or body temperature instability is thus recognized.

C. Institute **continuous transcutaneous PO$_2$ and PCO$_2$ monitoring.**
D. Because apnea is usually a symptom of a serious disorder, especially in a term infant, **all patients** should at the least have an evaluation of the following:
   1. **Arterial blood gases**
   2. **Chest x-ray**
   3. **CBC, Hct**
   4. **Blood glucose, electrolytes, calcium**
   5. **Cultures of blood, urine, secretions, and spinal fluid**
E. Further studies are performed as indicated.
   1. **CNS.** EEG, cranial CT scan, or echoencephalogram
   2. **Reflex abnormality.** Barium swallow, esophageal pH study
   3. **Heart disease.** ECG, echocardiogram
   4. **Pneumogram**

IV. Treatment

A. **Immediately**
   1. Correct any abnormality of ventilation or oxygenation.
      a. Intubate and give ventilatory assistance if necessary.
      b. Provide supplemental oxygen—keep transcutaneous oxygen (PtcO$_2$) normal.
   2. Treat any other underlying disorder (anemia, hyperthermia, electrolyte imbalance, sepsis).
B. **Later**
   1. Symptomatic treatment: tactile stimulation prn.
   2. Drug therapy
      a. Theophylline, 5 mg/kg IV, then 1–3 mg/kg q8h PO or IV. Monitor blood levels after third dose and daily.
      b. Caffeine citrate, 20 mg/kg PO, followed by 5–10 mg/kg daily.
   3. Apneic spells caused by gastroesophageal reflux may respond to positional and dietary (thickened feedings) therapy or use of metoclopramide, 1 mg/kg qid. If spells are life-threatening and clearly due to reflux, fundoplication is indicated.
   4. Recurrent apnea may require a home monitoring program.

Bleeding Disorders

I. **Definition.** Abnormal hemostasis as evidenced by bleeding from venipuncture or surgical incision sites, or blood in the stool or urine in the absence of trauma.

II. **Etiology**
   A. **Vitamin K deficiency**
   B. Disseminated intravascular coagulation (DIC) resulting from:
      1. **Sepsis**
      2. **Shock**
      3. **Necrotizing enterocolitis**
      4. **Hypoxia**
      5. **Renal vein thrombosis**
   C. **Inherited clotting disorders** (e.g., hemophilia, von Willebrand's disease, immune disorders)
   D. **Liver disease**
   E. **Platelet abnormalities**
   F. **Maternal drugs** (phenytoin [Dilantin], phenobarbital, salicylates, sodium warfarin [Coumadin], quinine, quinidine, sulfonamides, thiazides, indomethacin, tolbutamide, calcium channel blockers, digitalis)
   G. **Consumption coagulopathy, hemorrhage, or thrombosis:** surgical, cephalohematoma, intraventricular, retroperitoneal, rupture of spleen or liver

III. **Diagnosis**
   A. **History** of maternal medications, family history of bleeding disorders
   B. **Sick infant:** most likely DIC, infection, or liver disease
   C. **Well infant:** most likely vitamin K deficiency, familial clotting disorders, or immune deficiencies
   D. **Physical findings**
      1. Petechiae, ecchymoses, mucosal bleeding, oozing from venipuncture sites: platelet abnormality
      2. Enlarged spleen: infection, erythroblastosis
      3. Jaundice: liver diseases or infection
      4. Large bruises: clotting factor deficiency, DIC, vitamin K deficiency
      5. Retinal hemorrhages: TORCH infection
   E. **Laboratory tests**
      1. **Apt test** should be performed on blood in the stool or gastric aspirate if it is the only evidence of bleeding, since the blood may be maternal in orgin.
      2. **Platelet count and smear.**
      3. **Prothrombin time (PT).**
      4. **Partial thromboplastin time (PTT).**
      5. **Fibrinogen and fibrin split products** are measured if liver disease or DIC is suspected.
      6. **Bleeding time** if other tests are normal.

Ch 6. Troubleshooting Neonatal Emergencies 33

Table 6-1. Differential diagnosis of bleeding in the neonate

Clinical evaluation	Laboratory studies			Likely diagnosis
	Platelets	PT	PTT	
Sick infant	D	I	I	DIC
	D	N	N	Platelet consumption (infection, necrotizing enterocolitis, renal vein thrombosis)
	N	I	I	Liver disease
Well infant	D	N	N	Immune thrombocytopenia, occult infection, thrombosis
	N	I	I	Vitamin K deficiency
	N	N	I	Hereditary clotting disorder
	N	N	N	Trauma, qualitative platelet abnormality

Key: PT = prothrombin time; PTT = partial thromboplastin time; D = decreased; I = increased; DIC = disseminated intravascular coagulation; N = normal.
Source: Modified from B. E. Glader, Bleeding Disorders in the Newborn Infant. In A. J. Schaffer and M. E. Avery (eds.), *Diseases of the Newborn*. Philadelphia: Saunders, 1977. Chap. 64.

IV. **Differential diagnosis** (see Table 6-1)

V. **Treatment**

   A. **Correction of specific deficiencies**

      1. **Platelets.** 1 U/3kg will raise platelet count above 50,000/cmm.

      2. **Clotting factors.** Fresh frozen plasma, 10 ml/kg q8–12 h. Cryoprecipitate is used if larger amounts are needed.

      3. **Vitamin K.** 1 mg IV.

   B. DIC (see p. 38)

   C. **Consumption coagulopathy,** massive hemorrhage. Correct underlying disorder and transfuse necessary clotting elements and blood.

   D. **Maternal drugs.** Give vitamin K and fresh frozen plasma (FFP) as necessary.

Bradycardia

I. **Definition.** Heart rate less than 85 in first week of life, less than 115 at 8–30 days.
II. **Etiology**
   A. **Hypoxia** is the most common serious cause of bradycardia.
      1. Airway obstruction: secretions, aspiration, plugged endotracheal tube
      2. Pneumothorax, hemothorax
      3. Pneumonia
      4. Ventilator malfunction
   B. **Metabolic acidosis, shock**
   C. **Sepsis**
   D. **Congenital heart disease**
      1. Congestive heart failure
      2. Arrhythmias
      3. Digoxin toxicity
   E. **Increased intracranial pressure**
   F. **Hypothyroidism**
III. **Diagnosis**
   A. **Immediately**
      1. Check adequacy of ventilation, tubes, ventilator.
      2. ECG.
      3. Chest x-ray.
      4. Arterial blood gases.
   B. **Later**
      1. Cultures of blood, urine, secretions
      2. Neurologic examination (is fontanelle tense?); head ultrasound
      3. T3, T4
IV. **Treatment.** Correct the underlying disorder.

Cardiac Arrest

I. **Definition.** Sudden and unexpected cessation of effective circulation in an infant who is not expected to die.

II. **Etiology**

A. **Airway obstruction**—secretions, aspiration, a plugged or displaced tube, or ventilator malfunction—is the most common cause of sudden cardiac arrest.

B. **Hypoxemia.** From prolonged inadequate ventilation, pneumonia, or pneumothorax.

C. **Hypovolemia.** Occult hemorrhage.

D. **Heart disease.** Especially heart failure, arrhythmias, shunting, and severe cyanotic heart disease. Persistent fetal circulation.

E. **Sepsis**

F. **CNS depression.** Anesthetics, narcotics

G. **CNS disease.** Intracranial hemorrhage, edema

H. **Electrolyte imbalance.** Especially bolus potassium treatment

I. **Stressful treatments**

1. Suctioning
2. Chest physiotherapy
3. Sudden change in ventilatory support, oxygen
4. Lumbar puncture
5. Extubation
6. Passage of nasogastric tube, feeding

III. **Diagnosis.** Diagnosis of the cause of the cardiac arrest must proceed simultaneously with resuscitation. Review of the circumstances immediately preceding the arrest will often uncover the cause.

IV. **Treatment.** Cardiopulmonary resuscitation requires a team effort and experience. The senior physician present should be in charge, delegating responsibility for various aspects of care.

A. **Position patient** to permit cardiac and respiratory assistance while maintaining access to airway. Place on a board.

B. **Intube** patient and give artificial ventilation with 100% oxygen.

1. Rate: 30–40/minute.
2. Caution: Excessive pressure will cause a pneumothorax.
3. Verify effectiveness by auscultation of chest.

C. **Connect ECG;** start timer.

D. **Begin closed chest massage.**

1. Place both hands around chest while facing infant. Compress the lower half of the sternum 0.5–1 inch with thumbs.
2. Maintain a rate of 100–120/minute.
3. Check effectiveness of massage by palpation of carotid, brachial, or femoral pulse.

4. Pause to note effectiveness of circulation when electrical activity is reestablished.

5. Do not pause longer than 15 seconds for assessment or for intubation.

E. **Establish venous access** if not already in place. Saphenous or femoral cutdown may be necessary. Continuing cardiac massage prohibits placement of a cervical central line at this point.

F. **Resuscitative drugs** (all IV)
   1. Sodium bicarbonate: 2 mEq/kg, in 2 minutes
   2. Calcium gluconate, 10%: 1–2 ml/kg, 1 ml/minute
   3. Glucose, 50%: 1–2 ml/kg, in 1 minute
   4. Atropine: .03 mg/kg push
   5. Epinephrine: 1 ml of 1:10,000 solution push
   6. Lidocaine: 1 mg/kg, push

G. **Treatment of arrhythmias.** Correction of hypoxia and acidosis is essential for catecholamines to work. Maintain ventilation and circulation. Treat as follows:
   1. Sinus bradycardia: epinephrine
   2. Multifocal (PVCs): lidocaine
   3. Ventricular fibrillation: epinephrine; defibrillation
   4. Ventricular tachycardia: lidocaine; defibrillation

Cyanosis

I. **Definition.** Blueness of the skin, particularly noticeable in the lips and nail beds, associated with low PaO_2.

II. **Etiology**
   A. **Cyanotic heart disease**
   B. **Respiratory distress**
   C. **Congestive heart failure**
   D. **Abnormal hemoglobin**
      1. **Methemoglobinemia** (PaO_2 is normal)
      2. **Polycythemia**

III. **Diagnosis.** Distinction between pulmonary and cardiac causes of cyanosis may be difficult. If the PaO_2 is greater than 150 mm Hg in 100% oxygen, cyanotic heart disease is excluded.
   A. **Cyanotic heart disease**
      1. PaO_2 is usually less than 50 mm Hg in 100% oxygen.
      2. Evidence of heart disease: murmur, ischemic or congested lung fields, cardiac enlargement, abnormal ECG.
      3. Echocardiogram, catheterization as indicated.
   B. **Respiratory distress.** PaO_2 is usually greater than 150 mm Hg in 100% oxygen.
      1. **Primary lung disease.** Respiratory distress, rales, rhonchi, and abnormal breath sounds, CO_2 retention; chest x-ray frequently diagnostic.
      2. **Airway obstruction.** Stridor and respiratory distress are the diagnostic features; may improve with prone position or change of neck position; chest x-ray may be positive.
      3. **Lung compression** (pneumothorax, diaphragmatic hernia, chylothorax). Respiratory distress, shift in cardiac impulse, asymmetric breath sounds, positive transillumination, diagnostic chest x-ray.
      4. **CNS or neuromuscular disorders.** Inadequate respirations, other signs of CNS abnormality. Chest x-ray is normal at first.
   C. **Congestive heart failure**
      1. Chest x-ray shows pulmonary congestion and cardiac enlargement.
      2. Evidence of heart disease by chest x ray, murmur, ECG, echocardiogram.
   D. **Abnormal hemoglobin.** Arterial PaO_2 is normal.

IV. **Treatment.** Most causes of cyanosis in neonates are serious or life-threatening abnormalities and demand immediate diagnosis and treatment.
   A. **Immediately**
      1. Administer 100% oxygen.
      2. Intubate airway and provide adequate ventilation.
      3. Chest x-ray.
      4. ECG.
   B. **Later.** Treatment of the underlying disease.

Disseminated Intravascular Coagulation

I. **Definition.** Disseminated intravascular coagulation (DIC) is a syndrome of **generalized bleeding** resulting from an abnormal activation of the blood-clotting mechanism in which there is consumption of all the clotting factors **(consumption coagulopathy)** and deposition of clots in the microvasculature.

Abnormality	Normal Values
Platelet count decreased	150–400,000/µl
Prothrombin time (PT) increased	11–16 sec
Partial thromboplastin time (PTT) increased	25–40 sec
Fibrinogen decreased	150–450 mg/dl
Fibrin split products elevated	<10 µg/ml

II. **Signs and symptoms**
   A. Bleeding from punctures, wounds, and drains
   B. Gastrointestinal bleeding
   C. Bruising

III. **Etiology**
   A. Sepsis
   B. Shock
   C. Hypoxia
   D. Obstetric complications
   E. Asphyxia
   F. Necrotizing enterocolitis
   G. Renal vein thrombosis
   H. Intestinal infarction
   I. Severe liver disease
   J. Vascular catheters

IV. **Diagnosis**
   A. Examine infant for signs of infection and abdominal complications
   B. Chest x ray for pneumonia
   C. Abdominal x ray for pneumatosis, free air, obstruction
   D. Culture of blood, urine, stool
   E. Arterial blood gases
   F. Ultrasound of abdomen for masses, renal vein thrombosis
   G. Liver function studies

V. **Treatment**
   A. **Treat underlying cause.** Clotting factors can seldom be restored if the causative pathology is not corrected.
   B. **Correct clotting factors** if infant is actively bleeding or if laboratory values are grossly abnormal:
      1. Platelet count less than 20,000
      2. PT more than 25 seconds

3. PTT more than twice control value
4. Fibrinogen less than 75 mg/dl
C. **Platelets.** Give platelet concentrate, 1 U/5 kg body weight.
D. **Give fresh frozen plasma,** 10 ml/kg, to replace prothrombin, fibrinogen, and various other clotting factors.
E. **Repeat** transfusions of platelets and plasma q12h and as necessary to keep the platelet count above 50,000 and the PT and PTT in the normal range.
F. Give **vitamin K,** 1.0 mg IV, to ensure adequate supply.
G. If bleeding persists, **exchange transfusion** with fresh whole blood or packed RBCs with fresh frozen plasma may be necessary.
H. If large-vessel **thrombosis** accompanies DIC, give **heparin,** 25 U/kg followed by 10–15U/kg/hour as a continuous infusion to keep PTT at 1.5–2.0 times normal.
I. **Transfuse fresh whole blood** or packed RBCs.

Edema

I. **Definition.** Fluid in the skin and subcutaneous tissues.

II. **Etiology**
   A. **Generalized edema**
      1. Hypoproteinemia.
      2. Fluid overload.
      3. Renal failure.
      4. Multiple organ failure may result in **sclerema,** a woody, hard, nonpitting fluid accumulation in the skin and subcutaneous tissues.
   B. **Focal edema**
      1. Venous obstruction
         a. Compression from increased intraabdominal pressure (as in repair of omphalocele)
         b. Spasm caused by indwelling catheter
         c. Thrombosis
      2. Wound infection
      3. Trauma
      4. IV infiltration
      5. Congenital lymphangioma, lymphedema

III. **Diagnosis**
   A. Review of history and examination
   B. Serum proteins, electrolytes, creatinine
   C. Venogram occasionally indicated

IV. **Treatment.** Correct the underlying disorder.

Fever

I. Definition. Core temperature (rectal) greater than 38°C.

II. Signs and symptoms
- **A.** Tachycardia
- **B.** Flushing
- **C.** Lethargy
- **D.** Metabolic acidosis
- **E.** Apnea
- **F.** Coma, seizures

III. Etiology
- **A.** Overheating by warmer or incubator, or by Bililites
- **B.** Sepsis
- **C.** Atropine overdose
- **D.** Intracranial hemorrhage
- **E.** Narcotic withdrawal
- **F.** Hyperthyroidism

IV. Diagnosis
- **A.** Check incubator for malfunction.
- **B.** Examine infant for signs of infection, abdominal complications.
- **C.** Review intake and output, medications.
- **D.** Culture blood, urine, stool.
- **E.** Consider spinal tap and culture.
- **F.** Arterial blood gases.

V. Treatment
- **A.** Cool infant by undressing and lowering ambient temperature.
- **B.** Treat cause as appropriate.

Hypercalcemia

I. **Definition.** Serum total calcium greater than 12.0 mg/dl or ionized calcium greater than 6.0 mg/dl.

II. **Signs and symptoms**
   A. Hypotonia and lethargy
   B. Poor feeding
   C. Hypertension
   D. Seizures
   E. Polyuria

III. **Etiology**
   A. **Hyperparathyroidism**
      1. Primary—may be familial
      2. Secondary to maternal hypoparathyroidism
   B. **Nonhyperparathyroid**
      1. Idiopathic
      2. Vitamin D intoxication
      3. Excessive calcium supplementation
      4. Blue diaper syndrome (tryptophan metabolism error)
      5. Fat necrosis

IV. **Diagnosis**
   A. **History**
      1. Familial hypercalcemia, renal stones
      2. Maternal vitamin D ingestion
      3. Birth trauma
      4. "Elfin facies"
   B. **Laboratory:** serum calcium, phosphorus, vitamin D, parathyroid hormone

V. **Treatment**
   A. **Immediately**
      1. IV fluids at 1.5 × maintenance level to increase calcium excretion (D5/1/2NS with 4 mEq KCl/dl)
      2. Furosemide (1 mg/kg q6h) to inhibit tubular resorption of calcium
      3. Phosphate (30–40 mg/kg/day) to maintain serum phosphorus level at 3–5 mg/dl
      4. Treatment for vitamin D intoxication
         a. Calcitonin (5–8 µ/kg q12h IV) to increase renal clearance of calcium
         b. Prednisone (2 mg/kg/day) to increase urinary calcium excretion
   B. **Later.** Total parathyroidectomy may be indicated in severe primary hyperparathyroidism.

Hyperglycemia

I. **Definition.** Blood glucose level greater than 124 mg/dl. Hyperglycemia is detected by **routine monitoring** of blood glucose, which should be performed in all premature infants.

II. **Signs and symptoms**

   A. **Intracranial hemorrhage** may result from **hyperosmolarity** in premature infants.

   B. **Dehydration** and **polyuria** result from **osmotic diuresis.**

   C. **Acidosis** and ketonuria occur if there is true diabetes.

III. **Etiology**

   A. Excessive administration of intravenous glucose

   B. Sepsis

   C. Surgical stress in premature infants

   D. Abnormal responses of the very small (<1000/gm) infant

   E. Ingestion of hyperosmolar formula

   F. Neonatal diabetes mellitus (rare)

IV. **Diagnosis**

   A. Review intake and output, IV contents, and oral formulas.

   B. Is there evidence of sepsis or postoperative complications?

   C. If diabetes mellitus is suspected, check electrolytes, pH, urine glucose, and ketones.

V. **Treatment**

   A. Glucose infusion rate is reduced until blood values return to normal.

   B. Insulin is not necessary unless diabetes is present.

Hyperkalemia

I. **Definition.** Serum potassium of greater than 6.0 mEq/liter.
   A. Serum potassium should be monitored regularly in all sick patients.
   B. ECG. Peaked T waves are seen when serum potassium reaches 6.5 mEq/liter. Higher values lead to shortening of the QT interval and widening of the QRS, which ultimately merges with the T wave.

II. **Signs and symptoms**
   A. Muscle weakness
   B. Ventricular fibrillation or cardiac arrest

III. **Etiology**
   A. Excessive intake
   B. Acidosis
   C. Renal failure
   D. Adrenal insufficiency

IV. **Diagnosis**
   A. Review intake and output.
   B. Arterial blood gases.
   C. Electrolytes, BUN, creatinine.

V. **Treatment**
   A. **Immediately** (if serum K > 7 mEq/liter or QRS is widened)
      1. Calcium gluconate 10%: 0.5–1.0 ml/kg IV in 2–5 minutes with ECG monitoring
      2. Sodium bicarbonate: 1.5–2.0 mEq/kg IV over 5–10 minutes
      3. Normal saline: 10 ml/kg IV
      4. Glucose: 0.5–1.0 gm/kg IV over 15–30 minutes
      5. Insulin: 0.1 U/kg SQ or IV
   B. **Later**
      1. Potassium exchange resins (Kayexalate) 0.5–1.0 gm/kg with 20% sorbitol per rectum
      2. Renal dialysis if appropriate
   C. **Asymptomatic** hyperkalemia with a normal ECG does not usually require specific therapy. Restoration of fluid balance and serum sodium and glucose levels and removal of potassium from IV solutions are sufficient.

Hypernatremia

I. **Definition.** Serum sodium concentration in excess of 150 mEq/liter.

II. **Signs and symptoms**
 A. Frequently none
 B. Irritability
 C. Restlessness
 D. Weight gain
 E. Edema
 F. Full pulse
 G. Tachypnea

III. **Etiology.** Hypernatremia in newborns, like hyponatremia, is usually iatrogenic. Causes include:
 A. Excessive loss of water (fever, use of a radiant heater)
 B. Excessive intake of sodium (administration of hypertonic saline)
 C. Diabetes insipidus

IV. **Diagnosis**
 A. **Review IV fluids.** Has the patient received isotonic saline as the sole intravenous replacement? Was hypertonic saline used?
 B. **Patient's weight.** Has there been a sudden decrease suggesting dehydration?
 C. **Urine osmolality,** specific gravity. Is there evidence of diabetes insipidus?

V. **Treatment**
 A. Estimate the water deficit.
 B. Replace deficit with half normal NaCl slowly (half correction at 24 hours) to avoid sudden shifts with convulsions. Switch to normal maintenance fluids (0.2 NS) when [Na$^+$] approaches normal.

Hypocalcemia

I. **Definition.** Serum total calcium less than 7.0 mg/dl or ionized calcium less than 4.0 mg/dl. **Calcium levels should be measured routinely** in all premature infants and in those with the predisposing factors listed under **Etiology.**

   A. Monitor at 6, 12, 24, and 48 hours of age and when symptomatic.

   B. ECG QT interval can be used for monitoring. A reading greater than 0.2 seconds indicates hypocalcemia.

II. **Signs and symptoms**

   A. Irritability

   B. Jitters

   C. Seizures

   D. Apnea

   E. Chvostek sign usually not present

III. **Etiology**

   A. **Early** (first 3 days of life)
   1. Maternal diabetes, toxemia, hyperparathyroidism
   2. Maternal deficiency of calcium or vitamin D
   3. Prematurity
   4. Asphyxia
   5. Sepsis
   6. Shock
   7. Hypoxia
   8. Respiratory distress syndrome
   9. Bicarbonate therapy
   10. Transfusion with citrated blood

   B. **Late** (after third day of life)
   1. High phosphate diet (cows' milk)
   2. Intestinal malabsorption
   3. Vitamin D deficiency
   4. Hypoparathyroidism
   5. Magnesium deficiency
   6. Renal disease
   7. Phototherapy with white light
   8. Furosemide therapy
   9. Intravenous lipid infusion
   10. High sodium intake

IV. **Diagnosis**

   A. Review antenatal and maternal history.

   B. If infant is premature and responds to treatment, more extensive evaluation may not be necessary.

C. Evaluate overall condition. Is there evidence of sepsis, respiratory compromise, or other serious condition?

D. Review intake and output, feeding formulas.

E. Monitor serum phosphate, BUN, creatinine.

V. Treatment

A. Risks of treatment

1. Rapid infusion of calcium can lead to **cardiac arrest**.
2. **Extravasation** of calcium solutions into the subcutaneous tissues can cause **severe tissue necrosis**.
3. Mixture of calcium with **bicarbonate** results in **precipitation** of calcium carbonate.
4. **Liver necrosis** has resulted from calcium infusion through an umbilical vein catheter.
5. **Intestinal injury** has resulted from infusion of calcium through an umbilical artery catheter.

B. Symptomatic hypocalcemia

1. Give 10% **calcium gluconate** (1 ml = 9 mg of calcium) intravenously, **1 ml/kg**, at the rate of 1 **ml/minute**. The dose may be repeated in 10 minutes if no response is observed.
2. **Monitor QT interval** during infusion, and carefully observe infusion site.
3. Add calcium gluconate to the IV fluid, 5–10 ml/kg/day, to maintain the serum level in the normal range.

C. Asymptomatic hypocalcemia (<7 mg/dl)

1. Add calcium gluconate to the IV fluids, 5–10 ml/kg/day (45–90 mg/kg) in continuous infusion (not bolus), or give orally if the infant is being fed.
2. Give low-phosphate formula (Similac PM 60/40, SMA, breast milk) when the baby is fed.
3. Continue treatment as long as necessary, monitoring serum calcium levels twice daily until normal.

D. Refractory hypocalcemia. Failure of response to intravenous calcium supplementation suggests:

1. Hypomagnesemia (normal magnesium level in newborn is 1.5–2.3 mEq/liter)
2. Renal insufficiency
3. Vitamin D deficiency
4. Hypoparathyroidism

Hypoglycemia

I. **Definition.** Blood glucose **less than 30 mg/dl.** Premature infants may be asymptomatic with levels as low as 20 mg/dl. Dextrostix values are unreliable under 40 mg/dl, so quantitative measurement must be obtained when Dextrostix result in less than 40 mg/dl.

II. **Signs and symptoms.** Symptoms may occur within the first few hours of life or at any time in the neonatal period. Unfortunately, neonates can have very low blood glucose levels without symptoms, so it is essential that blood levels be routinely monitored during the first few days of life in all infants at risk to prevent serious complications, particularly seizures, which are associated with a poor neurologic outcome.

   A. Early
   1. Lethargy
   2. Poor feeding
   3. Weak cry
   4. Tremors
   5. Poor muscle tone

   B. Late
   1. Seizures
   2. Apnea
   3. Cyanosis

III. **Etiology.** Hypoglycemia may result from reduced glycogen stores (RGS), excess insulin production (XSI), or abnormalities in glucose metabolism (AGM).

   A. **Common causes of neonatal hypoglycemia**
   1. Infant of diabetic mother (XSI)
   2. Intrauterine growth retardation (RGS)
   3. Prematurity (RGS)
   4. Sepsis (AGM)
   5. Shock (AGM)
   6. Asphyxia (AGM)
   7. Sudden cessation of high glucose infusion (XSI)
   8. CNS anomalies (AGM)

   B. **Rare causes of neonatal hypoglycemia**
   1. Adrenal insufficiency (AGM)
   2. Nesidioblastosis (XSI)
   3. Insulinoma (XSI)
   4. Beckwith syndrome (XSI)
   5. Leucine sensitivity (XSI)
   6. Maternal chlorpropamide therapy (XSI)
   7. Postexchange transfusion with high-glucose blood (XSI)
   8. Galactosemia, fructose intolerance, pyruvate carboxylase deficiency (AGM)
   9. Glycogen storage disease (AGM)

10. Hypopituitarism (AGM)
11. Aminoacidopathies (AGM)

I. Diagnosis
A. Immediately
1. Obtain quantitative blood sugar level prior to treatment and to confirm Dextrostix value or symptoms.
2. Review antenatal and maternal history.
3. Get blood, urine, cord, and spinal fluid cultures if sepsis is suspected.
4. Obtain arterial blood gases.

B. Later (if metabolic error or tumor is suspected)
1. Urine-reducing substances, amino acids, organic acids
2. Serum insulin
3. Serum enzymes for specific deficiencies

II. Treatment
A. Immediately
1. Draw quantitative blood glucose prior to treatment.
2. **Push** 25% glucose, 1 ml/kg IV, followed by 2 ml/kg over the next 10 minutes.
3. Begin continuous infusion of glucose at 10 mg/kg/minute.
4. Monitor blood glucose by Dextrostix q15min.
5. Adjust infusion rate to maintain Dextrostix readings above 45 mg/dl.

B. Later
1. Blood glucose should be monitored by Dextrostix every 4–6 hours for at least 24 hours after hypoglycemia is corrected.
2. For most infants, 10% D/W infusion is satisfactory for maintenance, but additional glucose may be necessary for several days or until infant can be fed by mouth.

Hypokalemia

I. **Definition.** Serum potassium of less than 3.5 mEq/liter. If hypokalemia is severe, ECG shows ST-segment depression and decreased T-wave amplitude.

II. **Signs and symptoms**
   A. Muscle weakness
   B. Abdominal distention and decreased intestinal motility
   C. Polyuria and polydipsia

III. **Etiology**
   A. Alkalosis
   B. Vomiting, diarrhea, GI suction
   C. Inadequate intake
   D. Renal tubular acidosis
   E. Diuretics

IV. **Diagnosis**
   A. Obtain **ECG**. Hypokalemia requires initial treatment if there are changes.
   B. Review intake and output, medications.
   C. Obtain arterial blood gases.
   D. Get urine pH.

V. **Treatment**
   A. Asymptomatic hypokalemia is corrected by adding KCl to IV solutions, 4 mEq/dl.
   B. Hypokalemia with ECG changes or symptoms requires more rapid IV infusion of KCl, but the rate should not exceed 0.3 mEq/kg/hour.
      1. Replacement solution should not be more concentrated than 80 mEq K/liter.
      2. Monitor the ECG continuously during infusion, and check serum [K^+] frequently.
   C. Treat underlying condition.

Hyponatremia

I. **Definition.** Serum sodium concentration less than 130 mEq/liter.
II. **Signs and symptoms**
   A. **Early**
      1. Vomiting
      2. Lethargy
      3. Pallor
      4. Hypothermia
      5. Dehydration
      6. Weight loss (sodium loss) *or*
      7. Weight gain (water excess)
      8. Edema
   B. **Late**
      1. Seizures
      2. Circulatory collapse: weak pulse, poor capillary refill, low blood pressure, cold pale skin
      3. Coma
III. **Etiology.** Hyponatremia results from either excessive loss of sodium or excessive intake of water.
   A. **Sodium loss**
      1. Vomiting
      2. Diarrhea
      3. Prolonged nasogastric drainage
      4. Intestinal fistula
      5. Intestinal obstruction
      6. Adrenal insufficiency, congenital hyperplasia
   B. **Water excess**
      1. **Water intoxication.** The intravenous administration of salt-free solutions is the **most common cause of hyponatremia in hospitalized patients.**
      2. Inappropriate ADH secretion (particularly postoperatively).
IV. **Diagnosis.** The objective is to determine whether the hyponatremia is caused by **salt loss or water excess,** and to assess its extent.
   A. **Review intake and output.** Most cases of hyponatremia are iatrogenic.
   B. Obtain levels of **urine electrolytes,** osmolality, and specific gravity.
   C. Obtain **patient's weight.** Has there been a sudden increase indicating water retention or a sudden decrease associated with abnormal sodium losses?
V. **Treatment**
   A. **Sodium loss**
      1. First, **calculate sodium deficit:**
         For a newborn: $(140 - [Na^+]) \times .65 \times BW = mEq\ Na^+$

2. If patient is **asymptomatic,** give normal saline in amount calculated to replace one-half of deficit in 8 hours, plus maintenance fluids.
3. **In an emergency** (seizures, coma, lethargy, [Na^+] less than 115) give 3% NaCl slowly (one-half of estimated need in 8 hours).

B. **Water excess**
1. **Asymptomatic** patient. Restrict fluids to less than half of normal maintenance volume, which is given as isotonic saline. A furosemide diuretic may also be given (Lasix, 1 mg/kg).
2. **Emergency** patient. Increase extracellular osmolarity to reverse the water shift. Give 3% NaCl, calculated by the same formula given previously. Give a diuretic.

Ch 6. Troubleshooting Neonatal Emergencies 53

Hypothermia

I. **Definition.** Core temperature (rectal) below 37.0°C. Onset of hypothermia in an infant who is in a constant temperature environment that is thermally neutral is a highly significant sign. Full evaluation is indicated to detect sepsis or a severe metabolic or hemodynamic abnormality.

II. **Signs and symptoms**
   A. Lethargy
   B. Bradycardia
   C. Tachypnea
   D. Abdominal distention
   E. Edema/sclerema
   F. Metabolic acidosis
   G. Hypoglycemia
   H. Hyperkalemia

III. **Etiology**
   A. **Cooling.** Premature infants are unable to regulate body temperature. They must be kept in a **thermally neutral environment,** the temperature at which oxygen consumption is minimal while core temperature is normal.
      1. **Thermally neutral environmental temperatures** vary with age and weight, e.g., at 1 day of age:
         a. Weight: <1200 gm   >2500 gm
         b. Temperature: 34.0°C   32.1°C
      2. **Failure to keep an infant in a thermally neutral environment is the most common cause of hypothermia.**
   B. **Pathologic hypothermia** results from **altered flow states,** principally the following:
      1. Sepsis
      2. Intraabdominal catastrophe
      3. Multiple organ failure
      4. Heart failure
      5. Metabolic acidosis
      6. Neonatal asphyxia

IV. **Diagnosis** (same as for fever)
   A. Check incubator for malfunction.
   B. Examine infant for signs of infection, heart failure, abdominal complications.
   C. Review intake and output, medications.
   D. Culture blood, urine, stool.
   E. Consider spinal tap and culture.
   F. Obtain arterial blood gases.

V. **Treatment**
   A. **Treat the underlying disorder.**
   B. **Warm** infant **slowly** with ambient temperatures no greater than 1.5°C above abdominal skin temperature.

Jaundice

I. **Definition.** Hyperbilirubinemia developing during the first week of life is common and may be **physiologic** or **pathologic**.

  A. **Physiologic hyperbilirubinemia** occurs in a majority of normal infants and is presumed to be the cause of jaundice occurring in the first few days of life as long as the serum bilirubin level does not exceed 7, 9, or 11 mg/dl at 24, 48, or 72 hours of age, respectively. Premature infants often show a more rapid rise in serum bilirubin levels, reaching a maximum on day 5.

  B. **Pathologic hyperbilirubinemia** is suspected in any sick infant and in any neonate in whom the normal maximum values are exceeded. Investigation of possible causes is mandatory.

  C. **Kernicterus** is irreversible brain damage (with mental retardation and spasticity) resulting from hyperbilirubinemia.

   1. **Unconjugated bilirubin is highly toxic to the brain** if it is **unbound** to albumin. Hence it is critically important to prevent high levels of hyperbilirubinemia in the newborn.

   2. The **toxic threshold** level is **lower in prematures** and in the very **sick infant.**

  D. **Conjugated hyperbilirubinemia** (concentration of direct bilirubin > 1.5 mg/dl) is much less common than indirect hyperbilirubinemia but is **always pathologic.**

II. **Signs and symptoms**

  A. **Monitor serum bilirubin levels** in any infant who has:

   1. **Visible jaundice**—daily

   2. **Serious illness,** particularly asphyxia, sepsis, hypoglycemia, hypoxia, or acidosis—twice daily

   3. **Hemolytic jaundice**—every 4–6 hours until it declines

  B. **Hyperbilirubinemia is pathologic if:**

   1. **Jaundice** is noted before **36 hours of age**

   2. **Total serum bilirubin** is greater than **12 mg/dl**

   3. **Direct bilirubin** is greater than **1.5 mg/dl**

   4. **Jaundice persists** longer than **8 days** (2 weeks in a premature infant), even if bilirubin values are in the "physiologic" range

   5. **Serum bilirubin levels are increasing** at a rate of more than 5 mg/dl/day

  C. **Monitor bilirubin binding** by Sephadex filtration or fluorometry if normal threshold values are exceeded.

III. **Etiology**

  A. **Physiologic hyperbilirubinemia**

   1. Increased bilirubin load because of increased number and decreased survival of fetal red cells

   2. Increased resorption of bilirubin from the intestine

   3. Defective clearing of bilirubin from plasma

   4. Defective bilirubin conjugation because of maternal steroids or low levels of UDPGT

  B. **Hematologic disease** (indirect or direct hyperbilirubinemia)

   1. Fetal-maternal incompatibility—ABO, Rh, other

   2. RBC enzyme deficiencies—G6PD, pyruvate kinase

3. Spherocytosis
4. Polycythemia
5. Thalassemia
6. Sulfonamides

C. **Infection**
1. Bacterial—anywhere
2. TORCH

D. **Metabolic disorder**
1. Galactosemia
2. Crigler-Najjar syndrome
3. Hypothyroidism
4. Tyrosinosis
5. Lucey-Driscoll syndrome
6. Infants of diabetic mothers
7. Breast milk jaundice

E. **Prematurity**

F. **Intestinal obstruction**

G. **Enclosed hemorrhage** (e.g., adrenal, cephalohematoma)

H. **Biliary obstruction** (direct hyperbilirubinemia)
1. Biliary atresia
2. Choledochal cyst
3. Cystic fibrosis
4. Alpha$_1$-antitrypsin deficiency
5. Dubin-Johnson syndrome

I. **Hepatocellular injury** (direct hyperbilirubinemia)
1. Shock or hypoxia
2. Drugs
3. Sepsis
4. Hepatitis
5. Prolonged total parenteral nutrition

V. **Diagnosis.** Pathologic hyperbilirubinemia requires urgent diagnosis and treatment to prevent kernicterus or other sequelae.

A. **Clinical**
1. History. Review family history and perinatal events.
2. Physical examination. Look for enlarged liver or spleen and signs of intestinal obstruction, bleeding disorder, internal hemorrhage, shock, or sepsis.
3. Neurologic examination. Look for signs of kernicterus—hypotonia, lethargy, spasticity, opisthotonos.

B. **Laboratory**
1. Serial bilirubin levels, direct and indirect.
2. Coombs' test, typing, Rh for mother and infant; if Coombs' test is positive, identify antibody.

3. If direct bilirubin is under 1.5 mg/dl, evaluate RBCs (morphology, reticulocyte count, and fragility).
4. If direct bilirubin is over 1.5 mg/dl, suspect sepsis or biliary obstruction and order the following:
   a. TORCH screen and urine CMV cultures
   b. Bacterial cultures of blood, urine, spinal fluid
   c. Liver function tests (SGOT, SGPT, alkaline phosphatase, LDH)
   d. Serum alpha$_1$-antitrypsin level
   e. CT scan of liver, biliary ducts
   f. Biliary scan (DISIDA) for patency of biliary tree

V. Treatment

A. Indirect (unconjugated) hyperbilirubinemia

1. Treatment begins when serum bilirubin level approaches 10 mg/dl in a premature infant, 15 mg/dl in infants weighing over 2500 gm.
2. Treat underlying cause if identified.
3. Give phototherapy with fluorescent light (Bililite).
   a. Protect eyes.
   b. Give extra fluid for increased insensible loss.
   c. Monitor temperature continuously.
4. Exchange transfusion is indicated when lesser measures fail and bilirubin levels approach toxic levels: 10 mg/dl in a 1000-gm infant and 20 mg/dl in a full-term infant.
   a. The threshold for exchange is lower in sick infants.
   b. Unbound bilirubin is an indication for exchange.
   c. Early exchange is indicated in erythroblastosis when there is significant anemia or rapidly rising bilirubin.

B. Direct (conjugated) hyperbilirubinemia

1. Infection or metabolic abnormalities are treated if identified.
2. Biliary exploration is often necessary to make a diagnosis, since obstruction cannot be differentiated from hepatitis by laboratory tests in most cases.
   a. DISIDA scan demonstration of no bile excretion is an indication for operative treatment.
   b. Biliary atresia can be treated successfully by portoenterostomy in about 50% of infants if the operation is done in the first 2 months of life.
   c. Choledochal cyst is managed by excision and portoenterostomy.
3. Hepatitis is treated symptomatically.

Jitters

I. **Definition.** Rapid, low-amplitude, nonpurposeful movements resembling a startle reaction, occurring in response to physical or auditory stimulation.

II. **Differential diagnosis.** Jitters must be differentiated from seizures (see p. 62). In the jitters, unlike seizures:

   A. Gaze and eye movements are normal.

   B. There is no clonic jerking.

   C. There is no lateralization.

   D. The movements usually cease with passive flexion of a limb.

   E. The movements do not occur spontaneously, but in response to stimulation.

III. **Etiology.** In most infants the cause of the jitters is not apparent and the symptom disappears spontaneously. The infant may have a diabetic mother. Several serious abnormalities may present as jitters:

   A. Hypocalcemia

   B. Hypoglycemia

   C. Hypoxia

   D. Drug withdrawal

   E. Postasphyxia

   F. Theophylline toxicity

IV. **Diagnosis**

   A. Review maternal history for drug withdrawal, diabetes, and asphyxia.

   B. Perform neurologic examination and observation to differentiate from seizures.

   C. Check serum calcium, blood glucose, and arterial blood gases as indicated.

V. **Treatment.** Treatment is that of the underlying disorder. If investigations are negative, no treatment is needed.

Lethargy

I. **Definition.** Decreased activity: poor feeding, prolonged sleeping (normal premature infants sleep 80–90% of the time), decreased motor activity when awake.

II. **Etiology**
   A. Sepsis
   B. Metabolic acidosis
   C. Hypoglycemia
   D. Hypercalcemia
   E. Hyponatremia
   F. Hypoxia
   G. Hypothermia
   H. Hyperthermia
   I. Occult seizures (postictal)
   J. Intracranial bleeding
   K. Hyperammonemia
   L. Oversedation
   M. Shock

III. **Diagnosis.** True lethargy is often a sign of a serious disease or a surgical complication. Prompt evaluation is necessary.
   A. Arterial blood gases
   B. Blood glucose, electrolytes, calcium, ammonia
   C. Sepsis workup
   D. Chest x-ray
   E. Specific studies as indicated by the prior surgical procedure.

IV. **Treatment.** Correct the underlying disorder.

Oliguria

I. **Definition.** Urine output less than 0.5 ml/kg/hour.
II. **Signs and symptoms.** Usually none.
III. **Etiology**
   A. **Prerenal**
   1. Hypotension: sepsis, hemorrhage, operative
   2. Congestive heart failure (CHF)
   3. Asphyxia
   4. Dehydration
   B. **Renal**
   1. Decreased perfusion caused by hypoxia, sepsis, diarrhea, dehydration, hemorrhage, or shock
   2. Disseminated intravascular coagulation (DIC)
   3. Thromboembolic disease
   4. Nephrotoxins
   C. **Obstructive.** May occur at any level in the urinary tract.
IV. **Diagnosis**
   A. If **obstruction** is suspected:
   1. Catheterize the bladder.
   2. Obtain ultrasound examination of kidneys and bladder.
   B. If a **low flow state** is suspected:
   1. Verify low output by catheterizing bladder.
   2. Give fluid challenge (10 ml/kg in 1 hour) followed by furosemide (Lasix), 1 mg/kg IV. Failure of response suggests parenchymal failure.
   C. **Urine sodium** concentration of 30–90 mEq/liter indicates parenchymal disease.
V. **Treatment**
   A. **Obstruction:** surgical correction
   B. **Low flow state:** fluid administration, correction of underlying problem
   C. **Renal failure:** fluid, sodium, potassium restriction; dialysis as necessary

Respiratory Distress

I. **Definition.** Dyspnea, cyanosis, or abnormal arterial blood gases occurring in an infant who was previously ventilating well.

II. **Signs and symptoms**
   A. **Dyspnea.** Excessive respiratory effort is manifested by increased chest excursions or diaphragmatic movements, flaring of the alae nasi, and agitation.
   B. **Tachypnea**
   C. **Cyanosis**
   D. **Stridor**
   E. **Abnormal arterial or transcutaneous blood gases:** Rising PCO_2 or falling PO_2.

III. **Etiology** (see Chap. 10)
   A. **Airway obstruction**
      1. Retained secretions in major or minor airways with atelectasis
      2. Aspiration of gastric contents
      3. Obstructed endotracheal tube
      4. Tracheomalacia
      5. Vascular ring
   B. **Extrinsic lung compression**
      1. Pneumothorax
      2. Hydro- or hemothorax
      3. Pneumomediastinum (rarely symptomatic)
      4. Lobar emphysema
   C. Lung disease
      1. Hyaline membrane disease (HMD)
      2. Meconium aspiration
      3. Bronchopulmonary dysplasia (BPD)
      4. Pneumonia
   D. **Ventilator malfunction**
   E. **Heart disease**

IV. **Diagnosis**
   A. Immediately
      1. **Assess ventilation.** Is there full and equal air entry into both lungs?
      2. **Is endotracheal tube plugged?**
      3. **Is ventilator working properly?** Manually ventilate patient to be sure.
      4. **Transilluminate chest** if pneumothorax is suspected.
      5. Take **chest x-ray,** upright, to demonstrate air and fluid.
      6. Measure **arterial blood gases.** If it is possible to correct a ventilatory error, do that before obtaining gases.
   B. Later
      1. **Bronchoscopy** may be indicated if there is persistent airway obstruction.

2. **Cardiac evaluation.** ECG, echocardiogram, catheterization as needed.
3. **Barium swallow** if vascular ring or reflux is suspected.
4. **Soft tissue x-rays** of trachea.

V. Treatment

A. Immediately
   1. **Establish adequate ventilation by whatever means** required. Intubate patient if needed.
   2. **Administer 100% oxygen.** Remember to decrease concentration as soon as possible to prevent retrolental fibroplasia and lung damage.
   3. **Aspirate tension pneumothorax** if the patient is **in extremis.** Insert the needle in second to fourth intercostal space anteriorly. Use an Angiocath so that the expanding lung is not lacerated by the needle. Replace the catheter with a chest tube when the situation stabilizes.
   4. **Suction airway** or endotracheal tube to remove secretions.

B. **Later.** Correct underlying disorder.

Seizures

I. **Definition.** Various types of rhythmic muscular activities in neonates are classified as seizures. Repetitive limb motions may be tonic or clonic as in older children, but subtle eye or buccal movements are more common and are easily missed by the unskilled observer.

II. **Types of seizures**
   A. **Subtle:** "normal" activities **(50% of neonatal seizures)**
      1. Sucking, chewing, drooling, yawning
      2. Jerking of the eyes
      3. Cycling or swimming motions
      4. Fluttering of eyelids
      5. Tonic horizontal deviation of the eyes
      6. Tonic posturing of a limb
      7. Apnea
   B. **Focal clonic:** well-localized clonic jerking (good prognosis)
   C. **Tonic:** rigidity, posturing, tonic eye deviation. These are associated with structural brain damage and have a poor prognosis.
   D. **Multifocal clonic:** clonic movements of limbs in random fashion (poor prognosis)
   E. **Myoclonic:** synchronous jerks of the limbs indicating diffuse brain damage (poor prognosis)

III. **Etiology**
   A. **Brain damage (perinatal)**
      1. **Hypoxia**
         a. Most common cause of neonatal seizures.
         b. Causes include fetal distress, asphyxia neonatorum, and meconium aspiration.
         c. Seizures occur in the first 24 hours of life, are difficult to treat, and have a poor prognosis.
      2. **Intracranial trauma**
         a. Traumatic delivery
         b. Cerebral contusion; subarachnoid, subdural, or intraventricular hemorrhage
         c. Usually focal
      3. **Intracranial hemorrhage**
         a. Subarachnoid hemorrhage. Usually seen in premature infants with no history of trauma—second day (good prognosis).
         b. Subdural hemorrhage. Seen in large babies and related to breech deliveries. Usually occurs in first 2 days of life (uncommon).
         c. Intraventricular hemorrhage. Seen in premature infants, usually after hypoxia (poor prognosis).
   B. **Metabolic disorders**
      1. Hypoglycemia

2. Hypocalcemia
3. Hypomagnesemia
4. Hyponatremia
5. Hypernatremia
6. Hyperbilirubinemia
7. Pyridoxine deficiency
8. Aminoacidopathies
9. Hyperammonemia

C. **Infection**
   1. Bacterial meningitis
   2. Viral infections—congenital or acquired (rubella, CMV, herpes, coxsackie)
   3. Toxoplasmosis

D. **Drug withdrawal** (maternal addiction)—heroin, barbiturates

E. **Miscellaneous:** chromosomal abnormalities, cerebral dysgenesis, polycythemia, phakomatoses

F. **Unknown: 5–10%**

IV. **Diagnosis.** Seizures must be differentiated from apneic spells and jitters.

A. **Immediately**
   1. Maternal and perinatal history
   2. Neurologic examination
   3. Serum glucose, sodium, calcium, phosphorus, magnesium, bicarbonate, BUN, bilirubin, ammonia
   4. Arterial blood gases
   5. CBC
   6. Lumbar puncture—protein, glucose, blood, WBCs, culture

B. **Later**
   1. CT scan of skull
   2. TORCH titers—mother and child
   3. EEG
   4. Amino acid screen
   5. Pyridoxine level

V. **Treatment. If seizure activity is continuous, the first priority is to stop the seizures,** since they can cause brain damage by causing hypoxia, increased intracranial pressure, or decreased cerebral blood flow.

A. **Immediate treatment for continuous seizures**
   1. Establish **intravenous** line for medications, fluids.
   2. Maintain **ventilation**—intubate if necessary.
   3. If Dextrostix level is low (below 40), give intravenous 25% **glucose,** 2 ml/kg in 2 minutes and maintain blood glucose level with continuous drip of 10% D/W.
   4. If there is no hypoglycemia or no response, administer **phenobarbital** intravenously, 20 mg/kg, over several minutes.

5. Give phenytoin (Dilantin), 5–10 mg/kg, intravenously over 5–10 minutes if there is no response to the phenobarbital. The dose may be repeated 10 minutes later if necessary.

B. Elective treatment when seizures have stopped

1. Identify and treat the underlying disease if possible.
2. Give phenobarbital to prevent further seizure activity, 20 mg/kg loading dose, followed by 2.5–4.0 mg/kg/day to keep plasma levels in the 15–30 µg/ml range.
3. Phenytoin (Dilantin) may also be necessary.

Tachycardia

I. **Definition.** Heart rate of 200 or more. The normal newborn heart rate is 120 ± 16 at birth, 160 ± 20 after 1 week.

II. **Signs and symptoms**
   A. Irritability
   B. Fussiness
   C. Refusal to feed
   D. Respiratory distress
   E. Cyanosis or pallor

III. **Etiology**
   A. **Sinus tachycardia** is the most common form in a postoperative patient. It may be caused by any of the following:
      1. Stress
      2. Fever
      3. Hypovolemia
      4. Anemia
      5. Pain
      6. Theophylline toxicity
   B. **Congestive heart failure**
   C. **Arrhythmias**
      1. Paroxysmal atrial tachycardia (PAT). May be associated with structural malformations (transposition of the great arteries, tricuspid atresia, Ebstein's anomaly).
      2. Ventricular tachycardia. Associated with hypoxia, shock, electrolyte imbalance, digoxin toxicity, catecholamine toxicity, prolonged QT syndrome.

IV. **Diagnosis**
   A. Obtain ECG.
   B. Review intake and output, medications.
   C. Examine infant for signs of CHF, hypovolemia.

V. **Treatment**
   A. If the infant has sinus tachycardia, correct the underlying disorder.
   B. Seek cardiologic consultation if patient is in congestive heart failure or has an arrhythmia.

7 Ventilatory Assistance

I. **Indications.** Ventilatory assistance by means of a mechanical respirator is indicated whenever a child is unable to maintain satisfactory levels of arterial oxygen (PaO_2) or carbon dioxide ($PaCO_2$).

   A. **Causes of respiratory failure** in neonates
   1. Prematurity (CNS immaturity, apneic spells)
   2. Lung disease: hyaline membrane disease, meconium aspiration, pneumonia
   3. Sepsis
   4. CNS disease, intracranial bleeding
   5. Thoracic operations, particularly cardiac

   B. **Causes of respiratory failure in older children**
   1. Pneumonia, atelectasis.
   2. CNS trauma—inability to maintain ventilation.
   3. Prolonged operations.
   4. Underlying lung disease—cystic fibrosis, bronchopulmonary dysplasia.
   5. Chest trauma with unstable chest wall.
   6. Thoracic operative trauma, particularly cardiac surgery.

II. **Clinical signs of ventilatory failure**
   A. Agitation, restlessness
   B. Air hunger, retractions, flaring, use of accessory muscles
   C. Tachypnea
   D. Cyanosis, lethargy, and fatigue (late signs)
   E. Not moving air adequately

III. **Ventilators.** Both positive and negative pressure ventilators are available. Positive pressure respirators are either pressure controlled or volume controlled.
   A. **Negative pressure ventilators** (the iron lung) are theoretically preferable since they more nearly duplicate the normal respiratory mechanics. However, they require that the child be encased in a chamber, which is cumbersome and interferes with access for other treatments.
   B. **Pressure-controlled ventilators** deliver a continuous flow of warmed humidified gas past the patient's airway with intermittent controlled bursts of increased pressure that expand the lungs.
   1. **Essential characteristics**
      a. Control of pressure, flow, oxygen concentration, rate, and inspiratory:expiratory ratio
      b. Choice of modes: controlled ventilation, intermittent mandatory ventilation, and spontaneous
      c. Capacity to provide continuous positive airway pressure (CPAP) as selected

d. Delivery of warm and humidified gases

e. Pressure, temperature, and oxygen monitors and alarms

2. **Advantages.** Control over pressures and inspiratory:expiratory (I/E) ratio. Continuous flow permits easy, spontaneous respiration by the patient between ventilator breaths.

3. **Disadvantages.** Poor control of tidal volume and difficulty in delivering air when compliance is poor.

C. **Volume-controlled ventilators** deliver a selected volume of gas regardless of airway or lung resistance, within preset pressure limits.

1. **Advantages.** Volume is constant regardless of compliance.

2. **Disadvantages.** Control of inspiratory time is less meaningful, and the machines are more complicated and expensive than pressure-controlled respirators.

IV. **Setting up the ventilator.** Initial settings are those that provide ventilation as noted by respiratory excursion of the chest, air entry by auscultation, and adequate PaO_2. Prior manual ventilation usually gives clues to what is needed.

A. **Oxygen concentration,** or fraction of inspired oxygen **(FiO_2),** is set at 50–100%, depending on the severity of the respiratory distress. It is then reduced to keep PaO_2 in the normal range.

B. **Rate** is set appropriate to age and disease. For a neonate with normal lungs, the rate is 15–20 per minute.

C. **Inspiratory:expiratory ratio** is 1:4–6.

D. **CPAP.** Start at 4 and adjust.

E. If the patient tolerates the respirator poorly, reinstitute manual bag ventilation, adjust the ventilator, and try again.

V. **Controlled ventilation.** In most cases, complete control of ventilation is required initially.

A. **Pancuronium bromide (Pavulon),** 0.1 mg/kg, or morphine, 0.1 mg/kg, is given as needed for muscle relaxation if the patient "fights" the respirator and cannot be adequately ventilated.

B. **Oxygenation (PaO_2)** is controlled by the inspired oxygen concentration (FiO_2) and the efficiency with which it is delivered to the alveoli. The latter depends on inspiratory pressure, inspiratory duration, and CPAP.

1. PaO_2 can be raised by increasing the FiO_2 or the I:E ratio.

2. PaO_2 will increase and $PaCO_2$ decrease if inspiratory pressure is increased or rate is increased.

3. PaO_2 will increase and $PaCO_2$ increase if CPAP is increased.

C. **Carbon dioxide** elimination depends on minute ventilation, the product of tidal volume and rate. $PaCO_2$ can be decreased by increasing the peak inspiratory pressure, decreasing CPAP, or increasing the rate.

D. **Adequate ventilation,** as measured by arterial blood gases, should be achieved with the lowest possible inspiratory pressures and oxygen concentrations because of their known damaging effect on the lungs. High oxygen concentrations are also a cause of **retrolental fibroplasia** in neonates.

E. **Repeated adjustments** according to arterial blood gas determinations are necessary to achieve ideal ventilation.

VI. **Monitoring** is essential for every patient receiving ventilatory assistance.

A. **Arterial oxygen and carbon dioxide** must be monitored frequently at first while establishing the ventilatory parameters. An indwelling arterial catheter may be necessary initially, but use of transcutaneous monitors is satisfactory for long-term following.

B. **Chest x-ray** should be obtained initially to check the position and expansion of the lungs. It is repeated daily for the first few days and any time there is a significant unexplained change in the patient's condition.

C. **Ventilator function** must be continuously monitored to identify promptly problems that can be rapidly life-threatening: pressure (excessively high or low), inspired oxygen concentration, humidity, and temperature.

II. **Weaning from the ventilator.** There are many acceptable techniques, but most involve gradual decrease in the rate of ventilation (intermittent mandatory ventilation—IMV) until the patient is able to maintain normal gases while providing his own ventilation. The patient is then extubated and given supplemental oxygen.

III. **Complications of ventilatory assistance.** Ventilatory assistance is associated with a high incidence of complications. Both human and electronic monitoring are essential to its safe conduct.

A. **Pneumothorax, pneumomediastinum**
1. Signs and symptoms: Sudden clinical deterioration with cyanosis, air hunger, or agitation; unexplained deterioration of blood gases.
2. Diagnosis: Chest x-ray (upright or cross-table lateral) or transillumination.
3. Treatment: Tube thoracostomy; needle aspiration if urgent treatment required.

B. **Endotracheal tube in the bronchus**
1. Signs and symptoms: Poor breath sounds on one side; clinical deterioration with cyanosis, air hunger, or agitation; poor blood gases.
2. Diagnosis: Chest x-ray.
3. Treatment: Reposition the tube.

C. **Decreased cardiac output** due to decreased filling secondary to high pressure ventilation
1. Signs and symptoms: Falling blood pressure, tachycardia, poor peripheral perfusion, falling urine output.
2. Diagnosis: Trial of lower pressure ventilation.
3. Treatment: Decrease pressure, alter I:E ratio.

D. **Lung damage** from pressure, dessication, or oxygen
1. Signs and symptoms: Clinical and chemical worsening.
2. Diagnosis: Increasing opacification on chest x-ray.
3. Treatment: Restore oxygen and pressure toward normal (often not possible); humidify inspired gases.

E. **Airway trauma** from suctioning or the endotracheal tube
1. Signs and symptoms: Bleeding, increased secretions from the endotracheal tube.
2. Treatment: Improved technique, less frequent suctioning if possible. Bronchoscopy may be necessary.

F. **Pulmonary or tracheobronchial infection**
1. Signs and symptoms: Fever, leukocytosis, purulent secretions, deteriorating ventilation.

2. Diagnosis: Purulent secretions, positive culture of endotracheal tube aspirate.
3. Treatment: Antibiotics as indicated by sensitivity studies.

G. Obstruction of the endotracheal tube
1. Signs and symptoms: Difficulty ventilating patient, poor air exchange, increased pressure requirement, clinical and chemical deterioration. May be gradual or sudden.
2. Diagnosis: Inability to pass suction catheter beyond the end of the tube. Sometimes this test is negative because the obstruction is due to a one-way valve effect caused by dried secretions. If another explanation is not rapidly forthcoming, change the tube.
3. Treatment: Change the endotracheal tube.

H. Accidental extubation
1. Signs and symptoms: Clinical and chemical deterioration; breath sounds are not heard and chest does not expand when hand ventilation is attempted. Stomach may be distended.
2. Diagnosis: The patient cannot be ventilated properly. Reintubation is needed even if the diagnosis of accidental extubation cannot be confirmed.
3. Treatment: Reintubation.

I. Tracheal stricture
1. Signs and symptoms: Progressive difficulty in ventilation if the patient is receiving artificial ventilation, stridor and dyspnea if stricture occurs after extubation.
2. Diagnosis: Bronchoscopy.
3. Treatment: Tracheal dilatations. Rarely, tracheal reconstruction is necessary.

J. Ventilator failure, accidental disconnection
1. Signs and symptoms: Sudden clinical and chemical deterioration. Patient is not ventilating; manual ventilation is successful.
2. Diagnosis: Noted by examination of the equipment and performance of a trial of manual ventilation.
3. Treatment: Reconnect or replace ventilator as appropriate.

K. Ventilator alarm failure. Alarms sometimes malfunction or are turned off and forgotten. For this reason, clinical monitoring by an experienced nurse is essential, even when electronic monitors are in use. All alarms should be tested at least daily.

Bibliography

Bartlett, R. H. Respiratory Support. In K. J. Welch, et al. (eds.), *Pediatric Surgery.* Chicago: Year Book, 1986. P. 74.

Downes, J. J., et al. Chronic respiratory failure in infancy: Causes and survival. *Crit. Care Med.* 12:339, 1984.

Finholt D. A., Henry, D. B., and Raphaely, R. C. The "Leak" test: A standard method for assessing tracheal tube fit in pediatric patients. *Anesthesiology* 61:A450, 1984.

Indyk, L. Monitoring. In J. P. Goldsmith and E. H. Karotkin (eds.), *Assisted Ventilation of the Neonate.* Philadelphia: Saunders, 1981. P. 207.

Morgan, W. W. Ventilatory Management. In T. M. Holder and K. W. Ashcraft (eds.), *Pediatric Surgery.* Philadelphia: Saunders, 1980. P. 56.

Raphaely, R. C. Respiratory Support. In K. J. Welch, et al. (eds.), *Pediatric Surgery*. Chicago: Year Book, 1986. P. 68.

Sturgeon, C. L., et al. PEEP and CPAP: Cardiopulmonary effects during spontaneous ventilation. *Anesth. Analg.* 56:633, 1977.

Ziegler, M. M., et al. Sequelae of prolonged ventilatory support for pediatric surgical patients. *J. Pediatr. Surg.* 14:768, 1979.

8 Neonatal Nutrition

The goal of nutritional management is to enable the infant to achieve normal growth and development. Surgical patients have additional metabolic requirements imposed by the stress of the operation. They may also have limitations of absorptive capacity caused by derangements of intestinal anatomy. The following discussion is concerned primarily with premature infants, who make up the largest group of neonatal surgical patients.

I. **Requirements.** Growth requires that enough calories and essential nutrients be provided in a form that can be utilized by the infant, whether by the enteral or parenteral route. Intrauterine rates of accumulation of some substances, such as calcium, far exceed those that can be achieved postnatally with present methods.

A. **Calories**

1. **Amount required**

	kcal/kg/day
Maintenance, including basal metabolism plus activity and some cold stress	60
Growth	25
Total parenteral calorie requirement:	**85**
Feeding (specific dynamic action and fecal loss)	20
Total enteral feeding calorie requirement:	**105**

2. **Maintenance requirements** increase with age in the first 2–3 weeks to 75 kcal/kg/day, so growth may not occur in an older premature infant until he is fed a caloric intake of **120 kcal/kg/day** or more.

3. **Energy requirements** are increased by stress (cold, surgery, infection).

B. **Carbohydrate.** Approximately half (40–60%) of the total calories should be provided as carbohydrate (13–15 gm/kg/day). Lactose is the carbohydrate in breast milk and regular formulas, whereas sucrose and glucose are provided in special formulas for prematures.

C. **Protein.** The requirement is 2.2–4.0 gm/kg/day. Higher amounts result in acidosis and elevation of the BUN, ammonia, and urinary amino acid levels. Lower amounts result in poor growth. Tiny premature infants require high-whey, low-casein formulas because of their deficient metabolism of phenylalanine and methionine, which are high in cows' milk and casein.

D. **Fat.** The requirement is 4–6 gm/kg/day. Most formulas supply about 50% of the total calories as fat. Medium-chain triglycerides (MCT) are used for a significant fraction of fat in formulas for premature infants because long-chain fats are poorly absorbed due to decreased bile salt synthesis.

E. **Minerals**

Mineral	Requirement
Sodium	2–3 mEq/kg/day
Potassium	2 mEq/kg/day
Chloride	2 mEq/kg/day
Calcium	150 mg/kg/day
Phosphorus	75 mg/kg/day
Magnesium	3–4 mg/kg/day
Zinc	300 μg/kg/day
Copper	50 μg/kg/day

Table 8-1. Vitamin requirements

Vitamin	RDA[a]	Infant EDR[b]	Poly-Vi-Sol (1ml)	Tri-Vi-Sol (1ml)
Fat-soluble				
Vitamin A (IU)	1400	250	1500	1500
Vitamin D (IU)	400	200	400	400
Vitamin E (IU)	4.5	0.4mg/gm PUFA	5	
Vitamin K (μg)	12	5		
Water-soluble				
Ascorbic acid	35	10	35	35
Folacin (μg)	30	<50		
Thiamine (mg)	0.3	0.2/1000 kcal	0.5	
Riboflavin (mg)	0.4	<0.5/1000 kcal	0.6	
Pyridoxine (mg)	0.3	9μg/gm protein	0.4	
Niacin (mg)	6	4.4/100 kcal	8	
Vitamin B_{12} (μg)	0.5		2	

[a] Recommended daily allowance (adult).
[b] Estimated daily requirement.
Source: Modified from J. P. Cloherty and A. R. Stark, *Manual of Neonatal Care*. Boston: Little, Brown, 1985. P. 436.

Because they are poorly absorbed, calcium, phosphorus, zinc, and copper are provided in significantly larger amounts than required in infant formulas. The requirement for **iron** is unknown, but supplementation at the rate of 2 mg/kg/day is recommended after the age of 6 weeks.

F. **Vitamins** (see Table 8.1).

II. **Gastrointestinal function.** The ability to supply the necessary nutrients in the extremely small (750–1250 gm) premature infant by the enteral route is limited by the immaturity of the gastrointestinal tract as well as by the narrower ranges of tolerance of the metabolic and excretory systems.

   A. Because **suck** is poor in the tiny infant and **swallowing** function is immature, nursing or taking a bottle is impossible.

   B. **Stomach.** Although acid is produced at birth by infants as young as 28 weeks' gestation, the small size of the stomach and its slow emptying make feeding difficult.

   C. **Pancreas.** Secretion of trypsin and lipase is present by 30 weeks' gestation and seems adequate.

   D. **Liver.** Bile salt production is deficient, rendering lipolysis and absorption of long-chain fatty acids inefficient.

   E. **Intestine.** Absorption of vitamins, carbohydrates, and proteins is usually adequate, but premature infants tolerate an osmotic load poorly, developing distention and bleeding. Hyperosmolar feedings may be a cause of necrotizing enterocolitis.

III. **Enteral feeding.** The provision of nutrients by means of the intestinal tract, if possible, is clearly the ideal method.

   A. **Methods**

      1. **Breast or bottle** feeding is possible in most infants over 32 weeks' gestation. It is the preferred method.

2. **Gavage** feedings are indicated when the infant cannot suck, swallows poorly or has a poor gag reflex, or has heart failure. A small feeding tube is periodically passed through the nose or mouth into the stomach, and the feedings are instilled.
   3. **Continuous nasogastric feeding** may be preferable for the very small infant who does not tolerate intermittent gavage.
   4. **Continuous jejunal tube feeding,** via a polymeric silicone (Silastic) catheter passed through the pylorus, is indicated if the stomach does not empty properly or if there is massive gastroesophageal reflux in a small infant with functional intestine.
   5. **Gastrostomy** is sometimes indicated if the infant has severe neurologic damage and will need tube feedings for a prolonged period.
   6. **Jejunostomy** is an alternative to gastrostomy in which a soft catheter is placed in the jejunum and brought out through an opening on the abdomen. Continuous feeding is required.
B. **Formulas** (see Table 8-2 and 8-3).
   1. **The normal newborn** infant can be successfully fed by maternal nursing or by use of any of the standard proprietary formulas.
   2. **The small premature infant** requires formulas that are low in casein, high in calories (24 instead of 20/oz), have MCT as the source of fat, and have supplemental calcium and phosphorus.
   3. **Caloric supplements** are provided as necessary by adding MCT or glucose polymers (Polycose) to the formula.
C. **Postoperative feeding** is a subject of considerable debate and individual variation in approach. Every surgeon has his own preferences.
   1. The premature infant's intestine adapts slowly to feeding, particularly if it has been distended or injured from prior disease or surgery (e.g., atresia, gastroschisis). Feedings should initially be dilute and given in small amounts, gradually increasing either the volume or concentration as preferred.
   2. One method that has been successful is to start with 3–5 ml/kg of water or electrolyte solution q2h. If this is tolerated (low gastric residuals) one-fourth strength special formula is given, and the concentration increased to one-half strength after a day or two. Volumes of feedings are then gradually increased until the required amount is being accepted. Concentration is then gradually increased as tolerated. This process may take a week or two.
   3. A full-term baby will tolerate regular formulas readily and does not need a gradual and prolonged schedule, provided the intestine is normal.
D. **Problems.** Feedings are stopped and the infant is evaluated for other serious disorders, such as sepsis or necrotizing enterocolitis (NEC), if any of the following signs are noted. Usually these are merely signs of too aggressive feeding—a too rapid increase in the rate or osmolarity of the feeding.
   1. **Increasing gastric residuals**
   2. **Vomiting and distention**
   3. **Diarrhea**
   4. **Blood or glucose** in the stool
Parenteral nutrition (see Chap. 9). Peripheral or central **total parenteral nutrition** (TPN) is used whenever the infant is unable to be **adequately nourished** by the preferred intestinal route. With present-day methods, **even the smallest infant** can

Table 8-2. Formula comparison

Formula	kcal/30ml	gm/dl			mg/liter			mEq/liter			Osm
		Protein	Fat	CHO	Ca	P	Fe	Na	K	Cl	
Breast milk	20	1.1	3.8	6.8	330	150	0.2	7	13	11	300
Regular infant formulas											
Similac 20	20	1.6	3.6	7.3	510	390	1.5	11	20	15	300
Enfamil	20	1.5	3.7	7.0	530	440	1.5	10	17	14	290
Similac 24	24	2.2	4.3	8.5	730	560	1.8	16	28	21	360
Enfamil 24	24	1.8	4.5	8.3	640	530	1.5	12	21	16	340
Similac 27	27	2.5	4.8	9.6	810	620	2	17	32	23	410
Humanized formulas											
Similac PM 60/40	20	1.6	3.8	6.9	400	200	2.6	7	15	7	260
SMA	20	1.5	3.6	7.2	440	320	1.3	6	14	10	300
SMA 24	24	1.8	4.3	8.6	530	390	1.5	8	17	12	360
Premature formulas											
Similac Special Care	24	2.2	4.4	8.6	1440	720	3	15	26	18	300
Enfamil Premature	24	2.4	4.1	9.0	950	480	1.3	14	23	18	300
Specialized formulas											
Isomil	20	2.0	3.6	6.8	700	500	12	13	18	15	250
Prosobee	20	2.0	3.6	6.9	630	500	13	9	21	16	200
Nursoy	20	2.1	3.6	6.9	630	440	13	13	19	10	NA
Nutramigen	20	2.2	2.6	8.8	660	495	12	13	17	13	340
Pregestimil	20	1.9	2.7	9.1	660	440	12	13	19	16	348
Portagen	20	2.4	3.2	5.8	660	495	13	13	20	16	NA

Source: Modified from J. P. Cloherty and A. R. Stark, *Manual of Neonatal Care.* Boston, Little, Brown, 1985. Pp. 430–435.

Table 8-3. Component sources in commercial formulas

Formula	Protein source	Fat source	CHO source
Regular infant formulas			
Similac 20	Nonfat milk	Coconut and soy oils	Lactose
Enfamil	Nonfat milk	Coconut and soy oils	Lactose
Similac 24	Nonfat milk	Coconut and soy oils	Lactose
Enfamil 24	Nonfat milk	Coconut and soy oils	Lactose
Similac 27	Nonfat milk	Coconut and soy oils	Lactose
Humanized formulas			
Similac PM 60/40	Nonfat milk	Coconut and corn oils	Lactose
SMA	Nonfat milk	Coconut, soy, and safflower oils; oleo	Lactose
SMA 24	Nonfat milk	Coconut, soy, and safflower oils; oleo	Lactose
Premature formulas			
Similar Special Care	Nonfat milk	MCT; corn and coconut oils	Lactose, corn syrup
Enfamil Premature	Nonfat milk	MCT; corn and coconut oils	Lactose, sucrose
Specialized formulas			
Isomil	Soybeans	Coconut and soy oils	Corn syrup, sucrose
Prosobee	Soybeans	Coconut and soy oils	Corn syrup
Nursoy	Soybeans	Coconut, soy, and safflower oils; oleo	Sucrose
Nutramigen	Hydrolyzed casein	Corn oil	Sucrose, tapioca
Pregestimil	Hydrolyzed casein	MCT; corn oil	Glucose, corn syrup, tapioca
Portagen	Hydrolyzed casein	MCT; corn oil	Sucrose, corn syrup

Source: Modified from J. P. Cloherty and A. R. Stark, *Manual of Neonatal Care.* Boston: Little, Brown, 1985. Pp. 430–435.

be adequately nourished. Although trial and error is characteristic of premature infant feeding, when the trials are too many and the progress is too slow, parenteral nutrition is indicated.

Bibliography

Coran, A. G. Nutrition of the surgical patient. In K. J. Welch, et al. (eds.), *Pediatric Surgery.* Chicago: Year Book, 1986. P. 96.

9 Total Parenteral Nutrition

I. **Indications.** Parenteral nutrition is indicated whenever adequate nutrition cannot be provided by the enteral route. Intestinal catastrophes such as short bowel syndrome or gastroschisis are typical surgical indications for TPN. The most common indication in the neonatal nursery is extreme prematurity.

II. **Central TPN.** A catheter is placed in the right atrium via the internal jugular, subclavian, or femoral vein. Hypertonic glucose is the calorie source.
   A. **Indications**
      1. Infants in whom intravenous nutrition will be required for a **long time.**
      2. **Very small premature** infants or others in whom peripheral **venous access has become impossible.**
      3. Those in whom nutritional requirements cannot be met by the peripheral intravenous route because of special circumstances such as renal or cardiac disease.
   B. **Central TPN is more hazardous than peripheral TPN** because of the need for operation, the presence of a catheter in the atrium, and the risks of thrombosis and infection. Hence, it should not be used unless peripheral nutrition is impossible.
   C. **Catheter placement** is an operative procedure, but it may be done in the neonatal intensive care unit. The radiopaque Silastic catheter is tunneled under the skin so that the entry into the vein is separated from the skin exit point. The Broviac catheter has a Dacron cuff that is sutured to the fascia in the tunnel to prevent accidental removal.
   D. **Nothing may be added to the solution** because of the **risk of infection.** Standard solutions prepared by the pharmacy should be used unless there are unique requirements.
   E. **Half** of the calculated requirement is given at a steady rate by infusion pump the **first day,** three-fourths the second, and full volume the third day in older children. The progression is slower in the **premature infant.** Blood and urine glucose must be monitored during this time and the infusion rate adjusted as necessary to allow gradual adaptation.
   F. **Essential fatty acids** must be given to patients who receive TPN for more than 2 weeks. Small doses of lipid solution (10 ml/kg) or fresh frozen plasma are given twice weekly.
   G. **Catheter care** is a critical aspect of central TPN. Infection is a constant hazard that is best minimized by strict aseptic precautions during alternate-day dressing changes by an experienced nurse. The line should be broken only once daily at the time of hanging the new solution. The line is not used for drawing blood samples, transfusions, or drug administration.

III. **Peripheral TPN.** The development of a nontoxic fat emulsion to replace the hypertonic glucose solution made possible the delivery of TPN through a peripheral vein. (High volumes of 10% glucose solution can be used but are not always tolerated.)
   A. **Indications.** The inability to maintain adequate nutrition by the enteral route. Accessible veins are required, and the predicted duration of therapy should be short.

Table 9-1. Composition of pediatric parenteral nutrition solutions

Component (per 1000 ml)	Central TPN		Peripheral TPN	
	Children 2.5/20	Premature Infants 2/20	Children 2/10	Premature Infants 2/10
Amino acids (gm)	25	20	20	20
Dextrose (gm)	200	200	100	100
Na (mEq)	40	20	40	20
K (mEq)	40	20	40	20
Cl (mEq)	50	25	48	25
Ca (mEq)	25	25	25	25
P (mM)	15	15	15	15
Mg (mEq)	5	2.4	7.5	2.4
Ac (mEq)	53	35	47	35
Trace elements (ml)	2	2	2	2
Multivitamins (ml)	5	5	5	5
Osmolarity (mOsm)	1443	1363	895	823
Calories/ml	0.78	0.76	0.42	0.42
Rate (ml/kg/day)	125	125	120	120
Intralipid (ml/kg/day)	a	a	35	30
Calories (kg)[b]	98	95	90	84

[a] Lipids are given twice weekly, 10 ml/kg, to supply essential fatty acids.
[b] When given at the recommended rates.

- **B. Hazards** of peripheral parenteral nutrition are those of the intravenous cannula: **thrombosis, phlebitis,** and **infiltration,** and those associated with the fat emulsion: respiratory distress, fever, rash, hyperlipidemia, platelet dysfunction, and fatty change in the liver.
- **C. Catheter** selection. A standard Angiocath or "butterfly" can be used, but if a Silastic catheter can be threaded into the vein, the catheter will last much longer.
- **D. Standard solutions** are recommended, but breaking the line or making additions to the solution is not as hazardous as with central TPN. The lipid solution is "piggybacked" onto the amino acid–dextrose solution as near to the entry site as possible, and both solutions are infused at a steady rate by infusion pumps.
- **E.** Total parenteral nutrition is **poorly tolerated** if given before the second postoperative day or the third day of life. Ten percent glucose and amino acid solution is then begun in half the normal volume, increasing over several days to full amounts.
- **F. Lipid infusion** is begun **after the first week of life** at the rate of 0.5 gm/kg/day given over 12–16 hours and increased by 0.5 gm/kg each day as tolerated to a maximum of 3.0 gm/kg/day. Serum is visually checked daily for lipemia, and infusion is slowed if it is cloudy, stopped if it is opaque.

IV. Solutions. Standard solutions are prepared by the pharmacy and should be used if possible to minimize the hazards of infection and miscalculation. The compositions of the solutions used at the New England Medical Center are listed in Table 9-1.

V. Metabolic monitoring

A. Central TPN

1. All **blood** and **urine tests** should be performed before TPN is begun and according to the following schedule:

Test	Each shift until stable, then weekly	Daily, first 3 days	Weekly	Every 2 weeks
Urine glucose, specific gravity, ketones	X		X	
Dextrostix	X		X	
Na, K, Cl, Ca, BUN, pH		X	X	
Glucose		X	X	
Magnesium			X	
Phosphorus			X	
Total protein			X	
CBC, platelets			X	
Blood culture			X	
Serum and urine osmolality			X	
Liver function tests				X
Bilirubin				X

2. Body weights are measured and recorded daily. No weight gain is seen for several days in very sick patients, but subsequently gain should average 0.5–1.0% of body weight per day. Greater weight gains usually signify fluid accumulation.

3. Children on long-term TPN should have zinc, copper, and manganese levels measured monthly.

B. Peripheral TPN.
The monitoring schedule is the same as for central TPN plus:

1. Check serum for **lipemia** daily.
2. Perform liver function tests weekly.
3. Measure **triglyceride** and **cholesterol** levels weekly.

VI. Complications

A. Metabolic disorders

1. **Hyperglycemia** with hyperosmotic diuresis causing **dehydration** and electrolyte imbalance may occur in infants on central TPN who do not initially tolerate the glucose load. Close monitoring of urine and blood glucose levels at the beginning of therapy is necessary to prevent this complication. Reducing the glucose infusion and gradually increasing it is all that is needed in most infants. Insulin administration is seldom necessary.

2. **Hypoglycemia** is a theoretical complication of sudden cessation of TPN that rarely occurs. Nevertheless, gradual "tapering" is the method of discontinuing therapy.

3. **Hypocalcemia**, hypercalcemia, and high or low phosphorus levels have been seen but are seldom significant. Treatment is alteration in the fluid composition.

4. **Metabolic acidosis** may result from the amino acid load in very premature infants and those with renal or hepatic disease.

5. **Hyperammonemia** is rarely seen with current amino acid mixtures but can result if fluid with too high an amino acid concentration is given or if there is severe liver disease.
6. **Hyperlipidemia** is common in infants receiving lipid solutions. It usually responds to a temporary decrease in the infusion rate.
7. **Liver damage** frequently occurs in infants receiving long-term TPN, whether central or peripheral. Cholestatic jaundice and fat deposition are seen, as well as deposition of a brown pigment. Gallstones may develop. In most patients, liver function returns to normal after cessation of TPN.
8. **Fatty acid deficiency** and deficiencies of copper, zinc, or other trace metals may occur if these substances are omitted from the formula.

B. **Infection** is the most common serious complication of TPN.
1. The central catheter is both a **portal of entry** for bacteria and a **foreign body** in the bloodstream upon which bacteria can colonize if bacteremia occurs.
2. Central parenteral nutrition solution is a **nutrient medium** for *Candida*, but bacterial infections are more common.
3. The incidence of infection parallels **duration** of therapy.
4. Strict **aseptic precautions** during the insertion of the line and during each dressing change significantly decrease the risk of infection, as does limiting the use of the catheter to TPN. Institution of a TPN program with trained nurses as the sole persons changing dressings greatly decreases the infection rate.
5. Bloodstream infection is rarely seen with **peripheral TPN,** but **phlebitis** can occur and be severe.

C. **Line problems** are related to care in placement and fixation.
1. The tip of the catheter must be identified by x-ray as located in **the atrium** at the time of insertion. Placement of the tip in the superior or inferior vena cava is associated with a high incidence of thrombosis. Overinsertion may result in placement of the catheter tip in a hepatic vein with development of a liver abscess.
2. **Accidental dislodgment** of the catheter may occur if it is not properly fixed to the chest wall. The use of the Broviac catheter has greatly decreased this complication.
3. **Hydrothorax** has resulted from misplacement of the central catheter (usually subclavian), particularly when it is inserted percutaneously.
4. Catheter breakage, leaking, and clotting occasionally occur.

Bibliography

Coran, A. G. Nutrition of the surgical patient. In K. J. Welch, et al. (eds.), *Pediatric Surgery.* Chicago: Year Book, 1986. P. 96.

Coran, A. G. Total intravenous feeding of infants and children without the use of a central venous catheter. *Ann. Surg.* 179:445, 1974.

Dudrick, S. J., et al. Long-term parenteral nutrition with growth, development, and positive nitrogen balance. *Surgery* 64:134, 1968.

Dudrick, S. J., et al. Can intravenous feeding as the sole means of nutrition support growth in the child and restore weight loss in an adult: An affirmative answer. *Ann. Surg.* 169:974, 1969.

Filler, R. M., et al. Long-term parenteral nutrition in infants. *N. Engl. J. Med.* 281:589, 1969.

Leape, L. L., and Valaes, T. Rickets in low birth weight infants receiving total parenteral nutrition. *J. Pediatr. Surg.* 11:665, 1976.

II Neonatal Surgical Diseases

10   Respiratory Distress

I. Definition. The term *respiratory distress* refers to difficulty breathing, as evidenced by tachypnea, nasal flaring, stridor, air hunger, retractions, or cyanosis.

II. Pathophysiology. Respiratory distress results from hypercapnia or hypoxia. There are **three major categories** of disorders that produce respiratory distress: abnormalities of **ventilation**, impaired **diffusion**, and **shunting**.

  A. Ventilatory abnormalities include all the structural malformations that prevent adequate amounts of air from reaching the alveoli for exchange of oxygen and CO_2.

    1. Airway obstruction may be present at any level from the nose (choanal atresia) to the bronchi (bronchomalacia) and may be either intrinsic (subglottic hemangioma) or extrinsic (vascular ring). Stridor (noisy breathing) results from turbulent air flow due to the obstruction.

    2. Decreased lung volume may result from external compression, as from pneumothorax or diaphragmatic hernia, from replacement of lung tissue by tumor or cyst, or from congenital failure of development (agenesis or hypoplasia).

    3. Impaired function of **respiratory muscles** may reflect inadequate muscle development, as in eventration of the diaphragm, a birth injury (e.g., of the phrenic nerve), or disorders of the CNS.

  B. Impaired diffusion results from alveolar failure caused by developmental abnormalities (hyaline membrane disease), aspiration, atelectasis, pneumonia, or congestive heart failure.

  C. Shunting within the heart (right to left) from septal defects and other anomalies permits poorly oxygenated blood to enter the arterial circuit, decreasing the PaO_2.

III. Clinical presentation. The age of presentation and the rapidity of progression of symptoms give clues to the cause of the respiratory distress.

  A. Onset of symptoms shortly after birth indicates a major malformation, one that is potentially life-threatening. Babies with diaphragmatic hernia, tracheal agenesis, hypoplastic lungs, and phrenic or vocal cord paralysis are symptomatic from birth. Hyaline membrane disease causes symptoms soon after birth.

  B. Sudden onset of symptoms in an infant who was **previously well** suggests a mechanical event such as pneumothorax or aspiration.

  C. Restlessness may be the first sign of respiratory distress coming on in a previously asymptomatic baby. It is a subtle sign, often unnoticed by the unwary or inexperienced practitioner. **Tachypnea** follows, then true **dyspnea**, with **flaring** of the alae nasi, **retractions, grunting,** and finally, **cyanosis.**

  D. Stridor is the pathognomonic sign of airway obstruction anywhere from the larynx to the carina. **Wheezing** indicates bronchial obstruction. **Opisthotonos** indicates airway compression, frequently seen in patients with a vascular ring.

IV. Diagnosis

  A. History and physical examination give important clues to the adequacy of ventilation and whether there is airway obstruction. Auscultation of the lungs is frequently misleading, however, since breath sounds are easily transmitted from the opposite side. **An infant with a significant pneumothorax may have apparently normal breath sounds.**

B. **Chest x-ray** is obtained promptly in any infant with respiratory distress. The infant is never "too sick" for a portable chest x-ray. It gives critically important information about the lungs and the airway and often readily separates surgical from nonsurgical causes of respiratory distress. **Upright** films are more accurate than supine films for discriminating between diaphragmatic hernia and lung cysts or between lobar emphysema and pneumothorax.

C. **Passage of a tube** through the nares eliminates the possibility of choanal atresia. Passage into the stomach rules out esophageal atresia.

D. **Laryngoscopy** is performed as an emergency if there is airway obstruction. Upper airway obstruction can often be relieved by passage of an endotracheal tube.

E. **Bronchoscopy** is indicated in all infants with **stridor** even if there is no significant respiratory distress. It is the simplest and most accurate method for making a specific diagnosis and for identifying those infants who require corrective surgery. One should not assume that noisy breathing is caused by laryngomalacia.

F. **Soft tissue x-rays** of the neck give important clues to airway diameter and external compression.

G. **Esophagogram** is indicated if a vascular ring is suspected.

H. **Arterial blood gas** determinations are helpful in management and in separating cardiac from pulmonary cyanosis but seldom contribute to etiologic diagnosis.

I. **Cyanosis** from cardiac causes can usually be differentiated from pulmonary cyanosis by having the infant breathe 100% oxygen. Cardiac cyanosis does not improve significantly with 100% oxygen, while pulmonary cyanosis does.

V. **Differential diagnosis.** Most abnormalities of ventilation are mechanical in origin and often require surgical treatment. Diffusion defects are usually best treated by medical means.

  A. **Airway obstruction**
  1. Nasopharynx
     a. Absent nares
     b. Choanal atresia
     c. Encephalocele
     d. Teratoma
  2. Mouth
     a. Macroglossia
     b. Pierre Robin syndrome
     c. Hypopharyngeal cysts
     d. Lingual thyroid
  3. Larynx
     a. Vocal cord paralysis
     b. Laryngomalacia—congenital laryngeal stridor (CLS)
     c. Laryngotracheal hemangioma
     d. Laryngotracheal lymphangioma
     e. Laryngotracheoesophageal cleft

4. Neck
    a. Cystic hygroma
    b. Goiter
5. Trachea
    a. Subglottic stenosis
    b. Subglottic cyst, hemangioma
    c. Tracheomalacia
    d. Tracheal stenosis
    e. Tracheal atresia
    f. Vascular ring
6. Bronchi: bronchomalacia

B. Reduced lung volume
1. Diaphragmatic hernia
2. Agenesis of the lung
3. Pneumothorax
4. Chylothorax
5. Lobar emphysema
6. Lung cysts
7. Cystic adenomatoid malformation

C. Impaired muscle function
1. Phrenic nerve injury
2. Eventration of the diaphragm
3. Absent abdominal muscles
4. Spinal paralysis

D. Impaired diffusion
1. Hyaline membrane disease
2. Aspiration
    a. Meconium aspiration
    b. Esophageal atresia
    c. Tracheoesophageal fistula (TEF)
    d. CNS disease
3. Atelectasis
4. Pneumonia
5. Pulmonary hemorrhage
6. Interstitial emphysema
7. Wilson-Mikity syndrome
8. Transient tachypnea of the newborn
9. Congestive heart failure

Treatment. Specific treatment is discussed in subsequent sections on the various disorders. A few general principles are worth noting.

A. **Endotracheal intubation** may be necessary, both to diagnose airway obstruction and to treat it, as well as to give assisted ventilation. Common errors are use of a tube that is too large and putting the tube in too far. Position of the tube must be verified by chest x-ray.
B. **Assisted ventilation** must be given with special care in patients with diaphragmatic hernia and those with lobar emphysema, in which even moderate pressure can rupture the lung and produce a rapidly fatal tension pneumothorax.
C. **Tension pneumothorax** can be treated emergently with a needle-catheter (Angiocath) followed by insertion of a chest tube.
D. **Beware of fatigue.** Even if arterial oxygen and carbon dioxide are well maintained, the infant who is working to breathe will eventually tire. Then his extra respiratory effort will decline, he will retain carbon dioxide and go into respiratory failure. Ventilatory assistance should be given before this happens.

Bibliography

Ashcraft, K. W., and Holder, T. Airway Malformations and Obstructions. In T. M. Holder and K. W. Ashcraft (eds.), *Pediatric Surgery*. Philadelphia: Saunders, 1980. P. 183.

Holder, T. M., Leape, L. L., and Ashcraft, K. W. Congenital Malformations of the Trachea, Bronchi, and Esophagus. In M. M. Paparella and D. A. Shumrick (eds.), *Otolaryngology* (2nd ed.). Philadelphia: Saunders, 1980.

11 Airway Obstruction

I. **Definition.** A large number of diverse disorders result in obstruction of the airway and cause respiratory distress. Fortunately, most of them respond to surgical treatment or disappear as the infant matures.

II. **Pathophysiology**
   A. **Resistance to flow** is increased by the reduction in the size of the airway. In a high flow state, air flow is reduced at a rate proportional to the fourth power of the reduction of the radius of the lumen.
   B. The **work of breathing** is increased since extra pressure must be generated by the muscles of respiration to move air against a higher resistance.
   C. **Muscle fatigue** from excessive respiratory work ultimately leads to decompensation with hypoxia and hypercapnia (CO_2 retention).

III. **Clinical presentation**
   A. **Dyspnea** is the cardinal symptom of airway obstruction. The infant struggles to breathe and is apprehensive, restless, and sweaty.
   B. **Stridor** indicates obstruction in the larynx or trachea.
   C. **Wheezing** is a sign of bronchial obstruction.
   D. **Opisthotonos** seems to relieve tracheal compression and is often seen in patients with a vascular ring.
   E. **Cyanosis** is a late sign of airway obstruction and indicates that the child is **decompensated**—unable to move sufficient air to maintain oxygenation.

IV. **Diagnosis**
   A. **Physical examination** may reveal the abnormality. If examination of the face and mouth is unremarkable, but the infant has stridor, the obstruction is at or below the larynx.
   B. **Chest x-ray** is obtained to assess the lungs and intrathoracic airway but is usually normal.
   C. **Soft tissue x-rays** of the neck may reveal tracheomalacia or a subglottic narrowing.
   D. **Laryngoscopy** is performed if the cause of obstruction is not evident on physical examination. If the infant is in severe distress and decompensating, passage of an endotracheal tube may be required. Difficulty in passing a tube is a sign of laryngeal or subglottic stenosis and an indication for immediate bronchoscopy.
   E. **Bronchoscopy** is indicated in all infants with stridor as well as those with unexplained respiratory distress.
   F. **Arterial oxygen and CO_2 determination** will indicate whether the infant is compensating for the obstruction.

V. **Management**
   A. **Visible obstruction**
      1. **Absent nares.** This exceedingly rare but obvious disorder causes respiratory distress because neonates are obligatory nasal breathers. An oral airway bypasses the obstruction. Tracheostomy may be required before begin-

ning plastic reconstruction of the nose. These infants often have other serious anomalies.

2. **Choanal atresia** is not obvious on examination but readily demonstrated by the failure of a tube to pass through the nose into the pharynx. An oral airway bypasses the obstruction until an adequate channel is created surgically.

3. **Encephalocele or teratoma** may present through a cleft palate or in the hypopharynx as a globular mass, sometimes skin-covered. Excision is required after CT evaluation of its central connections.

4. **Macroglossia** accompanies Beckwith's syndrome, congenital hypothyroidism, and other anomalies. Airway obstruction can often be managed by positioning, but an oral airway or tracheostomy may be required.

5. **Pierre Robin syndrome,** hypoplastic mandible with cleft palate, results in airway obstruction by the tongue. Prone positioning is often sufficient therapy, but sometimes an oral airway is needed. For severe cases, forward positioning of the tongue with a suture from the base of the tongue to the hyoid bone or use of a steel "skewer" has been recommended. Alternatively, temporary tracheostomy can be used. A feeding gastrostomy may also be necessary.

6. **Cystic hygroma** can obstruct the airway by **compression** of the larynx or trachea, by cysts that **occlude** the larynx or subglottic airway, and by **elevation** and **infiltration** of the tongue, obstructing the oral cavity. Surgical excision is required, often combined with temporary tracheostomy.

7. **Goiter** is rare in infants and even more rarely causes airway obstruction. Partial thyroidectomy may be required.

B. **Pharyngolaryngeal obstruction**

1. **Hypopharyngeal cyst** may not be evident on routine examination. If pedunculated, it can swing up behind the uvula and be missed. Excision is curative and usually simple.

2. **Lingual thyroid** presents as a firm mass at the base of the tongue, the foramen cecum. It may be the sole thyroid present, representing a failure of caudal migration. Excision is required to cure or prevent airway obstruction. Replacement therapy is necessary.

3. **Vocal cord paralysis** may be congenital or may result from birth or surgical injury to the recurrent laryngeal nerve. If it is bilateral, tracheostomy is required. Fixation of the cords in abduction can be performed surgically at a later date if there is no spontaneous return of function.

4. **Laryngomalacia** (congenital laryngeal stridor) is by far the most common cause of stridor in infancy. The abnormally soft laryngeal cartilage folds in on itself during inspiration, creating an **"omega-shaped" epiglottis.**

    a. The diagnosis can only be made by **indirect laryngoscopy** (with a right-angle or fiberoptic instrument). Examination with a standard laryngoscope stabilizes the base of the larynx, eliminating the omega-shaped collapse, so the diagnosis is missed. The stridor is typically inspiratory but may be biphasic.

    b. Laryngomalacia, while distressingly noisy, seldom causes significant airway obstruction or requires treatment. As the infant matures, the cartilage stiffens and the stridor disappears. This may take up to a year or two, however. Rarely, tracheostomy is required.

5. **Laryngeal hemangioma** is not as common as subglottic hemangioma but can be just as difficult to treat. If there is significant airway obstruction,

tracheostomy is necessary. Hemangiomas often respond to systemic steroids in infancy.

C. Tracheal obstruction

1. **Laryngotracheoesophageal cleft** is a very rare variant of tracheoesophageal fistula that extends into the larynx. Choking and aspiration with feedings are the presenting symptoms. The diagnosis must be thought of at the time of bronchoscopy or it is easily missed as the instrument is passed into the trachea. Surgical repair and temporary tracheostomy are needed.

2. **Subglottic stenosis** may be congenital or, more commonly, acquired as a result of use of an endotracheal tube that is too large.

    a. The airway is narrowest at the cricoid cartilage. Pressure from an oversized tube can rapidly cause necrosis, which heals with scar formation, narrowing the airway.

    b. Dilatations are usually sufficient treatment, but they must be repeated over a period of several months. Laser excision and tracheal fissure with or without a cartilage graft have also been used successfully.

3. **Subglottic cyst, hemangioma.** These rare lesions can present formidable therapeutic challenges. The subglottic region is an area of predilection for hemangioma in the airway. Tracheostomy is usually required. Cysts are excised. Most hemangiomas will spontaneously disappear, a process that can sometimes be hastened by the use of systemic corticosteroids. Laser treatments are also effective.

4. **Tracheomalacia** is a relatively common cause of neonatal airway obstruction. It is usually associated with other major anomalies, such as esophageal atresia or agenesis of the lung. The diagnosis will be missed if the infant is not breathing spontaneously while the trachea is being examined with the bronchoscope. Collapse of the trachea with anteroposterior apposition occurs with expiration. Minor degrees of tracheomalacia require no treatment, but in a severe case temporary tracheostomy is needed.

5. **Tracheal stenosis** below the subglottic region is rare. Dilatations, stenting, and incision and grafting with autogenous cartilage have been successfully employed.

6. **Tracheal atresia.** This condition is exceedingly rare and, so far, uncorrectable. Severe malformations of the bronchi and lungs are usually present as well.

7. **Vascular rings** result from abnormal dissolution of primitive vascular aortic arches. They are often asymptomatic and undiagnosed.

    a. **Symptoms** occur when the arteries compress the esophagus or airway causing dysphagia, stridor, and respiratory distress. If the obstruction is severe, opisthotonos may be seen.

    b. Numerous possibilities exist for formation of a vascular ring. Those most likely to cause symptoms are **double aortic arch, aberrant right subclavian artery,** and **right aortic arch with ductus arteriosus.**

    c. **Esophagogram** demonstrates a characteristic indentation with most symptomatic vascular rings. Angiography gives precise definition of the anatomy.

    d. **Operative division** is curative and almost always possible. Persistent symptoms may result from **tracheomalacia** at the site of vascular compression.

8. **Bronchomalacia** is usually associated with other pulmonary anomalies, such as agenesis of the lung. Collapse of the bronchi during spontaneous

respiration at bronchoscopy establishes the diagnosis. Continuous positive airway pressure ventilation (CPAP) is required until the bronchi stiffen as they mature.

Bibliography

Ashcraft, K. W., and Holder, T. M. Airway Malformations and Obstructions. In T. M. Holder and K. W. Ashcraft (eds.), *Pediatric Surgery*. Philadelphia: Saunders, 1980. P. 183.

Burroughs, N., and Leape, L. L. Laryngotracheoesophageal cleft: Report of a case successfully treated and review of the literature. *Pediatrics* 53:516, 1974.

Canty, T. G., and Hendren, W. H. Upper airway obstruction from foregut cysts of the hypopharynx. *J. Pediatr. Surg.* 10:807, 1975.

Cogbill, T. H., et al. Primary tracheomalacia. *Ann. Thorac. Surg.* 35:538, 1983.

Cohen, D. Tracheopexy: Aorto-tracheal suspension for severe tracheomalacia. *Aust. Paediatr. J.* 17:117, 1981.

Cotton, R. Management of subglottic stenosis in infancy and childhood. *Ann. Otol. Rhinol. Laryngol.* 87:649, 1978.

Cotton, R. T., and Richardson, M. A. Advances in head and neck surgery in children. *Head Neck Surg.* 3:424, 1981.

de Lorimier, A. A. Congenital Malformations and Neonatal Problems of the Respiratory Tract. In K. J. Welch et al. (eds.), *Pediatric Surgery*. Chicago: Year Book, 1986. P. 631.

Healy, G. B., et al. Treatment of subglottic hemangioma with the carbon dioxide laser. *Laryngoscope* 90:809, 1980.

Holder, T. M., Leape, L. L., and Ashcraft, K. W. Congenital Malformations of the Trachea, Bronchi, and Esophagus. In M. M. Paparella and D. A. Shumrick (eds.), *Otolaryngology* (2nd ed.). Philadelphia: Saunders, 1980.

Johnson, D. G. Lesions of the Larynx and Trachea: Tracheostomy. In K. J. Welch, et al. (eds.), *Pediatric Surgery*. Chicago: Year Book, 1986. P. 622.

Koufman, J. A., Thompson, J. N., and Kohut, R. I. Endoscopic management of subglottic stenosis with the CO_2 surgical laser. *Otolaryngol. Head Neck Surg.* 89:215, 1981.

Kveton, J. F., and Pillsbury, H. C. Conservative treatment of infantile subglottic hemangiomas with corticosteroids. *Arch. Otolaryngol.* 108:117, 1982.

Nakayama, D. K., et al. Reconstructive surgery for obstructing lesions of the intrathoracic trachea in infants and small children. *J. Pediatr. Surg.* 17:854, 1982.

Schwartz, M. Z., and Filler, R. M. Tracheal compression as a cause of apnea following repair of tracheoesophageal fistula: Treatment by aortopexy. *J. Pediatr. Surg.* 15:842, 1980.

Weider, D. J., and Parker, W. Lingual thyroid: Review, case reports and therapeutic guidelines. *Ann. Otol. Rhinol. Laryngol.* 86:841, 1977.

12 Pneumothorax

I. **Definition.** *Pneumothorax* means air in the pleural space. It occurs in 1–2% of newborns. *Tension pneumothorax* is pneumothorax under pressure, a rapidly fatal condition in a neonate.

   A. **Spontaneous pneumothorax** occurs in hyaline membrane disease, meconium aspiration, fetal distress, and pneumonia, and occasionally in infants with apparently normal lungs.

   B. **Iatrogenic** causes of pneumothorax are much more common.

   1. Intubation
   2. Resuscitation
   3. Excessive ventilatory pressure
   4. Suctioning
   5. Continuous pressure ventilation
   6. Insertion of a central venous catheter
   7. Bronchoscopy
   8. Tracheostomy
   9. Postoperative conditions

      a. Thoracotomy—leaking in and around chest tube
      b. Recurrent TEF
      c. Lung resection—bronchial leak

II. **Pathophysiology**

   A. **Spontaneous pneumothorax** and pneumothorax caused by artificial ventilation result from **alveolar rupture.** Air dissects into the interstitium of the lung, thence to the pleural surface, forming a subpleural bleb that ruptures into the pleural space. **Postoperative** and instrumental pneumothorax result from a wound in the pleura that communicates with the outside.

   1. **The partial vacuum** (negative pressure) in the pleural space sucks air through any opening.
   2. The **lung collapses** because of its natural **elasticity,** no longer held up by the partial vacuum in the pleural space.
   3. If the infant is on a **respirator,** positive pressure ventilation forces air through an alveolar leak into the pleural space.
   4. Collapse of the lung reduces air exchange causing **respiratory distress and cyanosis,** with symptoms proportional to the extent of the pneumothorax.

   B. **Tension pneumothorax** results from a continuing air leak causing positive pressure in the pleural space.

   1. **A one-way valve effect** is created by the softness of tissues, preventing escape of air, which accumulates, compressing the lung.
   2. Pressure causes the lung to **collapse** and to **displace** the flexible **mediastinum** of the newborn infant to the opposite side, compressing the opposite lung.

3. **Venous return is inhibited** by angulation of the great veins by the mediastinal displacement as well as by the increased intrathoracic pressure.
4. **Cardiac output falls,** followed by hypotension and arrest.

III. **Clinical presentation**
   A. **Sudden onset of respiratory distress** suggests pneumothorax in any newborn infant, whether or not lung disease is present and whether or not he is receiving ventilatory assistance. Pneumothorax and obstruction of the endotracheal tube are the main causes of sudden deterioration of an infant on a respirator.
   B. **Tachypnea, retractions, and cyanosis** rapidly occur. If tension pneumothorax develops, apnea, bradycardia, and cardiac arrest may follow in rapid succession.
   C. **Physical examination** shows asymmetry of the chest and shift of the cardiac impulse. **Decreased breath sounds are difficult to recognize in neonates** because of the ready transmission of sounds from the other side of the chest.
   D. **Pneumothorax may also accumulate** slowly, with gradually increasing symptoms, or may even be asymptomatic if it is small in amount. **Hypoxia and hypercapnia** as reflected by arterial blood gas monitoring may be the only signs.

IV. **Diagnosis**
   A. **Upright chest x-ray** is diagnostic. A small pneumothorax will be missed on a supine film.
   B. **Transillumination** with a fiberoptic light source is an immediately available method of diagnosing pneumothorax and is accurate unless the infant is very small or has massive chest-wall edema. A transilluminator should be available in every neonatal intensive care unit.

V. **Treatment**
   A. **No treatment** is needed for a **small pneumothorax** (10–20%) if the infant is **asymptomatic,** is not on a ventilator, and has no lung disease, and if there is no evidence of continuing air leak. Serial chest x-rays must be obtained until resolution.
   B. **Chest tube** insertion is necessary in all others with pneumothorax, both to relieve symptoms and to control further leakage (see Chap. 108).
   C. **Needle aspiration** is performed as an emergency procedure if tension pneumothorax is present. An angiocath is used to avoid laceration of the lung.
   D. **Operative treatment** is necessary if there is a major postoperative leak from the trachea or bronchus, conditions rarely seen in neonates.

Bibliography

Banagale, R. C., Outerbridge, E. W., and Aranda, J. V. Lung perforation: A complication of chest tube insertion in neonatal pneumothorax. *J. Pediatr.* 94:973, 1979.

Hall, R. T., and Rhodes, P. G. Pneumothorax and pneumomediastinum in infants with idiopathic respiratory distress syndrome receiving continuous positive airway pressure. *Pediatrics* 55:493, 1975.

Rich, H. R., Warwick, W. J., and Leonard, A. S. Open thoracotomy and pleural abrasion in the treatment of spontaneous pneumothorax in cystic fibrosis. *J. Pediatr. Surg.* 13:237, 1978.

13 Lobar Emphysema

I. **Definition.** Infantile or congenital lobar emphysema is a disease of the neonatal period or early infancy in which a lobe of the lung becomes hyperinflated and is unable to exchange air. The left upper and right middle lobes are most frequently affected.

  A. **Congenital heart disease** with left to right shunt is present in 20–50% of patients.

  B. **Boys** are affected twice as commonly as girls.

  C. The etiology of the air trapping varies. **Bronchomalacia**, bronchial **compression** (from a dilated branch of the pulmonary artery), and primary **alveolar fibrosis** have been found. Mechanical ventilation with malposition of the endotracheal tube may cause lobar emphysema.

II. **Pathophysiology.** Overexpansion of a lobe not only inhibits its function, but also affects the surrounding structures.

  A. **Atelectasis** of the neighboring lobes decreases air exchange on the ipsilateral side.

  B. **Mediastinal shift** and **herniation** of the emphysematous lobe to the other side compresses the lung on the opposite side.

  C. **Overexpansion** of the chest wall and **flattening of the diaphragm** decrease the efficiency of the ventilatory muscles.

III. **Clinical presentation**

  A. **Respiratory distress** is the characteristic symptom of infantile lobar emphysema: air hunger, tachypnea, and cyanosis.

  B. **Physical findings** include hyperexpansion, hyperresonance, and decreased breath sounds on the affected side. Pneumothorax may be suspected.

  C. **Rarely,** a fulminant, **rapidly progressive course** is seen in the young infant, requiring prompt intervention for salvage.

  D. **Intubation** and ventilatory assistance may make the patient **worse** by further overdistending the emphysematous lobe.

  E. Mild degrees of infantile lobar emphysema may be **asymptomatic**. In most children, progression of the air trapping ultimately leads to respiratory distress.

IV. **Diagnosis**

  A. **Chest x-ray** establishes the diagnosis. Typical findings are as follows (Fig. 13-1):

    1. **Overexpansion** of a single **lobe** with decreased vascular and bronchial markings
    2. **Compensatory atelectasis** of the adjacent lobes
    3. **Herniation** of the affected lobe across the anterior mediastinum
    4. **Mediastinal shift** away from the emphysematous lobe
    5. **Flattening** of the **hemidiaphragm**

  B. The presence of **bronchovascular markings** differentiates infantile lobar emphysema from pneumothorax or lung cyst.

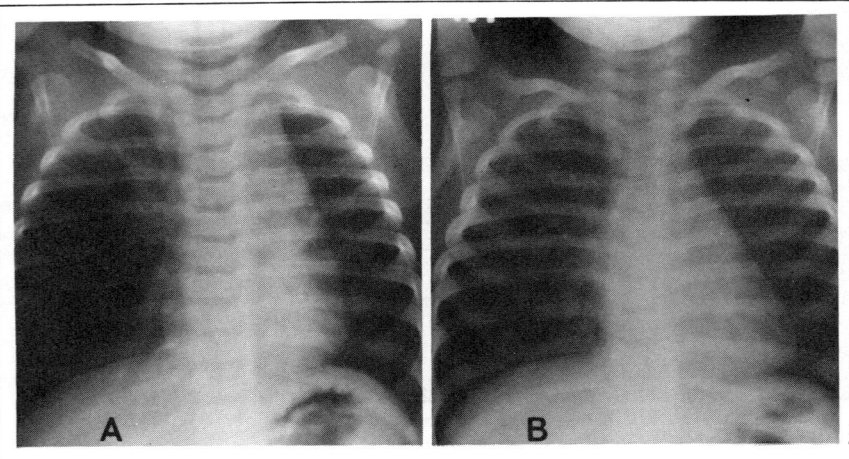

Fig. 13-1. Lobar emphysema. A. Classic roentgenographic findings of middle lobe emphysema: radiolucency of the affected lobe, compensatory atelectasis in adjacent lobes, mediastinal shift, flattening of the diaphragm. B. Normal chest x-ray following middle lobectomy. (From L. L. Leape, Thoracic Surgical Problems in Infants and Children. In S. H. Ellis (Ed.), *Thoracic Surgery*. Philadelphia: Lippincott/Harper & Row, 1983.)

- **C. Bronchogram** and **bronchoscopy** are **not necessary** for diagnosis and are hazardous if respiration is already compromised.
- **D. Cardiac catheterization** may be indicated if there is evidence of associated severe congenital heart disease.

V. Problems

- **A. Sudden expansion** of the lobe can lead rapidly to respiratory insufficiency and require emergency operation.
- **B. Tension pneumothorax** can develop from rupture of the overinflated lobe. This is particularly likely to happen if the patient is receiving positive pressure ventilation. Immediate tube thoracostomy is required.

VI. Indications for operation

- **A. Symptomatic** patients should undergo lobectomy.
- **B. Asymptomatic** patients require close observation. If a cardiac abnormality is present, its correction may lead to gradual disappearance of the lobar emphysema.
- **C. Nonoperative treatment by selective intubation** of the opposite bronchus may result in decompression of the affected lobe if overventilation is the cause.

VII. Preoperative preparation

- **A. If the infant is otherwise well,** no special preparation is necessary other than maintaining adequate ventilation and ensuring that blood is available.
- **B. If the infant is in cardiac failure,** an effort should be made to improve cardiac function medically. If unsuccessful, cardiac corrective surgery may be advisable prior to lobectomy.

VIII. Operative care.
Lobectomy is curative and well tolerated in infants. A specific obstructing mechanism is seldom identified.

K. **Postoperative care.** Routine.
L. **Complications.** Rare. Occurrence of lobar emphysema in another lobe has been reported.
M. **Prognosis.** Excellent.

Bibliography

Cooney, D. R., Menke, J. A., and Allen, J. E. Acquired lobar emphysema: A complication of respiratory distress in premature infants. *J. Pediatr. Surg.* 12:897, 1977.

De Lorimier, A. A. Congenital Malformations and Neonatal Problems of the Respiratory Tract. In K. J. Welch et al. (eds.), *Pediatric Surgery*. Chicago: Year Book, 1986. P. 631.

Eigen, H., Lemen, R. J., and Waring, W. W. Congenital lobar emphysema: Long-term evaluation of surgically and conservatively treated children. *Am. Rev. Respir. Dis.* 113:823, 1976.

Hislop, A., and Reid, L. New pathological findings in emphysema of childhood. 2. Overinflation of a normal lobe. *Thorax* 26:190, 1971.

Leape, L. L., and Longino, L. A. Infantile lobar emphysema. *Pediatrics* 34:246, 1964.

Ledesma, J., and Girdany, B. R. Congenital lobar emphysema: A case report with a thirty-two-year follow up. *Ann. Radiol.* 15:181, 1971.

Lewis, J. E. Pulmonary and Bronchial Malformations. In T. M. Holder and K. W. Ashcraft (eds.), *Pediatric Surgery*. Philadelphia: Saunders, 1980. P. 196.

Miller, K. E., Edwards, D. K., and Hilton, S. Acquired lobar emphysema in premature infants with bronchopulmonary dysplasia: An iatrogenic disease? *Radiology* 138:589, 1981.

Murray, G. F. Congenital lobar emphysema. *Surg. Gynecol. Obstet.* 124:611, 1967.

Tapper, D., et al. Polyalveolar lobe: Anatomic and physiologic parameters and their relationship to congenital lobar emphysema. *J. Pediatr. Surg.* 15:931, 1980.

14 Lung Cysts

I. **Definition.** Cysts of the lung are most commonly discovered in the neonatal period but may occur at any age. Four major types are recognized.

   A. **Bronchogenic cysts** arise from the foregut and develop from abnormal branching of the primitive tracheobronchus.

   1. Histologically, the wall of the cyst contains cartilage, mucous glands, elastic tissue, and smooth muscle.

   2. Most bronchogenic cysts are solitary and located in the mediastinum, but they can occur anywhere in the chest or neck and more than one may be present in a patient.

   B. **Simple cysts** arise from sequestered primitive pulmonary tissue and are usually symptomatic in the neonatal period or early infancy. They usually communicate with the airway.

   C. **Cystic adenomatoid malformation (CAM)** is a hamartomatous developmental abnormality of the lung affecting a lobe or the entire lung. Solid and cystic elements are usually present. Most are symptomatic in the neonatal period.

   D. **Pneumatoceles** result from pulmonary infection, primarily staphylococcal. Improved diagnosis and effective antibiotic treatment have greatly reduced the incidence of this disease.

II. **Pathophysiology.** Respiratory insufficiency may develop from reduction of functioning lung tissue. There are several mechanisms.

   A. **Sudden expansion** of a large cyst may compress the normal lung. This is most likely to happen with simple cysts and pneumatoceles.

   B. **Rupture** of a cyst may result in tension pneumothorax.

   C. **Bronchial compression** by the cyst can result in atelectasis or air trapping with localized emphysema.

   D. **Infection** may result from retention of secretions caused by bronchial compression or may occur in the cyst itself.

III. **Clinical presentation.** Symptoms from a lung cyst depend on its size, the location, whether it communicates with a bronchus, and whether there is infection.

   A. Many lung cysts are **asymptomatic** and are discovered on chest x-ray obtained for another reason.

   1. Huge solitary cysts are usually simple lung cysts.

   2. Small solitary cysts are usually bronchogenic cysts.

   3. Multiple cysts usually represent cystic adenomatoid malformation or pneumatoceles, rarely bronchogenic cysts.

   B. **Acute respiratory distress** in an infant may be caused by bronchial compression from a bronchogenic cyst. It can be caused at any age by sudden expansion of the cyst or rupture with development of tension pneumothorax. Symptomatic bronchogenic cysts in infants are often subcarinal in location.

   C. **Recurrent or nonclearing pneumonia** is a common mode of presentation of bronchogenic cysts. Infection may result from bronchial compression or from infection in the cyst itself. Pus may drain into other lobes causing abscesses or bronchiectasis.

IV. Diagnosis

- **A. Chest x-ray** is diagnostic in most patients, but in others the findings may be obscured by surrounding infection.
- **B. CT scan** will often differentiate cysts from tumors. It is particularly helpful in assessing mediastinal lesions.
- **C. Bronchoscopy** is seldom necessary for diagnosis and can be hazardous in the symptomatic patient. If the cyst is centrally located, bronchoscopy at the time of thoracotomy may assist in planning the resection.

V. Differential diagnosis.
Radiologic findings of a rounded contour and a detectable cyst wall permit accurate diagnosis in most patients. Common diagnostic errors and their distinguishing characteristics include the following:

- **A. Pneumothorax.** Central collapse of the lung; no cyst wall.
- **B. Lobar emphysema.** Lung markings in the hyperlucent area.
- **C. Diaphragmatic hernia.** Scaphoid abdomen; nasogastric tube identifies intrathoracic location of stomach.
- **D. Tumor.** Presence of cystic areas indicates CAM.

VI. Indications for operation

- **A. Symptomatic cysts** require prompt removal, often as an emergency.
- **B. Asymptomatic cysts** should also be removed because of the risk of infection, sudden expansion, or rupture.
    1. In infants sudden expansion or rupture is more likely, so operative excision should be carried out promptly even if the child appears perfectly well.
    2. In older children, excision may be performed electively.

VII. Preoperative preparation.
Eradication of superimposed pneumonia or infection of the cyst before its excision is desirable but may not be possible if there is bronchial obstruction.

VIII. Operative care

- **A.** The **objective** of the operation is to remove the cyst and nothing else. While lobectomy is usually necessary, in most patients the unaffected lobes can be preserved.
- **B. Pneumonectomy,** if necessary, is well tolerated even by infants.

IX. Postoperative care. Routine

X. Complications

- **A. Bronchial leak** with pneumothorax.
- **B. Empyema** if cyst is infected and the pleural space is inadequately drained.
- **C. Respiratory insufficiency is rarely seen** after excision of a lung cyst. In infants, lung growth will compensate for removal of even a large amount of lung tissue.
- **D. Scoliosis** develops in infants following **pneumonectomy** because of unequal intrathoracic pressures. Early splinting minimizes deformity. Spinal fusion may be necessary.

Bibliography

Buhain, W. J., and Brody, J. S. Compensatory growth of the lung following pneumonectomy. *J. Appl. Physiol.* 33:898, 1973.

Frenckner, B., and Freyschuss, U. Pulmonary function after lobectomy for congenital lobar emphysema and congenital cystic adenomatoid malformation: A follow up study. *Scand. J. Thorac. Cardiovasc. Surg.* 16:293, 1982.

Haller, J. A., et al. Surgical management of lung bud anomalies: Lobar emphysema, bronchogenic cysts, cystic adenomatoid malformations, and intrapulmonary sequestration. *Ann. Thorac. Surg.* 28:33, 1979.

Lewis, J. E. Pulmonary and Bronchial Malformations. In T. M. Holder and K. W. Ashcraft (eds.), *Pediatric Surgery.* Philadelphia: Saunders, 1980. P. 196.

McBride, J. T., et al. Lung growth and airway function after lobectomy in infancy for congenital lobar emphysema. *J. Clin. Invest.* 66:962, 1980.

Miller, R. K., Sieber, W. K., and Yunis E. J. Congenital adenomatoid malformation of the lung: A report of 17 cases and review of the literature. *Pathol. Annu.* 15:387, 1980.

Nishibayashi, S. W., Andrassy, R. J., and Woolley, M. M. Congenital adenomatoid malformations: 30-year experience. *J. Pediatr. Surg.* 16:704, 1981.

Ramenofsky, M. L., Leape, L. L., and McCauley, R. G. K. Bronchogenic cyst. *J. Pediatr. Surg.* 14:219, 1979.

Sieber, W. K. Lung cysts, Sequestration, and Bronchopulmonary Dysplasia, in K. J. Welch, et al. (eds.), *Pediatric Surgery.* Chicago: Year Book, 1986. P. 645.

Wolfe, S. A., Hertzler, J. H., Philippart, A. I. Cystic adenomatoid dysplasia of the lung. *J. Pediatr. Surg.* 15:925, 1980.

15 Diaphragmatic Hernia

I. **Definition.** Herniation of the abdominal viscera through a congenital defect in the diaphragm results in severe respiratory distress soon after birth. The most common form of herniation, and the most serious, is through the foramen of **Bochdalek,** a posterolateral defect in the diaphragm resulting from failure of closure of the pleuroperitoneal canal in the eighth to tenth week of fetal life. Eighty-five percent occur on the left side, and most patients are symptomatic within hours after birth. The cause is unknown.

II. **Pathophysiology.** The developing lung is compressed by intestine (and sometimes the spleen, kidney, and liver as well) inhibiting development and displacing all intrathoracic structures to the opposite side (Fig. 15-1).

   A. **There is severe hypoplasia** of the lung with marked reduction in alveolar surface for gas exchange as well as reduced pulmonary vasculature.

   B. **Displacement of the heart** to the opposite side may also result in hypoplasia of the contralateral lung.

   C. **The muscular layers of the pulmonary arteries** appear to be thickened, increasing pulmonary vascular resistance. They are more reactive to hypoxia.

III. **Clinical picture**

   A. **Severe respiratory distress** occurs within minutes after birth if there has been extensive compression of the lung. Dyspnea, cyanosis, and tachypnea demand early attention. The earlier the onset of symptoms, the greater the degree of pulmonary hypoplasia and the worse the prognosis.

   B. **In less severe hernias** there may be no symptoms initially, but as the baby swallows air the intestines distend and compress the lung, causing respiratory distress.

   C. **Survival** is directly related to the age at onset of symptoms. Infants whose symptoms begin after 8 hours of age have a survival rate of better than 90%, while those with onset of respiratory distress within the first 8 hours of life have only a 1 in 3 chance of surviving. These babies require the earliest possible surgical correction.

   Congenital diaphragmatic hernia is the most urgent neonatal emergency. Rapid identification and prompt transfer for surgical treatment are essential if these infants are to have any chance of surviving.

   D. **Asymptomatic diaphragmatic hernias** are occasionally seen. Usually these are right-sided. The patient does not become symptomatic for days or even months. Presumably this is because the position of the liver prevents early herniation of the intestines. There is some association of the late development of right-sided hernias with neonatal streptococcal infection.

IV. **Diagnosis**

   A. **Respiratory distress within the first hours of life** should lead to suspicion of a diaphragmatic hernia.

   B. **Physical examination** may show a **scaphoid abdomen** and shift of the heart sounds to the opposite side. Breath sounds are absent or diminished. The presence or absence of bowel sounds is unreliable as a clue since they are easily transmitted from the abdomen in many other conditions.

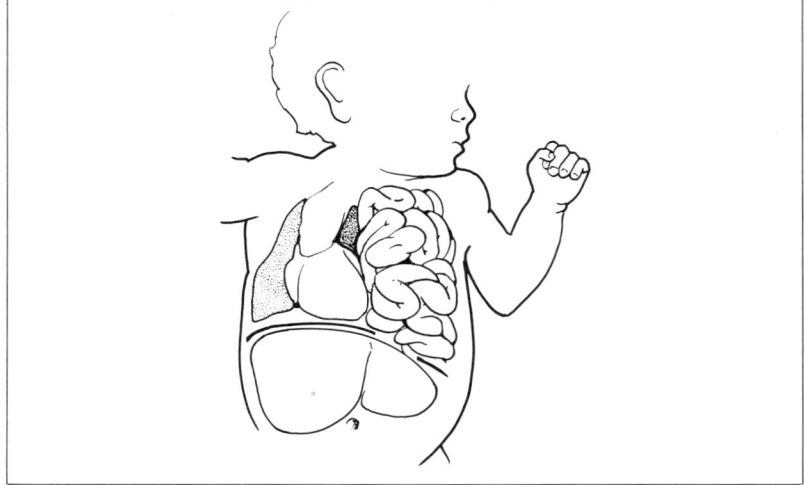

Fig. 15-1. Diaphragmatic hernia. Pathologic anatomy of typical posterolateral (Bochdalek) diaphragmatic hernia. Not only is the ipsilateral lung compressed by the abdominal viscera, but shift of the mediastinum causes compression of the opposite lung as well.

- C. **Chest x-ray** may not show much air in the first hour if the intestines have not yet filled. It may appear as if there is a mass in the chest. A repeat film in 15–30 minutes will usually demonstrate air and permit diagnosis. An **erect** film should always be obtained to differentiate congenital **cysts** or **cystic adenomatoid malformation,** rare conditions that may be mistaken for a diaphragmatic hernia.
- D. If in doubt, **passage of a nasogastric tube** into the stomach will demonstrate the location of the stomach in the chest.
- E. **Arterial blood gas** determinations are unnecessary for diagnosis but if obtained will show a progressive severe hypoxia, hypercapnia, and acidosis.

V. **Problems**
- A. **Respiratory acidosis, hypoxemia, and hypercapnia** result from inadequate exchange of oxygen and carbon dioxide because of the deficiency of functioning lung tissue.
- B. **Metabolic acidosis** rapidly develops as the peripheral tissues are perfused with inadequately oxygenated blood.
- C. **Persistent fetal circulation (PFC)** may result from failure of pulmonary vasodilation, which normally takes place after birth. PFC is exacerbated by the hypoxia, hypercapnia, and acidosis. This right-to-left shunt contributes to the peripheral hypoxemia and acidosis.
- D. **Damage to the hypoplastic lung** also results from the hypoxia, hypercapnia, and acidosis, producing interstitial hemorrhage, edema, and deposition of a pseudohyaline membrane, which further compromises gas exchange.
- E. **Tension pneumothorax** may occur if the infant is ventilated with high pressure. Many patients do not respond to resuscitative measures. This may lead to use of excessive pressure during ventilation and cause additional injury to the hypoplastic lung as well as rupture of alveoli.

VI. Indications for operation.
The presence of a diaphragmatic hernia is the indication for operation. There is no nonoperative treatment. There is no neonatal condition in which the need for immediate operation is more pressing and clear-cut.

VII. Preoperative preparation

A. Preparation for transfer
1. **Delay in treatment** is the most common error in management and may alter the outcome in an otherwise salvageable patient.
2. **Resuscitation is frequently impossible** in congenital diaphragmatic hernia until the hernia is reduced and the lung is ventilated.
3. **A nasogastric tube** (not an infant feeding tube), **size 14F**, should be inserted and placed on suction to prevent increasing distention of the intestine with further compromise of the lungs.
4. **Heat loss must be prevented,** for hypothermia causes acidosis and increased oxygen demand.
5. **Venous or arterial catheters should not be inserted,** nor should arterial blood gas determinations be obtained. These efforts invariably take more time than expected, contribute little to the patient's management, and only delay transfer for definitive treatment.
6. **Bicarbonate** administration may moderate the acidosis but is of limited value until adequate ventilation can be accomplished.
7. An **endotracheal tube** should be inserted even if the infant appears to be ventilating adequately since it may be impossible to intubate the baby during transport if there is deterioration of respiratory function.
8. **Assisted ventilation,** if needed, should be rapid to decrease CO_2, but with **low pressure** (<35 cm H_2O) to avoid alveolar rupture and pneumothorax.
9. **Immediate transport** is essential. In most instances, time will be saved if the referring physician brings the baby in an ambulance rather than waiting for the transport team.

B. At the neonatal center
1. **Preoperative resuscitation** occurs in the operating room. The infant is taken there directly from the ambulance or helicopter. Rapid deterioration can occur without warning, and the infant may require immediate operation.
2. **An upright chest x-ray** should be obtained if one has not previously been taken.
3. The baby's **temperature** should be brought to normal if possible by use of a radiant heater, a warming blanket, and warmed ventilatory gases.
4. **Arterial and venous lines** are established, and baseline arterial blood gas determinations are performed. Improved ventilation by an experienced pediatric anesthesiologist may result in considerable improvement in oxygenation and acidosis. Bicarbonate is given (1 mEq/kg).
5. Although it is clearly worthwhile to spend some time to improve the patient's condition prior to operation, in many instances the infant's only hope for survival is prompt surgical correction of the hernia.
6. **The inability to elevate the blood PaO_2 to above 100 mm Hg** preoperatively by ventilation with 100% oxygen is an ominous prognostic sign.

VIII. Operative care
A. Anesthesia.
Because of the need to administer 100% oxygen, inhalation agents are inappropriate. Intravenous analgesia and muscle relaxants are used. Low-

pressure, high-frequency ventilation will result in optimal gas exchange with the least hazard of rupture of the immature lung and development of tension pneumothorax.

B. Technique

1. **An upper abdominal incision** gives rapid access, easy reduction of the hernia, and good exposure for repair of the diaphragmatic defect. It also permits examination of the abdominal viscera for other possible malformations. All patients have malrotation, for which treatment is seldom necessary.

2. **Insertion of a small catheter** alongside the viscera will break the suction and permit extraction of the intestines if reduction proves difficult.

3. **A hernial sac** is occasionally present. It should be removed from the chest and excised prior to closure of the defect.

4. **Primary closure** of the diaphragmatic defect is possible in most cases, using mattress sutures of heavy, nonabsorbable suture. If the defect is large, a Dacron mesh prosthesis may be necessary. A chest tube is brought out through a lateral stab wound.

5. **No attempt should be made by the anesthetist to expand the tiny ipsilateral lung after reduction of the hernia.** Positive pressure easily ruptures the hypoplastic alveoli, producing a continuing air leak and complicating postoperative management.

6. **Closure of the abdominal cavity is usually possible** even though it is smaller than normal. The muscle wall can be manually stretched if necessary. Milking the intestine free of its contents also will decrease its volume, if necessary. In rare cases in which closure is difficult or results in increased intraabdominal pressure, a single-layer skin closure or a **prosthetic patch** may be used.

7. **The chest tube is NOT connected to suction or water seal** but is plugged with a stopcock and syringe so that air may be removed or added as necessary postoperatively to center the mediastinum and maintain proper expansion of the contralateral lung. If the tube is connected to suction, or even to water seal, positive pressure ventilation will gradually overexpand the contralateral lung and drive air out of the operated side. The "cushion" of air maintained by leaving the operated hemithorax sealed prevents this.

8. **An umbilical artery catheter** should be placed to permit sampling of postductal arterial blood.

IX. Postoperative care. Proper postoperative management of these infants is one of the most difficult challenges in pediatric surgery. For the first 48 hours, they require constant care by physicians and nurses who are knowledgeable about the altered physiology and its treatment. There is no margin for error.

A. Patients may be grouped according to severity of disease (and prognosis) by the method described by Collins:

1. **Class 1** infants are not critically hypoxic and should survive with ordinary management. These infants have sufficient functioning lung tissue.

2. **Class 2** infants do not achieve a postductal arterial PO_2 above 100 mm Hg for at least 1 hour with maximal ventilation with 100% oxygen. These infants have inadequate functioning lung tissue and are incapable of survival regardless of treatment.

3. **Class 3** infants achieve a postoperative postductal arterial PO_2 above 100 mm Hg for at least an hour but then deteriorate. These babies appear to have a barely adequate amount of functioning lung but develop shunting with reestablishment of fetal circulation or sustain damage to the lung on the nonoperated side, which alters its gas-exchange capacity.

B. **The primary objective of postoperative care** is to enable babies in the marginal group (class 3) to survive by **prevention** of the two major lethal complications: **persistent fetal circulation** and **damage to the nonoperated lung**.
   1. **Persistent fetal circulation** results from pulmonary vasoconstriction, which causes right-to-left shunting through the ductus and the foramen ovale.
      a. Since the pulmonary vasculature is very sensitive to oxygen, CO_2, and pH, PFC is best prevented by avoiding hypoxia, hypercapnia, and acidosis, i.e., by adequate ventilation.
      b. **Prevention** of PFC is critical. Once it occurs, treatment is often ineffective.
   2. **Damage to the "good" lung** (the nonoperated side) also results from hypoxia, hypercapnia, and acidosis and from overdistention secondary to excessive ventilatory pressure or contralateral suction.
C. **Details of ventilatory management** are the most important factors in preventing PFC and damage to the nonoperated lung.
   1. **The patient must be paralyzed.** Without paralysis, the infant tends to "fight" the respirator, interfering with ventilation. Pancuronium bromide (Pavulon), 0.5–1.0 mg/kg q4h, is recommended.
   2. **Low-pressure ventilation** with little or no end-expiratory pressure (CPAP) and 100% oxygen is required. It is desirable to reduce the $PaCO_2$ to a level below normal (30–35 mm Hg) by overventilation.
   3. **No attempt should be made to wean** the patient from the ventilator for at least 36 hours, often longer in severe cases.
   4. **Bicarbonate** should be administered by bolus (1 mEq/kg) to combat metabolic acidosis but will be ineffective if adequate oxygenation of the blood cannot be accomplished.
   5. **The mediastinum is centered** to prevent overdistention of the "good" lung. Air is instilled or withdrawn from the operated side through the chest tube as necessary. Frequent chest x-rays (hourly for the first 4–8 hours, every 4 hours for the next 24 hours) are necessary to assess mediastinal position, as well as to detect an early pneumothorax.
   6. **Contralateral pneumothorax** is best prevented by low-pressure ventilation, but if it occurs it must be promptly treated by insertion of a chest tube. Prophylactic insertion of a chest tube on the unoperated side has been recommended to prevent this complication.
   7. **Close monitoring is essential.** Frequent determinations of PaO_2, $PaCO_2$, and pH are necessary to regulate ventilation. Electrolytes, hematocrit, and blood glucose should also be evaluated periodically.
   8. **Extracorporeal membrane oxygenation (ECMO)** has been employed with some success in infants with congenital diaphragmatic hernia who are unable to maintain adequate gas exchange postoperatively. Lung bypass may be necessary for several days to a week.

Complications

A. **Operative complications** include injury to the abdominal viscera during reduction of the hernia, injury to the adrenal gland by sutures placed to repair the diaphragmatic defect, and damage to the collapsed lung by ill-advised attempts to inflate it.

B. **Late postoperative complications** include persistent respiratory insufficiency, recurrent hernia, and infection of the prosthetic patch.

Prognosis. Most infants who do not survive are found to have associated severe congenital malformations, particularly of the heart. Survivors usually have no other abnormalities and can look forward to a normal life. Since the neonatal lung has a great ability to generate new pulmonary units, most survivors have little or no respiratory compromise in later life.

Bibliography

Anderson, K. D. Congenital Diaphragmatic Hernia. In K. J. Welch, et al. (eds.), *Pediatric Surgery*. Chicago: Year Book, 1986. P. 589.

Bartlett, R. H., et al. Extracorporeal membrane oxygenation of newborn respiratory failure: Forty-five cases. *Surgery* 92:425, 1982.

Cloutier, R., Fournier, L., and Levasseur, L. Reversion to fetal circulation in congenital diaphragmatic hernia: A preventable postoperative complication. *J. Pediatr. Surg.* 18:551, 1983.

Collins, D. L., et al. A new approach to congenital posterolateral diaphragmatic hernia. *J. Pediatr. Surg.* 12:149, 1977.

Collins, D. L. Diaphragmatic Hernia. In T. M. Holder and K. W. Ashcraft (eds.), *Pediatric Surgery*. Philadelphia: Saunders, 1980. P. 227.

German, J. C., et al. Pulmonary artery pressure monitoring in persistent fetal circulation (PFC). *J. Pediatr. Surg.* 12:913, 1977.

Gross, R. E. Congenital Hernia of the Diaphragm. In *Surgery of Infancy and Childhood*. Philadelphia: Saunders, 1953. P. 428.

Nguyen, L., et al. The mortality of congenital diaphragmatic hernia. Is total pulmonary mass inadequate, no matter what? *Ann. Surg.* 198:766, 1983.

Peckham, G. J., and Fox, W. W. Physiologic factors affecting pulmonary artery pressure in infants with persistent pulmonary hypertension. *J. Pediatr.* 93:1005, 1978.

Raffensperger, J. G., et al. The effect of overdistention of the lung on pulmonary function in beagle puppies. *J. Pediatr. Surg.* 14:757, 1979.

Ramenofsky, M. L. The effects of intrapleural pressure on respiratory insufficiency. *J. Pediatr. Surg.* 14:750, 1979.

Reynolds, M., Luck, S. R., and Lappen R. The "critical" neonate with diaphragmatic hernia: A 21-year perspective. *J. Pediatr. Surg.* 19:364, 1984.

Touloukian, R. J., and Markowitz R. I. A preoperative scoring system for risk assessment of newborns with congenital diaphragmatic hernia. *J. Pediatr. Surg.* 19:252, 1984.

Wohl, M. E. B., et al. The lung following repair of congenital diaphragmatic hernia. *J. Pediatr.* 90:405, 1977.

16 Esophageal Atresia and Tracheoesophageal Fistula

I. **Definition.** Esophageal discontinuity and communication with the trachea result from errors of embryogenesis occurring within the first 6 weeks of fetal life.
   A. There are **five** recognized variations (Fig. 16-1).
      1. **Esophageal atresia with distal tracheoesophageal fistula,** the most common form (85%)
      2. **Esophageal atresia with proximal fistula**
      3. **Esophageal atresia with proximal and distal fistulas**
      4. **Isolated esophageal atresia** (no fistula)
      5. **Isolated tracheoesophageal fistula** (no esophageal atresia)
   B. **Associated anomalies are frequently found.** Esophageal atresia may be part of the **VACTERL** syndrome (vertebral, anal, cardiac, tracheal, esophageal, renal, and limb anomalies).

II. **Pathophysiology**
   A. **Esophageal atresia (EA) with distal tracheoesophageal fistula (TEF),** the most common form, results in the following:
      1. **Inability to swallow** food or secretions.
      2. **Aspiration of saliva** as the proximal pouch fills up and spills over into the trachea. Respiratory distress, atelectasis, and pneumonia may result.
      3. **Abdominal distention** caused by air entering the GI tract through the tracheoesophageal fistula.
      4. **Aspiration of gastric acid juice,** which refluxes up the esophagus into the trachea through the tracheoesophageal fistula. This may cause a chemical pneumonia.
   B. **In isolated EA,** air cannot enter the intestinal tract, so the **abdomen is flat and airless.** Aspiration of saliva (but not gastric juice) can occur.
   C. **Isolated TEF** results in **aspiration of liquids** into the airway at the time of feeding. The patient may be asymptomatic between feedings.

III. **Clinical presentation**
   A. **Polyhydramnios** frequently accompanies esophageal atresia and may be detected before the baby is born, suggesting the diagnosis.
   B. The presence of **excessive secretions** is usually the first sign of esophageal atresia. The nurse may note that frequent suctioning is required to clear the airway.
   C. **Respiratory distress** and **cyanosis** develop as the infant repeatedly aspirates saliva, which spills over from the obstructed esophagus.
   D. **Vomiting of feedings** occurs if the diagnosis has not been made and the infant is fed.
   E. **Isolated TEF** is seldom diagnosed early in life. The infant has no breathing or swallowing difficulties but **chokes** at the time of feeding as liquid passes through the fistula. **Recurrent pneumonia** may be the presenting complaint in isolated TEF.

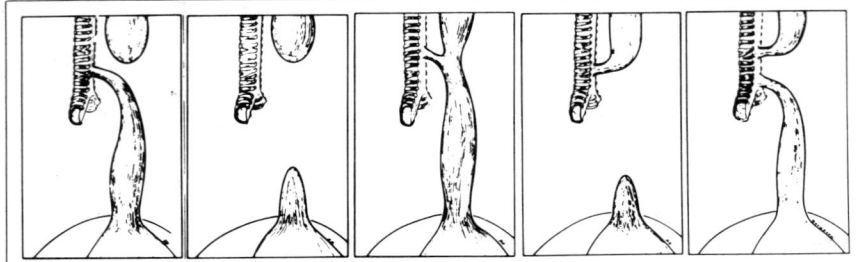

Fig. 16-1. Types of esophageal atresia and tracheoesophageal fistula (TEF). Left to right: Esophageal atresia with distal TEF. Esophageal atresia without TEF. TEF without esophageal atresia. Esophageal atresia with proximal TEF. Esophageal atresia with both proximal and distal TEF. (From L. L. Leape and T. M. Holder, Pediatric Surgery. In D. C. Sabiston (Ed.), *Textbook of Surgery*. Philadelphia: Saunders, 1981.)

IV. Diagnosis

A. **Failure of a nasogastric tube to pass** into the stomach is virtually diagnostic of esophageal atresia.

   1. This maneuver should be carried out in all babies with **unexplained polyhydramnios** and in any infant in whom the diagnosis of esophageal atresia is a possibility.

   2. **A large tube** (No. 14F rubber catheter) is used. A small feeding tube will coil in the blind esophagus, giving a false impression of complete passage into the stomach.

B. **Chest x-ray** will confirm the location of the catheter in the blind esophageal pouch (Fig. 16-2). A **lateral** film most accurately demonstrates pouch length. Contrast studies are unnecessary and may increase the risk of pulmonary complications.

C. **The presence of air in the stomach and intestinal tract** seen on chest x-ray confirms the presence of a TEF.

D. **Diagnosis of isolated TEF may be difficult.** Contrast esophagogram will sometimes demonstrate the fistula. **Bronchoscopy** is more reliable and should be carried out if the diagnosis is suspected.

V. Problems

A. **Prematurity** is commonly associated with esophageal atresia and complicates patient management. Ventilatory assistance may be required, as well as attention to other manifestations of immature organ systems, such as hypoglycemia, hypocalcemia, feeding problems, and jaundice.

B. **Aspiration pneumonia** often develops if the diagnosis is not promptly made or if treatment is delayed.

C. **Abdominal distention** may result from air forced into the intestine through a large tracheoesophageal fistula. If severe, it can lead to **respiratory embarrassment.**

D. **Associated anomalies,** found in 30–50% of patients, may influence treatment and outcome. **Cardiac** anomalies in particular may be severe and life-threatening. Approximately 10% of infants with esophageal atresia have **imperforate anus.**

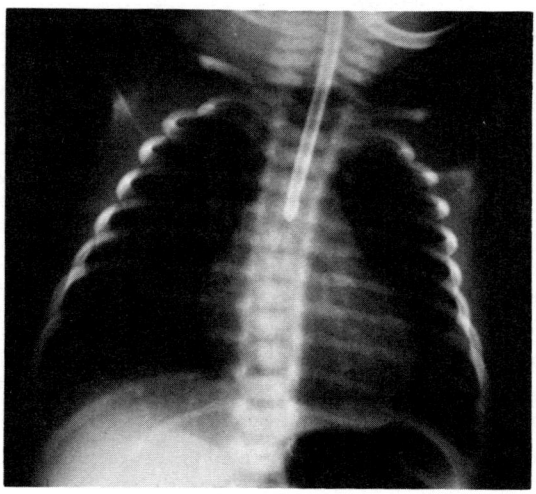

Fig. 16-2. Esophageal atresia. Chest x-ray demonstrates catheter arrested in the upper esophagus. (From L. L. Leape and T. M. Holder, Pediatric Surgery. In D. C. Sabiston (Ed.), *Textbook of Surgery*. Philadelphia: Saunders, 1981.)

    E. Long-gap atresia (typical in isolated esophageal atresia) poses a technical challenge to elongate the pouches so that a tension-free anastomosis may be achieved.

    F. Large tracheoesophageal fistula may result in **inadequate ventilation** because of air leak into the intestinal tract. Gastrostomy may aggravate this situation by making egress of air easier.

VI. Indications for operation. There is no nonoperative treatment for esophageal atresia or tracheoesophageal fistula; therefore, surgical repair is indicated unless the infant also has life-threatening uncorrectable anomalies of the heart or nervous system or has chromosomal abnormalities incompatible with life.

VII. Preoperative preparation

    A. First aid. The diagnosis of esophageal atresia should lead immediately to measures to decrease complications.

        1. A nasoesophageal sump catheter is inserted into the blind upper esophageal pouch and connected to high suction to clear swallowed saliva and minimize aspiration.

        2. The baby is placed in a chair at 60 degrees to minimize reflux of acid gastric juice up the esophagus and through the tracheoesophageal fistula into the lungs. Alternatively, he may be placed prone, but not supine.

        3. Intravenous fluids are given to replace losses.

        4. Antibiotics are given for presumed pulmonary infection.

    B. Timing of operation

        1. Uncomplicated EA with distal TEF in an otherwise healthy infant should be surgically repaired before complications develop—**within 24 hours.**

        2. Delayed operation is indicated for the following conditions:

            a. Pneumonia, sepsis, undefined symptomatic heart disease, or any condition that appreciably increases surgical risk.

b. **Severe prematurity.**

c. **Long gap atresia.** Delay of repair for 4–6 weeks enables the upper pouch to elongate, making end-to-end anastomosis possible in almost all patients.

3. **Staged operation (division of the TEF with later repair of the EA)** may be necessary if a definitive operation must be delayed and adequate ventilation cannot be achieved because of the size of the TEF, or if there is recurrent aspiration of gastric juice despite gastrostomy drainage.

C. **Supportive measures** maintain nutrition and help prevent complications if repair of EA must be delayed.

1. **Sump suction** of the proximal pouch to prevent spillover aspiration of saliva.

2. **Gastrostomy** for either:

   a. **Drainage of acid gastric juice** if an operation must be delayed for a week or longer (tiny premature infants)

   b. **Feeding** of the infant after a staged procedure and in isolated EA while awaiting elongation of the pouches

3. **Parenteral nutrition** via central catheter.

4. **Jejunal feedings** via a tube placed through the gastrostomy catheter at the time of gastrostomy may also be used.

5. **Ventilatory assistance** may be necessary, particularly if there is a large TEF or other lung disease.

6. In **long-gap atresia,** the patient may be nursed prone since there is no concern about reflux of acid into the lungs.

   a. **Gastrostomy feedings** may help distend and elongate the distal pouch.

   b. There is no evidence that **stretching** of the upper pouch by passage of bougies accomplishes more than the passage of time alone.

VIII. **Operative care**

A. **The retropleural approach,** through the right fourth interspace, permits easy access to the two ends of the esophagus while preventing intrapleural empyema if an anastomotic leak occurs.

B. **The thick proximal pouch is mobilized** as much as necessary to provide adequate length for a tension-free anastomosis. The thin distal pouch is not mobilized to avoid disturbing its tenuous blood supply.

C. **The TEF is divided,** and the tracheal opening is closed with fine absorbable sutures and covered with local connective tissue.

D. **End-to-end anastomosis** of the esophagus is performed in a single layer using six or eight 4-0 absorbable synthetic sutures tied on the outside.

E. **A catheter** is inserted through the mouth to the anastomosis and marked as a distance **guide for later suctioning.**

F. **Circular myotomy** is performed on the proximal pouch to give additional length if a tension-free anastomosis cannot be achieved without it.

G. **Gastrostomy** should be performed if the anastomosis is at all questionable.

H. **Repair of isolated TEF** is easier if bronchoscopy is carried out first, and a fine catheter is passed through the fistula for identification at the time of division. Most can be divided by a cervical approach.

I. **Esophageal replacement** by a gastric tube or colonic interposition is rarely required. It is indicated for a failed anastomosis which must be sacrificed because of disruption and severe sepsis.

Postoperative care

A. **Ventilatory management** is the prime consideration in the immediate postoperative period. Thoracotomy reduces thoracic excursions and causes diaphragmatic splinting. Repair of the TEF hampers clearing of secretions by the trachea, which is abnormal to begin with. Tracheomalacia may be present.

   1. **Frequent tracheal suctioning** is needed, using the premarked catheter as a guide.
   2. **Mechanical ventilation** via nasotracheal tube is frequently necessary for several days or more. Arterial blood gas determinations are obtained as necessary.
   3. **Chest x-rays** are obtained as needed, at least daily for the first several days and every other day until the chest tube is removed.

B. **Antibiotics** (ampicillin and gentamicin in usual doses) are given as prophylaxis for wound infection for the first 24 hours.

C. **Chest tube drainage** is to water seal. The tube is left in for 10 days, until danger of anastomotic leak has passed.

D. **Oral feedings** may begin on the second day unless there is concern about the anastomosis, in which case they should be withheld for 10 days. (The anastomosis is weakest at 5–7 days.)

E. **Dilatations of the anastomosis** are necessary in 5–10% of patients. The number of dilatations can be significantly decreased if they are begun **early** and performed **frequently**. Delay leads to the development of hard, mature fibrous tissue, which is difficult to dilate, greatly prolonging the duration of treatment.

   1. **The caliber** of the esophageal anastomosis **should be monitored** in every infant postoperatively. Because the infant drinks only liquid, dysphagia or other symptoms of stricture will not develop until the anastomosis gets very small (6–8F), by which time it will be difficult to dilate.
   2. The esophagus is calibrated by passage of **soft rubber catheters at 10–14 days postrepair.** It should accept a **14F** or larger catheter; if it does not, dilatation is indicated.
   3. **The caliber of the anastomosis is checked** with rubber catheters **every 2 weeks** for at least 6 weeks. If the anastomosis is growing with the patient, dilatations will not be needed.
   4. **If the anastomosis is not growing, dilatation** (with esophagoscopy under general anesthesia) is performed biweekly until it is no longer necessary.

F. **Gastroesophageal reflux** (GER) occurs in virtually every patient with esophageal atresia and may result in serious complications. **Prophylactic treatment** of GER reduces complications and is indicated for the first 6 months.

   1. Twenty-four-hour **upright positioning**—in a chair or prone on an inclined board
   2. **Thickening of all feedings** (1 tablespoon cereal per ounce of formula)
   3. **Cimetidine** (1 mg/kg qid) to prevent esophagitis

Complications

A. **Early complications**

   1. **Pneumothorax.** In the immediate postoperative period, pneumothorax results from incomplete evacuation of air at the time of the operation or from

leak around the chest tube at the skin entry site. Later, pneumonothorax may result from a leak in the esophagus or trachea.

2. **Anastomotic leak** results from excessive tension, too many or too tight sutures, or insufficient blood supply. A leak may occur at any time within the first 10 days.

   a. **Diagnosis.** The appearance of saliva or feedings in the chest tube is usually the first clue, but the only sign may be the accumulation of fluid in the upper thorax as noted by x-ray. A leak may be confirmed by giving the infant methylene blue–dyed saline to drink or by contrast esophagogram.

   b. **Treatment.** Esophageal anastomotic leaks will usually close spontaneously if feedings are discontinued and reflux is prevented by gastrostomy drainage. Parenteral nutrition is necessary.

3. **Anastomotic disruption** is a life-threatening event requiring immediate diagnosis and treatment.

   a. **Diagnosis.** Sudden deterioration of the infant with signs of sepsis suggests anastomotic disruption. Chest x-ray may show a pneumothorax, sometimes under tension. Esophagogram with water-soluble contrast demonstrates the leak.

   b. **Treatment.** Immediate tube thoracotomy may be sufficient treatment if sepsis is not severe, but in some patients reoperation is necessary. Reanastomosis is seldom possible, so closure of the distal esophagus and establishment of a cervical diverting esophagostomy may be necessary as life-saving measures.

4. **Tracheal leak** is a life-threatening complication resulting from infection, suction trauma, or improper suture technique. Immediate surgical repair is necessary. A pleural or muscle flap is used to reinforce the closure.

5. **Pulmonary insufficiency** may result from infection, lung trauma during operation, poor tracheal clearing of secretions, fluid accumulation, or infection. Ventilatory support, physiotherapy, and antibiotics are indicated.

B. **Late complications**

1. **Anastomotic stricture** results from excessive tension or ischemia. Anastomotic leak sometimes heals with stricture formation.

   a. **Early recognition and dilatation** greatly minimize stricture formation (see sec. **IX.E**). Aggressive treatment in the first few months of life prevents long-term disability.

   b. **Refractory stricture** may result from uncontrolled gastroesophageal reflux and require an antireflux operation for cure.

   c. **Steroid injections** in the stricture (triamcinolone, 1 mg) are sometimes helpful.

   d. **Rarely, resection and reanastomosis is necessary** for severe refractory strictures.

   e. **Dysphagia occurring after a prolonged asymptomatic period may not be due to anastomotic stricture.** Reflux esophagitis is more likely to be the cause.

2. **Foreign body obstruction** of the esophagus is a common complication, occurring at some time in at least half of patients with successful repair of esophageal atresia.

   a. **It is most common during the second and third years of life** when the child is able to eat large bites but unable to understand the consequences.

b. **Stricture is not necessary.** The anastomosis is an unyielding ring of scar tissue, even when adequate in caliber: A piece of meat or other insoluble food will get caught if it is just slightly larger.

c. **Esophagoscopy** is performed to remove the foreign body as well as to assess the adequacy of the anastomosis. Dilatation may be necessary.

3. **Complications of gastroesophageal reflux** may occur despite prophylactic treatment.

   a. **Recurrent pulmonary infections**

   b. **Apneic spells**

   c. **Esophagitis** with bleeding, dysphagia, or stricture formation

   d. **Refractory anastomotic stricture**

   e. **Vomiting with failure to thrive**

4. **Respiratory obstruction** may result from **tracheomalacia, tracheal stenosis,** or **compression** of the trachea by distention of the proximal esophagus at the time of feeding.

5. **Recurrent pulmonary infections** are a common problem following repair of EA. Possible causes include the following:

   a. **Tracheomalacia** and poor tracheal secretion clearing

   b. **Anastomotic stricture** with overflow aspiration

   c. **Gastroesophageal reflux**

   d. **Recurrent TEF**

6. **Recurrent TEF** may occur months or years after repair. The symptoms are choking and coughing with feedings (as with a primary isolated TEF). Since these symptoms are also seen with stricture, they may be misunderstood or ignored.

   a. **Diagnosis** is by thin-contrast cineesophagogram or bronchoscopy.

   b. **Surgical repair** may require reanastomosis of the esophagus or interposition of a muscle flap.

Prognosis. Following successful repair of esophageal atresia, aggressive postoperative management will prevent most complications. All patients have some esophageal dysmotility that requires food to be adequately chewed, but otherwise there should be no disability. Complications usually occur in the first year, after which all but a few children can lead a normal life.

Bibliography

Ashcraft, K. W., et al. Early recognition and aggressive treatment of gastroesophageal reflux following repair of esophageal atresia. *J. Pediatr. Surg.* 12:317, 1977.

Ashcraft, K. W., and Holder, T. M. Esophageal Atresia and Tracheoesophageal Malformations. In T. M. Holder and K. W. Ashcraft (eds.), *Pediatric Surgery.* Philadelphia: Saunders, 1980. P. 266.

Ashcraft, K. W., Leape, L. L., and Holder, T. M. Parenteral nutrition and esophageal anastomotic leak. *Arch. Surg.* 101:436, 1970.

Barry, J. E., and Auldist, A. The VATER Association: One end of a spectrum of anomalies. *Am. J. Dis. Child.* 128:769, 1984.

deLorimier, A. A., and Harrison, M. R. Long gap esophageal atresia: Primary anastomosis after esophageal elongation by bouginage and esophagomyotomy. *J. Thorac. Cardiovasc. Surg.* 79:138, 1980.

Filler, R. M., Rossello, P. J., and Lebowitz, R. L. Life-threatening anoxic spells caused by tracheal compression after repair of esophageal atresia: Correction by surgery. *J. Pediatr. Surg.* 11:739, 1976.

Holder, T. M., et al. Esophageal atresia and tracheoesophageal fistula. A survey of its members by the Surgical Section of the American Academy of Pediatrics. *Pediatrics* 34:542, 1961.

Holder, T. M., Leape, L. L., and Mann, C. M. Esophageal atresia, tracheoesophageal fistula and associated anomalies (hyperalimentation as an aid in treatment). *J. Thorac. Cardiovasc. Surg.* 63:838, 1972.

Janik, J. S., et al. Long-term follow-up of circular myotomy for esophageal atresia. *J. Pediatr. Surg.* 15:835, 1980.

Jolley, S. G., et al. Patterns of gastroesophageal reflux in children following repair of esophageal atresia and distal tracheoesophageal fistula. *J. Pediatr. Surg.* 15:857, 1980.

Livaditis, A., et al. Esophageal end-to-end anastomosis. *Scand. J. Thorac. Cardiovasc. Surg.* 6:206, 1972.

Louhimo, I., and Lindahl, H. Esophageal atresia: Primary results of 500 consecutively treated patients. *J. Pediatr. Surg.* 18:217, 1983.

Orringer, M. B., Kirsh, M. M., and Sloan, H. Long-term esophageal function following repair of esophageal atresia. *Ann. Surg.* 186:436, 1977.

Pieretti, R., Shandling, B., and Stephens C. A. Resistant esophageal stenosis associated with reflux after repair of esophageal atresia. *J. Pediatr. Surg.* 9:355, 1974.

Puri, P., et al. Delayed primary anastomosis following spontaneous growth of esophageal segments in esophageal atresia. *J. Pediatr. Surg.* 16:180, 1981.

Randolph, J. G. Esophageal atresia and congenital stenosis. In K. J. Welch, et al. (eds.), *Pediatric Surgery*. Chicago: Year Book, 1986. P. 682.

17 Omphalocele and Gastroschisis

Definition. Failure of embryologic closure of the abdominal wall during the eleventh week of fetal life results in protrusion of the viscera through an opening in or near the umbilical cord. The incidence is 1 in 3–10,000 live births.

A. Omphalocele. The opening is **in** the umbilical cord and may vary in size from 2 to 15 cm. There is a peritoneal sac in which the contents are mostly liver with varying amounts of intestine.

B. Gastroschisis. The opening is **next** to the umbilical cord, it is usually less than 5 cm in diameter, and there is **no sac**. Usually the small intestine and part of the colon eviscerate, rarely the liver, spleen, or small amounts of the stomach.

C. Related anomalies.

1. **Exstrophy of the cloaca.** Omphalocele in the lower abdomen with hindgut agenesis, imperforate anus, exstrophy of the bladder, and vesicointestinal fistula
2. **Pentalogy of Cantrell.** Epigastric omphalocele with cleft sternum, congenital heart disease, and absence of the central diaphragm and diaphragmatic pericardium

Pathophysiology

A. In **omphalocele, the sac** protects the viscera, so there is rarely intrauterine injury.

B. Absence of a sac in gastroschisis permits the intestines to float freely in the amniotic cavity.

1. **Nonfixation of the gut** permits rotation; **volvulus** may occur with venous compromise, ischemia, and edema.
2. **Exposure to amniotic fluid is irritating** to the herniated intestine, further adding to the injury from twisting.
3. As a result, the **gut appears swollen, edematous, leathery, semirigid, and matted together.** It may be shorter than normal.

C. The abdominal cavity is underdeveloped since many of the viscera have remained outside, particularly in gastroschisis.

D. Vaginal delivery may be impossible because of the added bulk of the external viscera.

Diagnosis. The diagnosis of omphalocele or gastroschisis is obvious at birth. **Prenatal diagnosis** may have been made by **ultrasound,** which is fairly reliable.

Problems

A. Hypothermia and hypovolemia may result from evaporative water loss caused by exposure of the intestine or sac.

B. Gangrene of part of the intestine may be present because of compromise of the blood supply.

C. Associated anomalies are present in 50% of patients with omphalocele.

1. Trisomy 13, 18, and 21.
2. Beckwith-Wiedemann syndrome (omphalocele, macroglossia, macrosomatia, facial nevus flammeus, indented ear lobes, microcephaly, and

hyperplasia of the kidney, pancreas, and liver). Severe **hypoglycemia** may occur.

3. **Cardiac, genitourinary, skeletal, and neurologic anomalies** are frequently found.
4. **Intestinal tract anomalies** include malrotation in all patients, Meckel's diverticulum, intestinal atresia, and duplication.

D. In **gastroschisis,** associated anomalies are **much less common.**

1. Many patients are **premature** infants.
2. All have **malrotation.**
3. **Meckel's diverticulum** and **intestinal atresia** may be seen, the latter sometimes resulting from volvulus of the unattached intestine.
4. **Short intestine** is sometimes present and may result in later **malabsorption.**

V. **Preoperative preparation**

A. **Preparation for transfer**

1. **A nasogastric tube** (14F or larger—**not** an infant feeding tube) should be inserted promptly and kept on suction to prevent dilatation of the intestine from swallowed air.
2. **The sac or intestines should be covered** to prevent loss of fluid and heat.
   a. **Sterile plastic sheeting** should be applied directly to the sac or bowel to serve as a vapor barrier.
   b. **Warm, dry dressings** covered by towels or blankets will further conserve heat.
   c. **Wet saline sponges should not be used** unless covered with plastic. Otherwise, they only serve as an efficient cooling agent as the moisture evaporates.
3. The infant's **entire body** except for the head can be placed in a **plastic bag** to prevent heat and moisture loss.
4. **Transport** should be in a **warm incubator.** Oxygen or assisted ventilation is seldom needed.
5. Insertion of intravenous or intraarterial lines is not necessary prior to transport if the infant is promptly and properly wrapped.

B. **Preparation at the neonatal surgical center**

1. Perform **physical examination** to discover associated anomalies.
2. Obtain **chest and abdominal x-rays.**
3. Administer **fluid resuscitation** intravenously if the patient is cold or hypovolemic. **Note:** Fluid balance and electrolytes are normal at birth. Resuscitation is needed only if pretransfer management has been inadequate or prolonged.
4. **Monitor blood glucose** if the patient has Beckwith-Wiedemann syndrome.
5. Take patients with **gastroschisis** to the operating room **as soon as possible** to minimize further intestinal damage and to decrease bacterial colonization.
6. **Omphalocele patients do not require immediate operation** because the sac protects the viscera. Take the time to assess the significance of any associated anomalies.

Ch 17. Omphalocele and Gastroschisis 119

I. Operative care

A. **Successful return** of the viscera and closure of the defect depends on two factors over which the surgeon has no control:

   1. **The discrepancy** in size between the large herniated **viscera** and the abnormally **small abdominal cavity**
   2. **The size of the defect** in the abdominal wall

B. **Primary closure** of the abdominal wall after reduction of the herniated viscera is the ideal. The following maneuvers are helpful:

   1. **Evacuation of the intestinal contents** antegrade out the rectum and retrograde into the stomach for removal by the anesthetist via the nasogastric tube
   2. **Manual stretching of the abdominal wall** from the spine to the edges of the defect

C. **Staged prosthetic closure should be performed if primary closure is impossible** or results in excessive intraabdominal pressure that compromises respiration or venous return (Fig. 17-1).

   1. **A "silo" extension** of the peritoneal cavity is created temporarily to allow the intestines to shrink and the abdominal wall to stretch.
   2. **Reinforced polymeric silicone (Silastic) sheeting** is used to protect the intestine (an artificial peritoneum) and is sewn to the full thickness of the abdominal wall with heavy sutures that will not cut through.
   3. **The prosthesis is removed** and the abdominal wall closed **at a second operation** under general anesthesia.

D. Before **operative closure,** the intestines are examined for atresias or other **anomalies. The edematous ischemic bowel** in gastroschisis does not readily accept sutures or heal well, so operative correction of any defects may be best deferred to a later time.

E. **A central line** should be inserted for parenteral nutrition in patients who will not be able to use their intestinal tract within a week or so (essentially all patients with gastroschisis and any patients with omphalocele requiring a prosthesis).

F. **Coverage** of an omphalocele or gastroschisis by **skin flaps** alone is no longer appropriate. This early method merely postpones the day when the muscles must be stretched to create an adequate abdominal cavity. It is much easier and faster to stretch the muscles in the first week of life.

G. **Nonoperative treatment** is also no longer appropriate except in patients with complicated omphalocele who are not candidates for any corrective surgery. The sac is painted with 0.25% silver nitrate solution or alcohol (not merbromin, which is toxic) to encourage the formation of a sterile eschar, which gradually contracts to produce skin coverage. Later muscle-wall repair is needed if the patient survives.

Postoperative care

A. **After primary closure** of an omphalocele or gastroschisis, the major concern is that the closure **may be too tight.**

   1. **Respiratory compromise** results from excessive pressure on the diaphragm. **Ventilatory assistance may be required** for several days. **In extreme cases,** reoperation and insertion of a prosthesis may be needed.
   2. **Venous stasis** results from pressure on the inferior vena cava, causing **edema and cyanosis of the lower extremities and perineum and decreased cardiac output.** Additional intravenous fluids must be given.

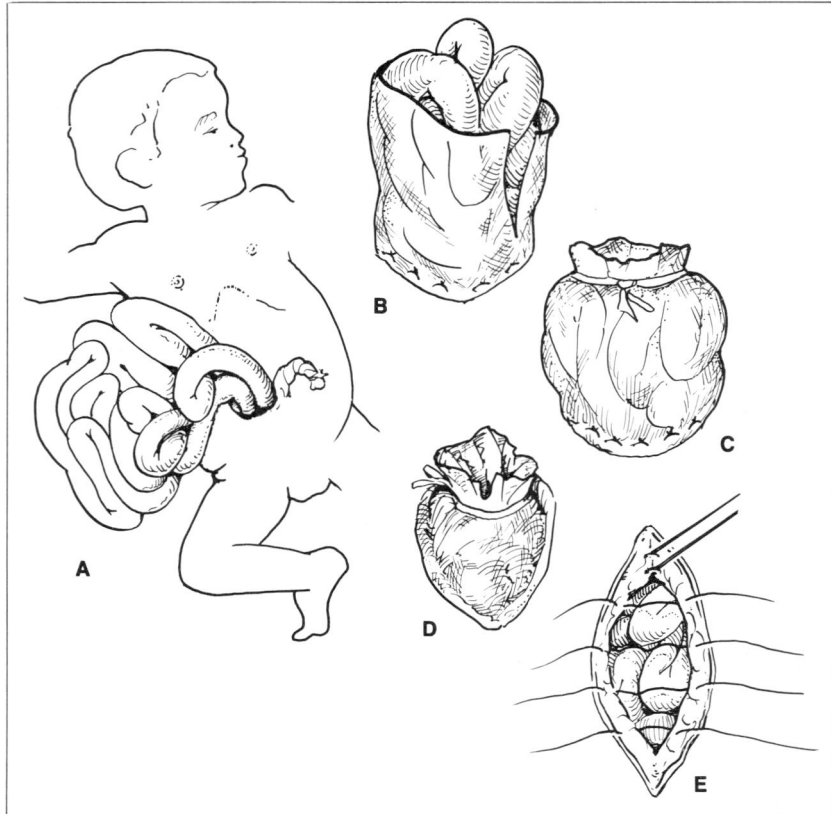

Fig. 17-1. Gastroschisis. A. Intestine herniated through periumbilical defect. B. Construction of a "chimney" of silastic sheeting and Dacron mesh. C. Daily reduction of size of prosthetic sac. D. Complete reduction of herniated viscera. E. Closure of abdomen after removal of prosthetic material.

- **B. Prosthetic closure** should not result in respiratory or vascular compromise but carries its own problems.
    1. **The prosthetic sac is twisted to reduce its size each day,** stretching the muscles as the intestine shrinks. This takes from 3–10 days, after which the risks of sutures pulling out and infection increase significantly.
    2. **Infection** must be prevented by:
        a. **Careful aseptic daily dressing changes**
        b. **Topical antibiotic ointment** applications to the suture line daily
        c. **Systemic antibiotic administration**
    3. **Nutrition** is maintained by intravenous total parenteral nutrition (TPN) during this process and until the intestine resumes function, which may take several weeks.

VIII. Complications

- **A. Infection of the prosthesis** is a feared and serious complication and can occur despite all precautions.

1. **Control may require removal** of the prosthesis and secondary healing by granulation. Fortunately, by the time this is necessary, there is usually enough of a pseudoperitoneal membrane to prevent evisceration.
2. **Later, staged closure** of the muscle is usually required.

B. **Intestinal obstruction** is common after closure of gastroschisis and some large omphaloceles, particularly if a prosthetic closure is required. **Reoperation should be delayed** for at least 3 weeks unless there is evidence of strangulation of bowel. Sometimes it takes 6 weeks or more for the bowel to function well enough to accept feedings.

C. **Malabsorption** may be caused by antenatal ischemic damage to the bowel and to the short intestine, compounded by prematurity.
1. **Feedings must be advanced slowly,** starting with dilute formula, gradually increasing volume and strength as tolerated. **Vitamin supplements** should be provided.
2. **Contrast radiograms** of the intestine should be obtained to rule out chronic partial obstruction.
3. **Prolonged hospitalization** is not unusual for these patients.

IX. Prognosis

A. **In omphalocele patients,** the ultimate outcome is usually determined by the severity of associated anomalies. In their absence, these patients do well once they recover from the operation.

B. The outcome in **gastroschisis patients** is usually dependent on the condition of the intestine—whether it is adequate to sustain nutrition. If it is, most of these babies can look forward to a normal life.

Bibliography

Allen, R. G. Omphalocele and Gastroschisis. In T. M. Holder and K. W. Ashcraft (eds.), *Pediatric Surgery*. Philadelphia: Saunders, 1980. P. 572.

Allen, R. G., and Wrenn, E. L. Silon as a sac in the treatment of omphalocele and gastroschisis. *J. Pediatr. Surg.* 4:3, 1969.

Berseth, C. L., et al. Longitudinal growth and late morbidity of survivors of gastroschisis and omphalocele. *J. Pediatr. Gastroenterol. Nutr.* 1:375, 1982.

Cantrell, J. R., Haller, J. A., and Ravitch, M. M. A syndrome of congenital defects involving the abdominal wall, sternum, diaphragm, pericardium and heart. *Surg. Gynecol. Obstet.* 107:602, 1958.

Filler, R. M., et al. Total intravenous nutrition, an adjunct to the management of infants with a ruptured omphalocele. *Am. J. Surg.* 121:454, 1971.

Greenwood, R. D., Rosenthal, A., and Nadas A. S. Cardiovascular malformations associated with omphalocele. *J. Pediatr.* 85:818, 1974.

Schuster, S. R. A new method for the staged repair of large omphaloceles. *Surg. Gynecol. Obstet.* 125:837, 1967.

Schuster, S. R. Omphalocele and Gastroschisis. In K. J. Welch et al. (eds.), *Pediatric Surgery*. Chicago: Year Book, 1986. P. 740.

18 Umbilical Anomalies

Definition. The umbilicus may be the site of several malformations: **hernia** (see Chap. 19), **granuloma, polyp, patent vitelline** (omphalomesenteric) **duct, patent urachus,** and urachal or vitelline **cysts** or **sinuses.** *Omphalitis* is infection of the umbilicus.

Pathophysiology

A. **Vitelline cysts and sinuses** result from failure of the vitelline duct to involute as it fuses with the body stalk to form the umbilical cord in the seventh week of embryonic life. This may be a fistula from the umbilicus to the midgut, a blind sinus, or a cyst.

B. **Urachal cysts and sinuses** are caused by failure of the allantois to involute. If there is an open connection with the bladder, it is a patent urachus.

C. Umbilical **polyp** is a mucosal remnant of the vitelline duct.

D. Umbilical **granuloma** is granulation tissue caused by incomplete healing of the umbilicus after separation of the cord.

E. **Omphalitis** in the newborn results from improper care of the umbilical stump or from insertion of catheters. In older children, omphalitis is usually caused by a persistent vitelline or urachal sinus.

Clinical presentation

A. A **patent vitelline duct** has a red mucosal opening; it drains intestinal contents if it is patent to the intestine. A shorter remnant (sinus) may drain mucoid material or become infected. A **cyst** develops from residual mucosa, which may occur along the incompletely involuted duct anywhere from the umbilicus to the intestine.

B. A **patent urachus** is a common anomaly, but it is usually asymptomatic unless the umbilical end is open, permitting drainage of urine. A sinus that is open only at the umbilicus may become infected. One open at the bladder may form a **bladder diverticulum. Urachal cysts** can grow to a large size before becoming symptomatic. Infection results in a large, tender infraumbilical mass.

C. An **umbilical polyp** is usually asymptomatic but may connect with a cyst, sinus, or band to the intestine.

D. **Umbilical granuloma** is noted as a pink-red mass in the umbilicus in the second or third week of life. Usually there is a small amount of semipurulent drainage from the raw tissue but no urine or intestinal contents.

E. **Omphalitis** presents as redness, swelling, and pain in the umbilicus, which readily spreads as cellulitis of the abdominal wall.

Diagnosis. Careful examination of the umbilicus and probing to demonstrate a fistula or sinus will usually indicate the diagnosis. Cysts may be palpable by rectal examination.

A. A **sinogram** (injection of radiocontrast material into an opening during fluoroscopy) will usually demonstrate a connection of a sinus with the intestine or bladder if it is present.

B. **Ultrasound or CT scan** best demonstrates a cyst.

Problems. Recurrent infections are common in cysts and sinuses.

VI. **Indications for operation.** Umbilical anomalies should be excised to forestall complications. Umbilical granuloma is treated by silver nitrate cauterization or excision in the office.
VII. **Preoperative preparation.** Routine.
VIII. **Operative care.** With the exception of a large vitelline or urachal cyst, umbilical anomalies can be removed through an intraumbilical incision. The entire tract or band must be removed. If it has been infected, the wound should be drained.
IX. **Postoperative care.** Routine. Many of these procedures are suitable for day surgery.
X. **Complications.** Wound infection is the most common complication.
XI. **Prognosis.** If excision is incomplete, recurrence is virtually assured. Otherwise, surgical removal is curative.

Bibliography

Bell, M. J. Umbilical and Other Abdominal Wall Hernias. In T. M. Holder and K. W. Ashcraft (eds.), *Pediatric Surgery*. Philadelphia: Saunders, 1980. P. 589.

Blichert-Toft, M., and Nielsen C. W. Congenital patent urachus and acquired variants. *Acta Chir. Scand.* 137:807, 1971.

Rich, R. H., Hardy, B. E., and Filler, R. M. Surgery for anomalies of the urachus. *J. Pediatr. Surg.* 18:370, 1983.

Shaw, A. Disorders of the Umbilicus. In K. J. Welch, et al. (eds.), *Pediatric Surgery*. Chicago: Year Book, 1986. P. 731.

Steck, W. D., and Helwig, E. B. Umbilical granulomas, pilonidal disease and the urachus. *Surg. Gynecol. Obstet.* 120:1043, 1965.

19 Umbilical Hernia

1. **Definition.** Herniation of intestine or omentum through a fascial defect in the umbilicus. It is a common defect, occurring 5–10 times more frequently in blacks than whites. The incidence is also increased in patients with Beckwith's syndrome, Hurler's syndrome, and trisomy 13 or 18.
2. **Pathophysiology.** Failure of the umbilical ring to contract completely as the intestines return to the coelomic cavity leaves a fascial defect at the exit of the umbilical cord. Ultimately, the fascial ring almost always closes, eliminating the hernia.
3. **Clinical presentation.** Umbilical hernias are usually noted soon after separation of the cord. There is an easily reducible soft bulge in the umbilicus. The hernia often "grows" as the intestine stretches the skin. Although a cause of distress to parents, umbilical hernias are almost never symptomatic, and incarceration is exceedingly rare. Spontaneous disappearance is the rule, often within the first year of life. **Operative repair is needed for only a small fraction of umbilical hernias.**
4. **Diagnosis.** The diagnosis is obvious on physical examination. The severity of the hernia depends on the size of the **fascial defect,** not the palpable subcutaneous mass.
5. **Problems.** Perforation, incarceration, or strangulation can occur, but they are rare.
6. **Indications for operation.** Since 95% of umbilical hernias will spontaneously disappear by age 5, operative repair is seldom indicated before then. The exceptions are the rare children who have pain or incarceration and those in whom the fascial defect is large. Spontaneous closure of a hernia with a fascial defect greater than **2 cm** is unlikely. Because of the risk of life-threatening complications during pregnancy, it is imperative that girls not reach maturity with an unrepaired umbilical hernia.
7. **Preoperative preparation.** Routine. This is a day-surgery operation.
8. **Operative care.** All umbilical hernias can be repaired through an intraumbilical incision with a subcuticular skin closure. Excision of redundant skin is not necessary even in huge hernias. A pressure dressing is applied to prevent hematoma formation.
9. **Postoperative care.** Routine.
10. **Complications.** Infection and bleeding are rare.
11. **Prognosis.** Excellent. Recurrence is almost unheard of.

Bibliography

Bell, M. J. Umbilical and Other Abdominal Wall Hernias. In T. M. Holder and K. W. Ashcraft (eds.), *Pediatric Surgery.* Philadelphia: Saunders, 1980. P. 589.
Blumberg, N. A. Infantile umbilical hernia. *Surg. Gynecol. Obstet.* 150:187, 1980.
Shaw, A. Disorders of the Umbilicus. In K. J. Welch, et al. (eds.), *Pediatric Surgery.* Chicago: Year Book, 1986. P. 731.
Walker, S. H. The natural history of umbilical hernia. *Clin. Pediatr.* 6:29, 1967.

20

Abdominal Masses

I. **Definition.** The finding of an abdominal mass in a newborn infant does not have the ominous significance that it does in an older child or adult. Only a small fraction are malignant, and many of those are curable. Over half arise in the genitourinary tract.

II. **Differential diagnosis of an abdominal mass in a neonate** (in order of frequency in each location):

   A. **Lateral**
      1. Multicystic kidney
      2. Hydronephrosis
      3. Hydroureter
      4. Renal vein thrombosis
      5. Mesoblastic nephroma
      6. Wilms' tumor
      7. Neuroblastoma
      8. Adrenal hemorrhage

   B. **Midabdominal**
      1. Mesenteric cyst
      2. Ovarian cyst
      3. Duplication of intestine
      4. Meconium ileus

   C. **Upper abdominal**
      1. Liver tumor
      2. Subcapsular hematoma of liver
      3. Choledochal cyst
      4. Splenic cyst
      5. Splenic hematoma

   D. **Lower abdominal**
      1. Bladder
      2. Hydrometrocolpos
      3. Urachal cyst
      4. Sacrococcygeal teratoma
      5. Anterior meningocele

III. **Diagnosis**

   A. **Physical examination** gives important clues to the identity of an abdominal mass, since most are asymptomatic. It is usually possible to narrow the diagnostic options to two or three, often to one, by examination alone.

1. **Specific location** in the abdomen is the most useful clue. Masses in the flank arise from the kidney or adrenal gland. Upper abdominal masses usually are related to the liver or spleen, while lower abdominal masses typically represent a distended bladder or uterus. Midabdominal masses, if freely movable, are most commonly mesenteric cysts or intestinal duplications.
2. **Large masses** may seem to fill the entire abdomen, making it impossible to determine the site of origin. A large neuroblastoma or mesoblastic nephroma may extend well beyond the midline and down into the pelvis.
3. **Hard masses** are typically tumors, particularly if the surface is nodular or irregular. Cysts are usually soft and smooth but can seem hard if tense.
4. **Mobility** of an abdominal mass is an important finding. Masses in retroperitoneal structures (kidney, adrenal), the liver, and retrorectal areas (meningocele, teratoma) are commonly fixed, while most other masses are movable.
5. **Rectal examination** will reveal an anterior meningocele or teratoma, as well as an enlarged bladder, vagina, or uterus. Imperforate hymen as a cause of hydrometrocolpos is evident on genital examination.

B. **Radiologic studies** are almost always indicated and result in diagnosis in most patients with an abdominal mass.
1. **Careful selection** is needed. The abundance and quality of the imaging modalities now available make it possible to make a fairly precise diagnosis with only one or two studies.
2. **CT scan** or magnetic resonance imaging **(MRI)** should be obtained in most newborns with an abdominal mass. They provide in a single study accurate information regarding the precise location of the mass, whether it is solid or cystic, its relationship to surrounding organs, and the presence of calcium (which may not be visible on plain x-rays). With contrast enhancement, details of the blood supply and the presence of tumor in the renal vein or vena cava are readily evaluated. Chest scan for metastases should be obtained at the same time in patients with tumors.
3. **Ultrasound** may be helpful as an initial screening examination to determine if a mass is present, but it seldom provides adequate information for preoperative assessment.
4. **Contrast x-rays (IVP, UGIS, BE)** are necessary if there is urinary or intestinal obstruction.
5. **Isotope scans** are seldom helpful; the detail provided is inferior to that of CT scan. The major value of isotope studies is in evaluating liver function in the jaundiced infant.

C. **Laboratory tests** include BUN and creatinine and "markers" if tumor is suspected: VMA and alpha fetoprotein. Liver function studies are obtained if liver disease is suspected.

IV. **Treatment.** Most neonates with an abdominal mass require operative treatment, both to establish the diagnosis and for definitive treatment. There are some exceptions, however.

A. **Nonoperative** treatment is appropriate for adrenal hemorrhage, most instances of renal vein thrombosis, splenic or hepatic hematomas, and neurogenic bladder.

B. **Operative** treatment is curative for most abdominal masses, including neuroblastoma and Wilms' tumor, which have higher cure rates in young patients. Severe bilateral hydronephrosis may be associated with sufficient renal destruction that survival is not possible, but that is rare. Specific therapy is discussed in the appropriate chapters.

Prognosis. The physician may be justifiably optimistic in discussions with the parents of a newborn with an abdominal mass. The vast majority can look forward to a normal life.

Bibliography

Koop, C. E. Abdominal mass in the newborn infant. *N. Engl. J. Med.* 289:569, 1973.
Leonidas, J. C., et al. Computed tomography in diagnosis of abdominal masses in infancy and childhood: Comparison with excretory urography. *Arch. Dis. Child.* 53(2):120, 1978.
Swischuk, L. E. Abdominal Masses and Fluid. In T. M. Holder and K. W. Ashcraft (eds.), *Pediatric Surgery*. Philadelphia: Saunders, 1980. P. 909.

21 Neonatal Ascites

I. **Definition.** Accumulation of fluid in the abdomen of a neonate is a sign of serious disease. Differentiation among the multiple possible causes begins with **paracentesis** and analysis of the fluid.

   A. **Serous fluid** with high or low protein concentration is associated with **nonsurgical causes** of ascites such as heart failure, liver failure, hemolytic diseases of the newborn (hydrops fetalis), congenital nephrotic syndrome, or congenital infection.

   B. **Urine, chyle, or bile** in the ascitic fluid indicates **obstruction** or **perforation** of the urinary tract, thoracic duct, or biliary tree, respectively. Operative treatment is usually required.

II. **Urinary ascites**

   A. **Urinary obstruction** is the underlying cause of almost all cases of urinary ascites. A discrete site of perforation is not found in 25%. **Posterior urethral valves** are responsible for obstruction in two-thirds of infants. Other causes include ureterocele, bladder neck obstruction, urethral atresia, and neurogenic bladder. Ascites may be present at birth.

   B. **IVP and voiding cystourethrogram** usually indicate the site of the obstruction if not the perforation. Serum creatinine and BUN are elevated.

   C. **Operative treatment** is indicated for all cases of urinary ascites. The site of perforation is repaired, if found, and the obstruction is relieved. Proximal decompression is usually called for. The prognosis is that of the underlying urinary tract disorder.

III. **Chylous ascites**

   A. The **etiology** of chylous ascites includes malformations or perforation of the thoracic duct, cystic hygroma, neoplasm, and obstruction of the intestinal lymphatics by malrotation or adhesive bands. In many instances the cause is unknown. Chylous ascites is rarely present at birth.

   B. **Ascitic fluid is clear at birth** or before the infant is fed but becomes milky once a fat-containing diet is consumed.

   C. **Upper gastrointestinal series** may reveal malrotation or other obstructive anomalies. **Lymphangiogram** may show lymphatic obstruction or leakage, but in most cases it is nondiagnostic.

   D. **Nonoperative treatment** is successful in most patients. The intestine is put to complete rest by use of **TPN**. Several weeks may be required. Fat-free feedings are given first, using medium-chain triglycerides supplementation.

   E. **Failure of medical therapy** or the demonstration of malrotation or lymphatic **obstruction** or **leakage** is the indication for surgical treatment. Unfortunately, in many cases no leak can be found at operation.

   F. **Recurrence** of ascites after the operation is not unusual, but the ascites almost always subsides eventually.

IV. **Biliary ascites**

   A. **Perforation** of the biliary tract is the cause of most cases of biliary ascites. The etiology is often obscure since most infants have no evidence of biliary obstruc-

tion. Inflammatory cholangitis may be responsible. Biliary ascites is rarely present at birth.
- **B. Radioisotope cholangiogram** may demonstrate free intraperitoneal bile drainage preoperatively.
- **C. Nonoperative treatment is usually fatal,** so every infant with biliary ascites should be operated on.
- **D. Biliary drainage** is usually all that is necessary. **Intraoperative cholangiogram** may demonstrate the point of leakage or obstruction. If a perforation or obstruction is found, it is repaired.
- **E. Survival is 80%** after operative treatment of biliary ascites.

Bibliography

Bernhoft, R. A., et al. Peritoneovenous shunt for refractory ascites. *Arch. Surg.* 117:631, 1982.

Guttman, F. M., et al. Experience with peritoneo-venous shunting for congenital chylous ascites in infants and children. *J. Pediatr. Surg.* 17:368, 1982.

Hansen, R. C., et al. Bile ascites in infancy: Diagnosis with 131 I–rose bengal. *Pediatrics* 84:719, 1974.

Hertel, J., and Pedersen, P. V. Congenital ascites due to mesenteric vessel constriction caused by malrotation of the intestines. *Acta Pediatr. Scand.* 68:281, 1979.

Kottmeier, P. K. Ascites. In K. J. Welch, et al. (eds.), *Pediatric Surgery.* Chicago: Year Book, 1986. P. 925.

Mann, C. M., et al. Neonatal urinary ascites: A report of 2 cases of unusual etiology and a review of the literature. *J. Urol.* 111:124, 1974.

Prevot, J., et al. Acute biliary peritonitis. *Prog. Pediatr. Surg.* 1:196, 1971.

Sanchez, R. E., et al. Chylous ascites in children. *Surgery* 69:183, 1971.

Schwartz, D. L., et al. Recurrent chylous ascites associated with intestinal malrotation and lymphatic rupture. *J. Pediatr. Surg.* 18:177, 1983.

Swischuk, L. E. Abdominal Masses and Fluid. In T. M. Holder and K. W. Ashcraft (eds.), *Pediatric Surgery.* Philadelphia: Saunders, 1980. P. 909.

Vasko, J. S., and Tapper, R. I. Surgical significance of chylous ascites. *Arch. Surg.* 95:355, 1967.

22 Neonatal Gastrointestinal Bleeding

I. **Definition.** Passage of blood from the GI tract, either as vomiting or guaiac-positive material or red blood in the stools, is not uncommon in the first few weeks of life. Massive hemorrhage is rare in newborns but requires aggressive treatment just as in older children.

II. **Differential diagnosis**
   A. **Hematemesis or tarry stools** indicates upper GI bleeding.
      1. Erosions of the nasopharynx from suctioning or tube passage
      2. Swallowed maternal blood during delivery
      3. Stress ulcer (gastric or duodenal)
      4. Cushing ulcer (meningitis, kernicterus, CNS tumor)
      5. Gastritis
      6. Esophagitis
      7. Clotting disorders
   B. **Bright red rectal bleeding in small amounts** is caused by a low colonic, rectal, or anal lesion.
      1. Anal fissure
      2. Necrotizing enterocolitis (NEC)
      3. Trauma
   C. **Maroon, dark red, or "currant jelly"** stools result from bleeding from the low ileum or colon.
      1. NEC
      2. Hirschsprung's enterocolitis
      3. Duplication
      4. Volvulus with strangulation
      5. Meckel's diverticulum
      6. Intussusception (very rare in newborns)
   D. **Occult blood** in the stools can come from a lesion anywhere from the nose to the anus. In neonates, possible causes are:
      1. Swallowed maternal blood
      2. Gastritis
      3. Peptic ulcer
      4. Esophagitis
      5. Clotting disorder
      6. Hemangioma
      7. Duplication
      8. Formula intolerance
      9. NEC

III. Diagnosis

A. **Perform a guaiac test** on the material to verify that it is indeed blood.

B. Perform **an Apt test** to determine if the blood is swallowed maternal blood.

C. **Examine the patient** for evidence of bleeding—lesions in the mouth, anal fissures, bruises or petechiae—and for other clues, such as abdominal distention, a mass, and tenderness.

D. **Aspirate the stomach** with a nasogastric tube to discover an upper GI source of bleeding if stools are guaiac-positive or black (but not if red blood is seen in the stools).

E. **Laboratory studies** depend on the presumed level of bleeding.

   1. **Bleeding studies** are indicated to exclude clotting abnormalities even when a focal lesion is encountered.
      a. CBC
      b. Platelet count
      c. Bleeding time
      d. Prothrombin time
      e. Partial thromboplastin time

   2. **Abdominal x-rays** may reveal signs of NEC or distended loops in Hirschsprung's disease, volvulus, or duplication.

   3. **Barium enema** is performed if a colonic source (other than NEC) is suspected from the clinical findings.

   4. **Upper GI series** contrast study is performed if the source of bleeding is thought to be proximal to the ligament of Treitz (patients with hematemesis or positive gastric aspirate and all those with occult bleeding).

F. **Sigmoidoscopy** is rarely of value in newborns. Anal lesions are seen better by direct examination.

G. **Esophagogastroscopy** is indicated in neonates with upper GI bleeding if the bleeding continues and the source is not evident from clinical and x-ray studies.

IV. Treatment

A. **Resuscitation** takes precedence over diagnosis if the bleeding is massive or if the infant has signs of hypovolemia. Use packed red cells and fresh frozen plasma to restore volume and red cell mass. Bolus therapy, 10 ml/kg, is given and repeated until pulse, color, and blood pressure are normalized.

B. Insert **a nasogastric tube,** both for diagnosis and to place the intestine at rest. If there is continuing upper gastrointestinal bleeding, saline lavage will often stop it. Iced saline must be used sparingly in newborns since it rapidly lowers body temperature.

C. **Monitor** the infant closely for signs of hypovolemia, acidosis, and rebleeding.

D. **Neutralization of acidity. Cimetidine** (10 mg/kg q4h IV) is given if the bleeding is from the upper tract. If gastric aspirate pH is below 5, add **aluminum hydroxide antacid,** 5–10 ml q2h, as necessary. Measure gastric pH hourly and titrate.

E. **Correct clotting abnormalities.**

V. Indications for operation

A. **Operation** is seldom indicated in the treatment of upper gastrointestinal bleeding in neonates. Rarely, uncontrolled gastritis or peptic ulcer may require operative treatment. If the transfusion requirement exceeds the calculated blood vol-

ume within a 48-hour period and bleeding continues, operative treatment is needed.
B. **Lower gastrointestinal bleeding** is more likely to require operation: NEC, volvulus, Hirschsprung's disease, duplication.
C. **Uncontrolled bleeding** from any source is an indication for operative treatment, provided clotting factors are normal.

Bibliography

Arensman, R. M. Gastrointestinal Bleeding. In K. J. Welch, et al. (eds.), *Pediatric Surgery*. Chicago: Year Book, 1986. P. 904.

Holcomb, G. W. Gastrointestinal Bleeding. In T. M. Holder and K. W. Ashcraft (eds.), *Pediatric Surgery*. Philadelphia: Saunders, 1980. P. 433.

23 Intestinal Obstruction

I. **Definition.** Obstruction of the intestine can be caused by malformations at any level of the intestinal tract from the pylorus to the anus. **In the neonatal period, bilious vomiting must be presumed to be due to intestinal obstruction until it has been conclusively eliminated.**

II. **Pathophysiology.** Obstruction causes increased intestinal secretion and decreased absorption, which results in the accumulation of intestinal contents within the lumen of the bowel. This leads to **intestinal dilatation and edema of the intestinal wall.**

   A. **Swallowed air** further adds to the dilatation of the intestine. If there is **massive distention,** pressure on the diaphragm may lead to **ventilatory failure.**

   B. Hyperperistalsis and fluid accumulation lead to **reversed peristalsis** and vomiting of intestinal contents.

   C. The **level of the obstruction** determines the severity of the physiologic derangement as well as how soon symptoms develop.

   D. **Low intestinal obstruction** (ileal atresia, meconium ileus, Hirschsprung's disease, imperforate anus) produces the most **profound alterations:**

   1. **Electrolyte imbalance.** Loss of gastric and intestinal juices results in subtraction acidosis and deficiencies of sodium, potassium, bicarbonate, and chloride.

   2. **Fluid loss** from vomiting and sequestration of fluid in the bowel lumen reduces circulating blood volume causing **hypovolemic shock.**

   3. **Metabolic acidosis** results from poor tissue perfusion caused by the hypovolemia.

   E. **High obstruction** (duodenal or proximal jejunal) causes less severe metabolic derangements.

   1. **Electrolyte imbalance** is largely the result of loss of gastric juice. Alkalosis develops, with deficiencies of sodium, chloride, and potassium.

   2. **Fluid loss is less severe,** although significant dehydration can result if the obstruction is undetected for days.

III. **Clinical presentation**

   A. **Vomiting and distention** are the common findings with all forms of intestinal obstruction. If the vomiting is bilious, the obstruction is distal to the ampulla of Vater.

   B. **Failure to pass meconium** is usual, but passage of meconium does not eliminate the possibility of obstruction. If meconium is noted, it is frequently pale and small in amount.

   C. **Abdominal distention** is mild and confined to the upper abdomen in patients with high intestinal obstruction, but massive and involving the entire abdomen in lower level obstruction. Passage of a nasogastric tube instantly relieves the distention in duodenal obstruction.

   D. An absent anal opening establishes the diagnosis of **imperforate anus.**

   E. If intestinal obstruction has been prolonged, or if there is volvulus, **hypovolemic shock, sepsis, or peritonitis** develops. Dehydration may be profound.

IV. Diagnosis. The diagnosis of intestinal obstruction is suspected in any newborn infant with **vomiting** and **distention**.

   A. **A large (14F) nasogastric tube** is placed to decompress the stomach, prevent further accumulation of intestinal air, and localize the stomach on x-ray examination.

   B. Palpable **"clay-like" loops** of intestine on abdominal examination are characteristic of **meconium ileus**.

   C. **Explosive release** of liquid fecal material after a negative rectal exam suggests **Hirschsprung's disease**.

   D. **Necrotizing enterocolitis** is suggested by sudden onset of distention, guaiac-positive stools, and hypovolemia in a tiny premature infant who **initially had no signs of intestinal obstruction**. **Intramural gas** in the bowel seen on plain x-rays of the abdomen is pathognomonic.

   E. **Medical causes** of intestinal ileus include **sepsis, hypothyroidism, maternal drugs,** and **increased intracranial pressure**.

   F. **Upright x-ray of the abdomen** is the most useful diagnostic study.

   1. **Gastric air bubble only indicates pyloric atresia** (very rare).
   2. **"Double bubble"** (dilated stomach and duodenum) indicates **duodenal atresia** (occasionally associated with annular pancreas). Contrast x-ray studies are seldom needed for diagnosis.
      a. **With air distally: duodenal stenosis or malrotation**
      b. **With lower abdominal distention: malrotation with volvulus** (air may or may not be present distally)
   3. **Two or three dilated intestinal loops indicate jejunal atresia.**
   4. **Multiple loops** of distended intestine filling the abdomen indicate obstruction in the ileum or colon. Since colon and small bowel look the same on plain x-rays, **contrast enema** is needed to make the specific diagnosis.

V. Differential diagnosis. The causes of low intestinal obstruction are distinguished by **contrast enema**.

Finding	Disorder
Microcolon (a fully patent colon with a tiny lumen)	Ileal atresia, meconium ileus (may also have "pellets" in right colon)
Narrowed left colon	Small left colon syndrome
Colonic obstruction	Colonic atresia
Dilated proximal colon with narrowed rectum and "transition zone"	Hirschsprung's disease
Normal colon with meconium mass in left colon	Meconium plug
Normal colon	Internal hernia
	Congenital bands
	Total-colon Hirschsprung's disease
	Ileus (nonmechanical obstruction)

VI. Problems. If the diagnosis of obstruction is made promptly, physiologic derangements are mild. Delay in diagnosis and treatment leads to progressively more serious complications.

   A. **Hypovolemic shock** may result from fluid accumulation in the bowel wall and lumen.

   B. **Metabolic acidosis** results from the hypovolemia. Poor tissue perfusion leads to anaerobic metabolism and buildup of acid metabolites.

C. **Strangulation** occurs if the blood supply is occluded by kinking or volvulus of the dilated loops of intestine. Infarction of the affected loops rapidly follows. Strangulation may also result from **midgut volvulus** due to **malrotation**.

D. **Enterocolitis** may develop in patients with Hirschsprung's disease because of ischemia and bacterial invasion due to prolonged intestinal distention.

E. **Perforation** of the intestine may result from infarction, enterocolitis, or overdistention alone.

F. **Overwhelming sepsis** develops if strangulation, perforation, or enterocolitis is present for more than a few hours.

G. **Disseminated intravascular coagulation** (DIC) may develop as a result of sepsis or intestinal infarction.

Indications for operation. All forms of mechanical intestinal obstruction require **operative treatment.** The **urgency** of operation depends on the level of obstruction, the presence of complications, and the need for resuscitation.

A. **Uncomplicated high obstruction** (duodenal atresia) does not require an emergency operation. Fluid and electrolyte imbalance is corrected first.

B. **Uncomplicated low obstruction** requires emergency operation to prevent complications. Fluid and electrolyte imbalance is restored toward (not *to*) normal. Four to eight hours' preparation may be necessary.

C. **Complicated obstruction (strangulated bowel, volvulus, actual or impending perforation,** or **overwhelming sepsis)** requires an operation as soon as perfusion is restored.

Preoperative preparation

A. **Uncomplicated intestinal obstruction**

 1. **Nasogastric tube** decompression relieves gastric distention and prevents aspiration and further abdominal distention.

 2. **Intravenous fluids** are given to replace losses. Normal saline with 10% glucose and 4 mEq KCl/100 ml is given (not lactated Ringer's solution unless acidosis is present).

   a. **At a minimum, the infant will need twice the normal daily maintenance amount** (the fluids required for that day as well as the preceding day). For a neonate this will total 200 ml/kg.

   b. **Fluids should be given rapidly at first** to restore circulating blood volume and urine output. One-half the deficit can be safely given in 4 hours.

   c. **The entire fluid deficit** should be made up in **12–16 hours.**

 3. **Electrolyte imbalance** may take longer to correct. Frequent monitoring of serum electrolytes guides therapy.

B. **Complicated intestinal obstruction** requires rapid **resuscitation** to permit operation as soon as possible.

 1. **Full correction** of the physiologic derangements is usually **impossible** until the cause is corrected by operation.

 2. **Blood volume restoration is the first priority.** Saline or Ringer's lactate solution is given, plus plasma or red cells as indicated. Adequate perfusion of all organs must be achieved before induction of anesthesia. **No patient should be operated on until blood volume is restored.**

   a. **Large quantities** of saline or lactated Ringer's solution are given rapidly.

b. **Bolus therapy** (10 ml/kg in 5 minutes) is the method of choice. Repeated boluses are given until there is evidence of return of perfusion (decreasing pulse, rising blood pressure, improved cutaneous circulation, and urine output).
3. **Adequate ventilation** must be established. Endotracheal intubation and ventilatory assistance may be necessary.
4. **Acidosis** should be corrected, or at least improved.
   a. **Restoration of perfusion** is the key to correcting acidosis. Give fluids!
   b. **Bicarbonate** should also be administered (1–2 mEq/kg).
5. **Electrolyte imbalance and fluid deficits** cannot be corrected fully before the operation.
6. **Fresh frozen plasma, platelets, and vitamin K** may be needed to correct coagulation abnormalities.
7. **Antibiotics** are given. Even if signs of sepsis are absent, poor perfusion lowers tissue resistance to bacterial invasion. Triple therapy is appropriate: ampicillin (100 mg/kg), gentamicin (2 mg/kg), and clindamycin (10 mg/kg).

IX. **Operative care.** The details of operative and postoperative care for each of the causes of neonatal intestinal obstruction are given in the sections that follow.

Bibliography

Hays, D. M. Intestinal atresia and stenosis. *Curr. Probl. Surg.* October 1969.
Holder, T. M., and Leape, L. L. The acute surgical abdomen in the neonate. *N. Engl. J. Med.* 278:605, 1968.

24 Duodenal Atresia and Annular Pancreas

I. **Definition.** Atresia of the duodenum results from a failure of recanalization after the "solid cord" stage of development of the proximal intestine. The atretic ends may be **completely separated** or may be connected by a fibrous cord. Forty percent of infants have a **diaphragmaic or "web" form** of obstruction. In others, atresia is incomplete—**stenosis.** The obstruction is distal to the ampulla of Vater in 80% of patients. **Annular pancreas** is always associated with atresia or stenosis and is clinically indistinguishable from them (Fig. 24-1).

II. **Pathophysiology.** Vomiting results in loss of gastric and duodenal secretions causing dehydration and deficiency of sodium, chloride, and hydrogen ions and of bicarbonate.

III. **Clinical presentation**

   A. **Polyhydramnios** is noted prenatally in approximately 50% of patients with duodenal atresia.

   B. **Vomiting** occurs early in duodenal atresia—usually on the first or second day of life. It is typically bilious.

   C. **Abdominal distention is not prominent** and is confined to the upper abdomen. Many infants with duodenal atresia have a scaphoid abdomen, so intestinal obstruction is not initially suspected.

   D. **Meconium passage** is noted in **30%** of patients.

   E. **Jaundice,** present in **40%,** is thought to be caused by increased enterohepatic recirculation of bilirubin.

   F. Vomiting in **duodenal stenosis** is delayed. The infant may be noted to be a poor feeder, vomit intermittently, and fail to thrive. **Recurrent aspiration pneumonia** may be a presenting finding.

IV. **Diagnosis.** The diagnosis of duodenal atresia is confirmed by x-ray examination of the abdomen. A single plain upright film will demonstrate the classic **"double bubble"** (Fig. 24-2). Contrast studies are unnecessary.

   A. If **air** is present in the intestine **beyond** the duodenum, the obstruction is incomplete, indicating **duodenal stenosis or malrotation.**

   B. **Malrotation with volvulus** must be suspected (and ruled out) if the abdomen is not scaphoid after passage of a nasogastric tube.

V. **Problems**

   A. **Dehydration** and **electrolyte imbalance**

   B. **Prematurity** (50%)

   C. **Associated anomalies:** trisomy 21 (33%); organ malformations (33%); cardiac, renal, CNS, and musculoskeletal

VI. **Indications for operation.** Unless other life-threatening conditions are present, operation is indicated in all of these infants since the malformation is completely correctable.

VII. **Preoperative preparation**

   A. The **general principles** of preparation of the neonate for operation apply (see Chap. 3).

141

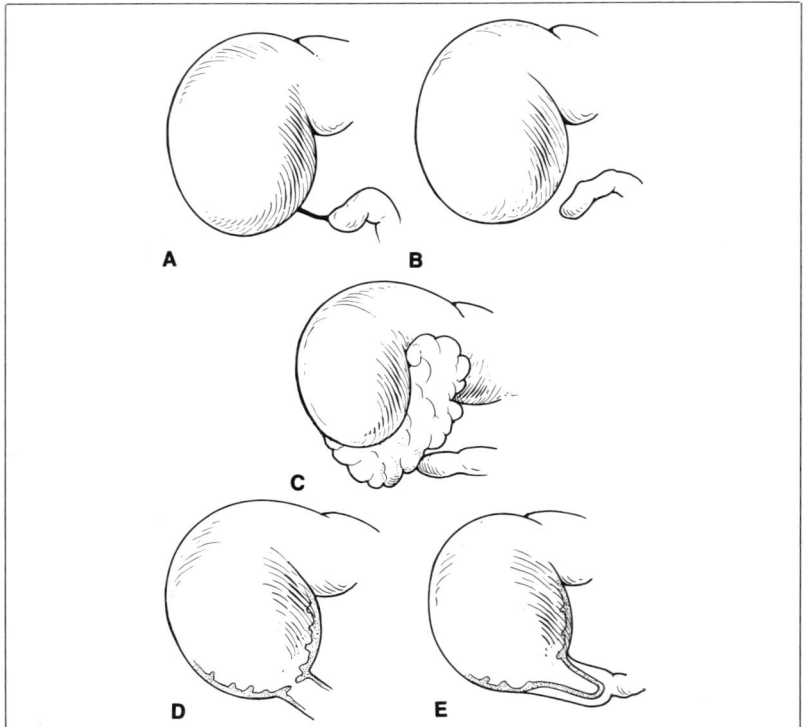

Fig. 24-1. Duodenal atresia. A. Massively dilated duodenum connected by a fibrous cord to distal intestine. B. Atresia with complete separation. C. Atresia associated with annular pancreas. D. Membranous or diaphragmatic form of duodenal atresia. There may or may not be an opening in the diaphragm. E. "Windsock" deformity: dilated mucosa prolapses into the segment beyond the apparent obstruction.

- **B. Fluid and electrolyte deficits must be corrected** (see **Chap. 23**).
- **C. Specific considerations** for patients with duodenal atresia:
    1. **Emergency correction is not required** unless malrotation is suspected; time can be taken to restore fluid and electrolyte balance.
    2. In long-standing partial obstruction from duodenal stenosis, **malnutrition may be severe.** Correction may require TPN for a week or more before the operation.

VIII. Operative care
- A. See **Chapter 4** for general principles.
- B. **End-to-end anastomosis** of the atretic ends eliminates concern about a "blind loop," although side-to-side anastomoses seem to work equally well.
- C. **Annular pancreas** is best handled by bypass anastomosis of duodenum to jejunum. The pancreas itself should not be incised.
- D. **Excision of the web** is appropriate for the diaphragmatic form of duodenal atresia, after precise identification of the ampulla of Vater.

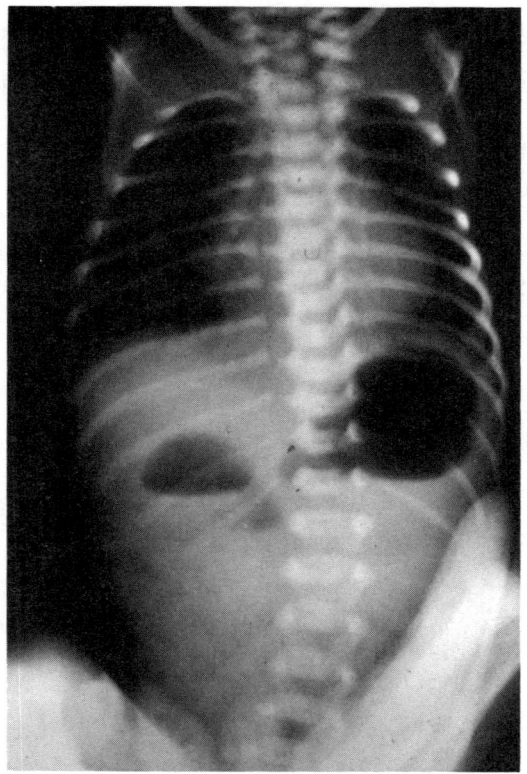

Fig. 24-2. Duodenal atresia. "Double bubble" sign is diagnostic. (From L. L. Leape and T. M. Holder, Pediatric Surgery. In D. C. Sabiston *Textbook of Surgery*. Philadelphia: Saunders, 1981.

   E. The **"windsock" deformity**—an elongated diaphragm—must be suspected and searched for in any patient with duodenal atresia in continuity. A catheter is passed proximally and distally to verify patency.
   F. **Gastrostomy** is performed if symptoms are long-standing and early recovery is not anticipated.
   G. **Placement of a central line** for TPN or insertion of a transanastomotic Silastic feeding tube into the jejunum may be indicated for postoperative nutrition in the severely depleted patient.
X. **Postoperative care**
   A. **Gastric decompression** is maintained until duodenal emptying occurs, after which feedings are begun and gradually advanced. Most patients can be fed within a week of the operation, but some take considerably longer.
   B. **TPN or jejunal feedings** are used as necessary.
   C. **Antibiotics are not indicated** since the operative field should be sterile and vascular compromise is not present.

X. Complications

A. Injury to the ampulla of Vater may occur if it is not positively identified in every operation for duodenal atresia. Increasing jaundice in the postoperative period is an indication for a liver isotope scan to evaluate bile excretion. Reoperation is necessary if obstruction is present.

B. Anastomotic stricture may occur, requiring reoperation. Delayed emptying of the duodenum is common after repair of duodenal atresia, so reoperation is rarely indicated before 3 weeks, and then only after radiologic demonstration of obstruction.

XI. Prognosis.
Ninety percent or more of infants operated on for duodenal atresia survive the operation. The ultimate mortality is largely determined by the presence of associated anomalies.

Bibliography

Free, E. A., and Gerald, B. Duodenal obstruction in the newborn due to annular pancreas. *Am. J. Roentgenol.* 103:321, 1968.

Madsen, C. M. Duodenal atresia: 60 years of follow-up (case report). *Prog. Pediatr. Surg.* 10:61, 1977.

Rowe, M. I., Buckner, D., and Clatworthy, H. W. Wind sock web of the duodenum. *Am. J. Surg.* 116:444, 1968.

Schnaufer, L. Duodenal Atresia, Stenosis and Annular Pancreas. In K. J. Welch, et al. (eds.), *Pediatric Surgery*. Chicago: Year Book, 1986. P. 829.

Touloukian, R. J. Intestinal Atresia and Stenosis. In T. M. Holder and K. W. Ashcraft (eds.), *Pediatric Surgery*. Philadelphia: Saunders, 1980. P. 331.

Wesley, J. R., and Mahour, G. H. Congenital intrinsic duodenal obstruction: A twenty-five year review. *Surgery* 82:716, 1977.

25 Malrotation

Definition. The term *malrotation* refers to a cluster of abnormalities of fixation of the colon to the posterior peritoneum. These result from incomplete rotation of the intestine as it returns to the abdominal cavity in the tenth week of gestation (Fig. 25-1).

Pathophysiology. (See Chap. 23.) **Intestinal obstruction** results from malrotation by one of three mechanisms:

A. **Duodenal obstruction** resulting from compression by **peritoneal bands** (Ladd's bands) crossing from the abnormally placed cecum in the right upper quadrant.

B. **Midgut volvulus.** Twisting of the entire midgut (jejunum to mid–transverse colon) on its mesentery because it lacks the normal broad base of fixation from the duodenojejunal junction to the right lower quadrant. Midgut volvulus may also result in vascular occlusion and **strangulation** of the midgut.

C. **Internal hernia** into or behind the malfixed mesentery (rare).

Clinical presentation

A. Seventy-five percent of patients with malrotation become symptomatic in the **first month of life.**

B. **Associated anomalies** include prune belly, vesicointestinal fissure, gastroschisis, omphalocele, and congenital diaphragmatic hernia (Bochdalek).

C. **Bilious vomiting,** similar to that seen in duodenal atresia, is the common presenting symptom in neonates.

D. **Abdominal distention** suggests volvulus.

E. **Shock, sepsis, and toxicity** indicate **strangulation** caused by compromise of mesenteric blood supply.

F. **Intermittent vomiting or abdominal pain** are the typical symptoms of malrotation in **older children.**

G. **Malabsorption** may occur as a result of lymphatic obstruction caused by chronic nonobstructing malrotation in older children.

Diagnosis. In newborn infants, the typical x-ray findings are a "**double bubble**" (dilated stomach and duodenum) **with air in the distal intestine** or lower abdominal distention. Volvulus may be associated with a gasless abdomen. In questionable instances and in older children with nonspecific symptoms, upper GI series will demonstrate duodenal dilatation and lack of fixation of the bowel at the ligament of Treitz. Barium enema will show the cecum in the right upper quadrant or further to the left side.

Problems

A. **In newborn** infants, it is not always easy to distinguish malrotation with potential or actual midgut volvulus from duodenal atresia or stenosis. If the abdomen is not absolutely scaphoid, volvulus should be suspected. In doubtful cases, a contrast study is indicated.

B. Midgut volvulus with strangulation infarction can result in **loss of all of the small intestine** except the duodenum, making enteral nutrition impossible.

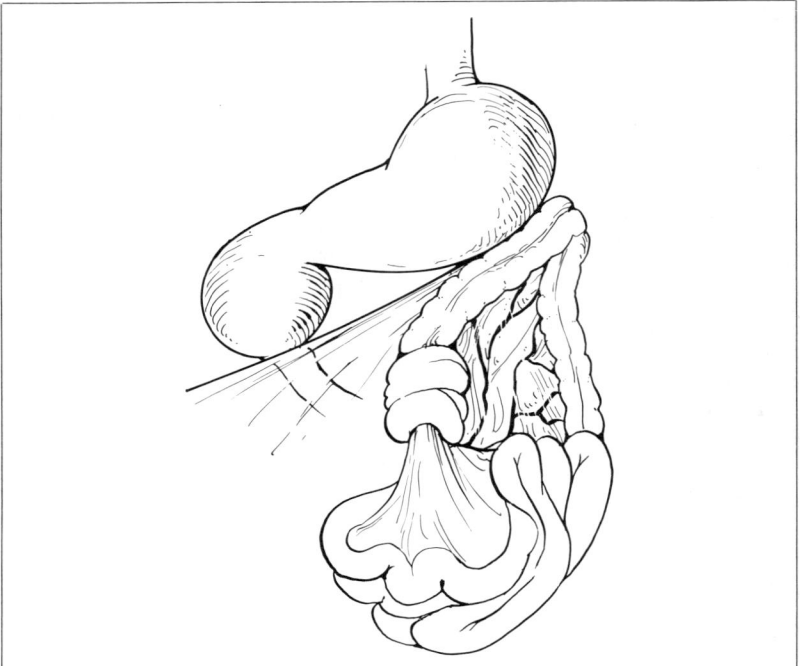

Fig. 25-1. Malrotation. Volvulus of midgut around unattached mesentery. The peritoneal bands from malposition of the colon cause partial obstruction of the duodenum.

VI. Indications for operation
  A. In **neonates,** signs of **intestinal obstruction** are the indication for operative repair of malrotation.
  B. **Asymptomatic malrotation** in older children discovered by x-ray alone **should not be repaired,** since as many as 3% of persons in the general population have some form of malrotation.
  C. **Recurrent abdominal pain or vomiting** is an indication for repair, both to relieve symptoms and to prevent the potential catastrophe of midgut volvulus.

VII. Preoperative preparation
  A. The **general principles** of preparation of the neonate for operations apply (see **Chap. 3**).
  B. **Fluid and electrolyte deficits must be corrected.** If midgut strangulation is present, rapid resuscitation is carried out with operation following as soon as possible (see **Chap. 23**).

VIII. Operative care
  A. See **Chap. 4** for general principles.
  B. The **volvulus is unwound** by a counterclockwise derotation. The intestine is carefully observed for viability. Frankly necrotic segments must be resected. In dubious cases, the ischemic segment is retained and reevaluated at a **second-look procedure** 24–48 hours later.

C. **Attachments** between the duodenum and colon are divided to free up the entire intestinal tract. "Traps" are closed.
D. **A variety of types** of incomplete and reversed rotation exist. These must be sorted out and the entire intestine freed to eliminate potential points of obstruction.
E. **Ladd's procedure,** division of the bands crossing the duodenum, is performed when appropriate.
F. **The base of the mesentery** is widened by incising the posterior peritoneum.
G. **Appendectomy** is performed to prevent later possible confusion if appendicitis were to develop.
H. **The small intestine is placed on the right** side and the colon on the left side of the abdomen.
I. **Suture fixation** of the bowel is not performed by most pediatric surgeons except for recurrent malrotation.

Postoperative care

A. **Gastric decompression** is maintained until duodenal emptying occurs, after which feedings are begun and gradually advanced.
B. **Parenteral nutrition** may be necessary for an extended period of time if there is malabsorption or if a long segment of ischemic intestine has been removed.

Complications

A. The **short bowel syndrome,** malabsorption caused by inadequate absorptive surface, occurs if a major part of the midgut must be removed (see Chap. 26). **Parenteral nutrition** via a central catheter may be required for many months, even years, if extensive resection has been required.
B. **Malabsorption** may also result from **ischemic damage** to the bowel, even if it is viable, or from **chronic lymphatic obstruction** caused by long-standing chronic volvulus. Parenteral nutrition is the treatment of choice.

Prognosis

A. The risk of **recurrent volvulus** is less than 5%.
B. **Short bowel malabsorption** may require lifelong parenteral nutrition, a feasible home-care procedure.

Bibliography

Andrassy, R. J., and Mahour, G. H. Malrotation of the midgut in infants and children. *Arch. Surg.* 116:158, 1981.
Bill, A. H. Malrotation and Failures of Fixation of the Intesitnal Tract. In T. M. Holder and K. W. Ashcraft (eds.), *Pediatric Surgery*. Philadelphia: Saunders, 1980. P. 346.
Bill, A. H., and Grauman, D. Rationale and technic for stabilization of the mesentery in cases of nonrotation of the midgut. *J. Pediatr. Surg.* 1:127, 1966.
Filston, H. C., and Kirks, D. R. Malrotation: The ubiquitous anomaly. *J. Pediatr. Surg.* 16:614, 1981.
Houston, C. S., and Wittenborg, M. H. Roentgen evaluation of anomalies of rotation and fixation of the bowel in children. *Radiology* 84:1, 1965.
Simpson, A. J., et al. Roentgen diagnosis of midgut malrotation: Value of upper gastrointestinal radiographic study. *J. Pediatr. Surg.* 7:243, 1972.
Smith, E. I. Malrotation of the Intestine. In K. J. Welch, et al. (eds.), *Pediatric Surgery*. Chicago: Year Book, 1986. P. 882.

Stauffer, U. G., and Herrmann, P. Comparison of late results in patients with corrected intestinal malrotation with and without fixation of the mesentery. *J. Pediatr. Surg.* 15:9, 1980.

Stewart, D. R., Colodny, A. L., and Daggett, W. C. Malrotation of the bowel in infants and children: A 15-year review. *Surgery* 79:716, 1976.

26 Jejunoileal Atresia

Definition. Congenital obstruction of the jejunum or ileum probably results from an in utero vascular accident that causes ischemia or necrosis of a segment of the bowel and its mesentery.

A. There are **five forms.**

1. Complete separation
2. Fibrous cord
3. Diaphragm or web
4. Multiple atresias and
5. "Apple peel" bowel, in which the distal microintestine is wrapped around a single ileocolic artery (Fig. 26-1)

B. Atresias occur with **equal frequency** in the jejunum and ileum. Incomplete obstruction, or **stenosis,** is present in about **20%** of atresias.

Pathophysiology (see Chap. 23)

Clinical presentation

A. Polyhydramnios is frequently present prenatally in instances of high jejunal atresia.

B. Vomiting is always bilious but may not occur until the second or third day of life if the obstruction is low.

C. Abdominal distention may be profound in low obstruction. As multiple loops fill with swallowed air, the abdomen becomes distended and tense.

D. Meconium passage is noted in some patients.

E. Jaundice is present in 20%, thought to be caused by enhanced enterohepatic recirculation of bilirubin.

F. Stenosis results in more subtle symptoms: poor feeding, intermittent distention, vomiting, or failure to thrive.

G. Dehydration and hypovolemic shock are more likely to be seen in patients with distal atresia. Profound internal fluid losses may develop before the diagnosis is made.

Diagnosis. Massive distention of the intestine with multiple air-fluid levels indicates distal obstruction. **Contrast enema** is necessary to differentiate the causes. (See Chap. 23.)

Problems (see Chap. 23). These patients are particularly likely to have hypovolemia and acidosis.

A. Prematurity commonly accompanies jejunoileal atresia and is most severe in those with the "apple peel" malformation.

B. Associated anomalies include meconium ileus, gastroschisis, and omphalocele.

Indications for operation. There is no nonoperative treatment. Operative correction should be carried out unless there are other, more serious life-threatening anomalies.

Preoperative preparation (see Chaps. 3 and 23).

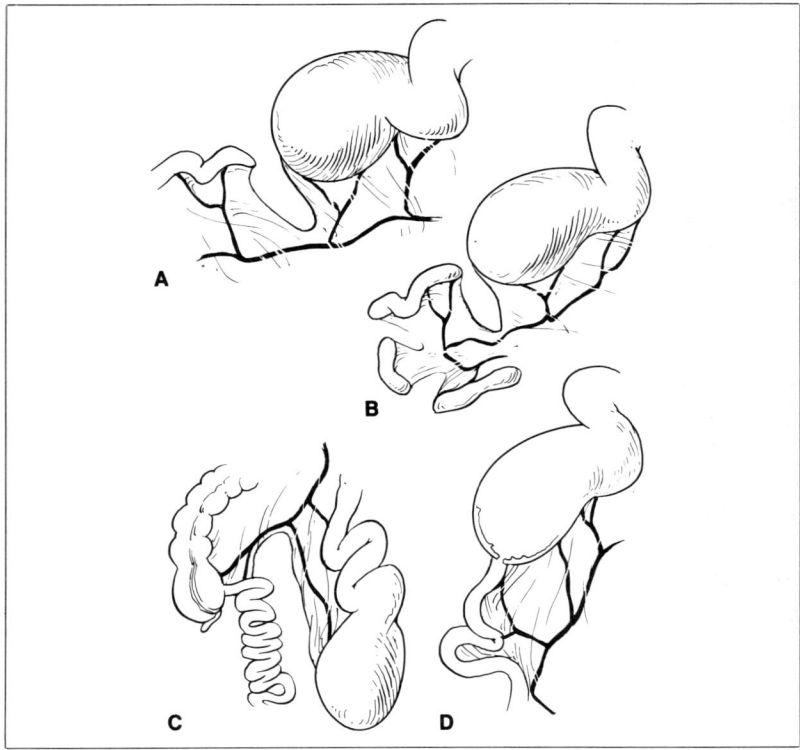

Fig. 26-1. Jejunoileal atresia. A. Complete separation with typical mesenteric defect. B. Multiple atresias with small sausage-like segments of intestine. C. "Apple peel" bowel. D. Diaphragmatic form of atresia.

VIII. Operative care. See Chap. 4 for general principles.

A. Complete examination of the entire intestine is essential for recognizing multiple atresias. Mineral oil or saline is instilled in the lumen and "milked" the length of the intestine to verify patency.

B. Resection, invagination, or "tailoring" of the hugely dilated proximal segment is necessary to permit effective peristalsis. If reduction is not carried out, the dilated segment acts as a functional obstruction.

C. End-to-back (bias-cut) anastomosis is carried out using a single layer of inverting sutures.

D. Gastrostomy may be necessary to facilitate drainage (which may be prolonged) and to gauge acceptance of feedings easily when they are begun.

E. A **central venous catheter** may be required for parenteral nutrition.

IX. Postoperative care

A. Parenteral nutrition should be given from the time of the operation since many of these patients are slow to "open up" and may not take adequate feedings for several weeks.

B. Gastric decompression is maintained until there is evidence of gastric emptying and intestinal activity.

Ch 26. Jejunoileal Atresia

C. **Feedings are advanced very slowly,** both in volume and in osmotic load, to permit the intestine to adapt. Predigested formula (Nutramigen) is given initially, one-fourth strength, slowly advancing the volume first and then the concentration as feedings are tolerated. If the length of the remaining intestine is short, this process may take months.

Complications

A. **Short-gut syndrome** is the term given to the complex malabsorption problem associated with inadequate intestinal absorptive surface. It is most commonly seen in patients with multiple atresias or "apple-peel" bowel, gastroschisis, and after abdominal catastrophes such as midgut volvulus with infarction.

1. **Normal length** of the small intestine in the newborn is approximately **200 cm.** Loss of up to three-fourths of the gut is tolerated amazingly well. If the ileocecal valve is intact, adequate intestinal absorption has been reported with as little as 15 cm of small intestine, but survival with less than 25 cm is rare. If the ileocecal valve is not present, 40 cm is needed.

2. **Feeding produces severe diarrhea,** steatorrhea, and dehydration. Initially, even small volumes of dilute formula will not be tolerated. Malnutrition results from inadequate absorption.

3. **Total parenteral nutrition (TPN) is essential** for these infants to survive. It should be started immediately postoperatively, used as necessary to achieve normal growth, and continued until weight gain can be achieved entirely with enteral feedings.

4. **Feedings are more likely to be successful if volume tolerance is first established** and then osmolarity is increased. This process takes many months and is fraught with failures, restarts, and frustrations. Regular formulas are not tolerated. A predigested formula such as Nutramigen or Pregestimil is better.

    a. **Dilute Nutramigen** (one-fourth strength) is offered initially, 5–10 ml per feeding, every 2 hours.

    b. **The volume is gradually increased** as tolerated to normal amounts (150 ml/kg/day).

    c. **Concentration** of the formula is gradually advanced, allowing a week or more for each increment. Formula concentration greater than three-fourths strength is often poorly tolerated, but increased volumes may be accepted and provide adequate caloric absorption.

    d. **Elemental diets** (Vivonex) may be tolerated when predigested formulas are not. Begin with a very dilute solution and increase gradually.

    e. **Bouts of diarrhea and dehydration are common** during this tedious process and require cessation of feeding, full-maintenance TPN, and starting over with dilute formula.

    f. **Eventually,** the infant is advanced to **standard formula** but often requires large volumes (50–100% above normal) to gain weight. Ultimately, a regular diet will be tolerated.

5. **Adaptation** of the intestine occurs gradually, with dilatation, increase in length, and villous hypertrophy.

6. **Intestinal adaptation takes many months.** It is not unusual for an infant with short-gut syndrome to be in the hospital for 1 to 2 years.

7. **Maintaining the morale** of the nursing staff and the parents is a major challenge. It is wise to inform everyone at the outset that the infant will survive and that it will take 1–2 years. This message needs frequent repeti-

tion. Continual optimism of the surgeon is essential and appropriate, for the vast majority do survive and live a normal life thereafter.

8. **Malabsorption of fat-soluble vitamins** and vitamin B_{12} is a common late effect of the short-gut syndrome. Careful monitoring and supplementation are necessary.

B. **Anastomotic stricture** may occur after repair of jejunoileal atresia. Reoperation should not be considered for at least 3 weeks, however, since effective intestinal activity is slow to occur even when all is well. The diagnosis must be confirmed by contrast x-rays prior to operation.

XI. **Prognosis.** More than 90% of patients with jejunoileal atresia survive. Mortality is usually related to prematurity or other organ malformations.

Bibliography

Benson, C. D., Lloyd, J. R., and Smith J. D. Resection and primary anastomosis in the management of stenosis and atresia of the jejunum and ileum. *Pediatrics* 26:265, 1960.

Boeckman, C. R., and Traylor, R. Bowel lengthening for short gut syndrome. *J. Pediatr. Surg.* 16:996, 1981.

de Lorimier, A. A., Fonkalsrud, E. W., and Hays, D. M. Congenital atresia and stenosis of the jejunum and ileum. *Surgery* 65:819, 1969.

de Lorimier, A. A., and Harrison, M. R. Intestinal imbrication for atresia and pseudo-obstruction. *J. Pediatr. Surg.* 18:734, 1983.

Dickson, J. A. S. Apple-peel small bowel: An uncommon variant of duodenal and jejunal atresia. *J. Pediatr. Surg.* 5:595, 1970.

Grosfeld, J. L. Jejunoileal Atresia and Stenosis. In K. J. Welch et al. (eds.), *Pediatric Surgery*. Chicago: Year Book, 1986. P. 838.

Grosfeld, J. K., Ballantine, T. V. N., and Shoemaker, R. Operative management of intestinal atresia and stenosis based on pathologic findings. *J. Pediatr. Surg.* 14:368, 1979.

Hays, D. M. Intestinal atresia and stenosis. *Curr. Probl. Surg.* October 1969.

Louw, J. H. Resection and end-to-end anastomosis in the management of atresia and stenosis of the small bowel. *Surgery* 62:940, 1967.

Nixon, H. H., and Tawes, R. Etiology and treatment of small intestinal atresia: Analysis of a series of 127 jejunoileal atresias and comparison with 62 duodenal atresias. *Surgery* 69:41, 1971.

Postuma, R., Moroz, S., and Friesen, F. Extreme short-bowel syndrome in an infant. *J. Pediatr. Surg.* 18:264, 1983.

Touloukian, R. J. Intestinal Atresia and Stenosis. In T. M. Holder and K. W. Ashcraft (eds.), *Pediatric Surgery*. Philadelphia: Saunders, 1980. P. 331.

Weber, T. R., Vane, D. W., and Grosfeld, J. L. Tapering enteroplasty in infants with bowel atresia and short gut. *Arch. Surg.* 117:684, 1982.

Weitzman, J. J., and Vanderhoof, R. S. Jejunal atresia with agenesis of the dorsal mesentery with "Christmas tree" deformity of the small intestine. *Am. J. Surg.* 111:443, 1966.

Wilmore, D. W. Factors correlating with a successful outcome following extensive intestinal resection in the newborn infant. *J. Pediatr.* 80:88, 1972.

27 Meconium Ileus

I. **Definition.** *Meconium ileus* is obstruction of the terminal ileum from abnormally viscous meconium caused by **cystic fibrosis**. It is seen in approximately 10% of children with cystic fibrosis, rarely seen in blacks, and virtually absent in Asians. Cystic fibrosis is **hereditary**, the result of an autosomal recessive trait, with a heterozygote incidence of 1 in 25.

II. **Pathophysiology.** Cystic fibrosis is a disease affecting all exocrine glands.
   A. **Abnormal intestinal and pancreatic secretions** produce meconium with a high protein content and abnormal mucoproteins, which make it much more viscous than normally. The meconium is thickest and most tenacious in the **distal ileum**, where the obstruction is most likely to occur (Fig. 27-1).
   B. Prenatal **volvulus** may result in perforation or infarction with aseptic **meconium peritonitis, intestinal atresia,** or **pseudocyst** formation. **Calcification** of the extravasated meconium may occur.

III. **Clinical presentation**
   A. The infant shows the typical findings of **low intestinal obstruction:** bilious vomiting, abdominal distention, and failure to pass stools.
   B. **Palpable "clay-like" masses** may often be felt in the abdomen, particularly on the right side. These are loops of distal ileum distended with inspissated meconium.
   C. **Polyhydramnios** occurs in 5–10% of cases.
   D. **Prematurity** is seen in 10–15%, but associated anomalies are rare.
   E. Approximately **5%** of children with meconium ileus **do not have cystic fibrosis;** the cause is unknown.

IV. **Diagnosis**
   A. Plain x-ray of the abdomen show **dilated loops** of intestine with air-fluid levels that tend not to shift with change in position and may be arranged in a **concentric pattern.** There may be a coarse granular appearance of the intestine caused by **bubbles** of air within the viscous meconium.
   B. **Calcifications** indicate prenatal meconium peritonitis.
   C. **Barium enema** shows a **microcolon,** sometimes with inspissated "pellets" of meconium in the terminal ileum or colon.
   D. An abnormal **sweat test** is diagnostic of cystic fibrosis. Unfortunately, the test is frequently not positive in the first few weeks of life, so it is of little value preoperatively. It is essential that the diagnosis ultimately be confirmed by sweat test, however.

V. **Problems**
   A. **Dehydration** and electrolyte imbalance occur if there is prolonged vomiting and treatment is delayed.
   B. Intestinal **ischemia** or **perforation** can result from volvulus of dilated loops of intestine.

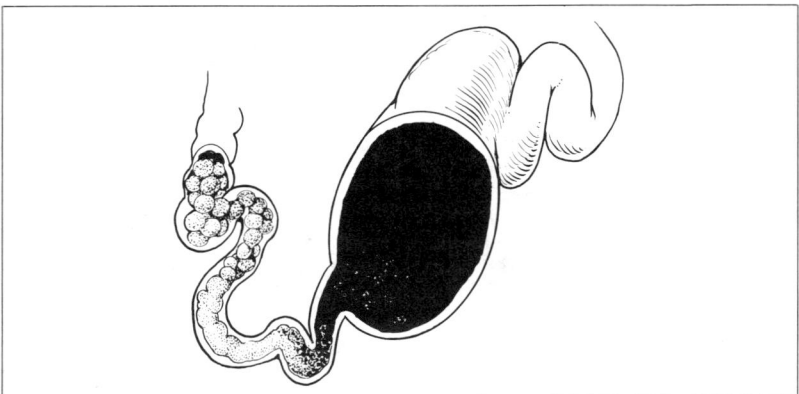

Fig. 27-1. Meconium ileus. Massive distention of ileum with thick, sticky meconium and inspissated "pellets" in terminal ileum and colon.

VI. Indications for operation

   A. An **emergency operation** is indicated in the infant with signs of decompensated intestinal obstruction—hypovolemic shock, acidosis—or signs of perforation or ischemia of the bowel.

   B. **Nonoperative treatment** is sometimes successful and is appropriate in patients who are compensated and have none of the previously mentioned complications.

VII. Nonoperative treatment.
Water-soluble contrast enema will sometimes loosen the obstructing meconium and relieve the intestinal obstruction. It works by its **hyperosmolarity,** which draws fluid into the intestine softening the meconium and separating it from the bowel wall.

   A. **Gastrografin** is the preferred agent. It is a hyperosmolar (1900 mOsm/liter) solution of meglumine diatrizoate with polysorbate 80 (Tween 80), a wetting agent.

   B. Several **precautions** are in order.

   1. **The infant must not have signs of bowel ischemia, sepsis, or hypovolemic shock.**

   2. The surgeon should be in attendance, with the **operating room ready,** in case there is perforation of the bowel requiring immediate operation.

   3. The infant must be **well hydrated** and have an intravenous line running, since the hyperosmotic solution can cause **vascular collapse** if the fluid it extracts is not replaced. Half-normal saline is administered, 4 ml for each milliliter of contrast retained after the enema.

   4. **Heat loss** from exposure in a cold x-ray suite must be prevented.

   C. If the obstruction is relieved, the patient is carefully observed for signs of persisting obstruction from an atresia or volvulus. Continuous nasogastric suction and intravenous fluids are needed.

   D. **Feedings** of Pregestimil together with **pancreatic enzymes** are begun when the intestine resumes function.

VIII. Preoperative preparation
(see Chaps. 3 and 23) **Fluid resuscitation** and correction of electrolyte imbalance and hypovolemia are carried out as for any intestinal obstruction.

I. Operative care. In the typical case of uncomplicated meconium ileus, the distal ileum is massively dilated with thick tenacious meconium, which becomes inspissated and forms pellet-like concretions distally near the ileocecal valve.

   A. The **objective** of the operation is to remove the obstructing meconium. This can be done in several ways.

   1. **Resection** of the dilated obstructed bowel with end-to-end anastomosis. This method requires an extensive resection and has a high incidence of leaks and strictures. It is **not recommended**.

   2. **Enterotomy, evacuation** of the meconium after softening with diluted **acetyl cysteine (2%), and closure** of the enterotomy. If it is possible to obtain complete relief of obstruction distally, this is the ideal method.

   3. **Enterotomy, evacuation, and ileostomy.** After irrigation with acetyl cysteine, the hugely **dilated part of the ileum is** tailored down, and end-to-side anastomosis with a decompressing **"chimney" ileostomy** is created. Distal irrigation with acetyl cysteine eventually loosens the meconium in the lower intestine.

   B. If there is **volvulus, pseudocyst formation, or atresia,** these must be resected, with reconstruction of the bowel, usually with a decompressive "chimney" ileostomy.

   C. Gastrostomy is performed for drainage and to facilitate feedings.

Postoperative care

   A. Ileostomy. Instill acetyl cysteine several times daily until the distal obstruction is relieved.

   B. Feedings. Begin Pregestimil when the proximal ileostomy starts to function. Add Viokase to the feedings to treat pancreatic enzyme deficiency.

   C. Verify the diagnosis **of cystic fibrosis** by a sweat test at several weeks of age.

   D. Administer **humidified air** and vigorous **pulmonary physiotherapy** from the first postoperative day to prevent pulmonary complications from cystic fibrosis.

   E. Close the ileostomy after intestinal function is well established, usually by 6 weeks.

Complications

   A. Anastomotic leak at the "chimney" ileostomy may result from poor suture technique, angulation of the bowel, compromise of blood supply, or rough catheter irrigation technique. Reoperation is necessary.

   B. Incomplete evacuation of meconium will lead to persistent obstruction, either proximally or distally. Repeated irrigations are the treatment. Reoperation is rarely needed.

   C. Adhesive obstruction can occur at any time in the postoperative period, most likely in the first 6 weeks.

   D. Pneumonia and atelectasis are much more common than in other neonates because of cystic fibrosis.

   E. Malabsorption may occur despite proper use of replacement pancreatic enzymes.

   F. *Meconium ileus equivalent* is the term applied to the fecal obstruction that occasionally occurs in the older child with cystic fibrosis. It is usually the result of an inadequate dose of pancreatic replacement enzymes.

Prognosis. The mortality following operation for meconium ileus is higher than that for other forms of neonatal intestinal obstruction, largely because of pulmonary complications.

Bibliography

Anderson, C. M., and Goodchild M. C. *Cystic Fibrosis: Manual of Diagnosis and Management.* Boston: Blackwell, 1976.

Bishop, H. C., and Koop, C. E. Management of meconium ileus: Resection, Roux-en-Y anastomosis and ileostomy irrigation with pancreatic enzymes. *Ann. Surg.* 145:410, 1957.

Bowring, A. C., Jones, R. F. C., and Kern, I. B. The use of solvents in the intestinal manifestations of mucoviscidosis. *J. Pediatr. Surg.* 5:338, 1970.

Chappell, J. S. Management of meconium ileus by resection and end-to-end anastomosis. *S. Afr. Med. J.* 52:1093, 1977.

Kalayoglu, M., et al. Meconium ileus: A critical review of treatment and eventual prognosis. *J. Pediatr. Surg.* 6:290, 1971.

Lloyd, D. A. Meconium Ileus. In K. J. Welch, et al. (eds.), *Pediatric Surgery.* Chicago: Year Book, 1986. P. 849.

Noblett, H. R. Treatment of uncomplicated meconium ileus by Gastrografin enema. *J. Pediatr. Surg.* 4:190, 1969.

Rickham, P. P., and Boeckman, C. R. Neonatal meconium obstruction in the absence of mucoviscidosis. *Am. J. Surg.* 109:173, 1965.

Rowe, M. I., Seagram G., and Weinberger, M. Gastrografin-induced hypertonicity. *Am. J. Surg.* 125:185, 1973.

Santulli, T. V. Meconium Ileus. In T. M. Holder and K. W. Ashcraft (eds.), *Pediatric Surgery.* Philadelphia: Saunders, 1980. P. 356.

28 Meconium Peritonitis

I. **Definition.** Meconium peritonitis results from **prenatal perforation** of the intestine. Since the contents are sterile, infection does not occur, but there is a chemical reaction resulting in fibrosis, granuloma formation, and calcification.

II. **Pathophysiology.** Possible causes of intrauterine intestinal perforation include a vascular accident (which also may cause atresia), meconium ileus, imperforate anus, intussusception, and volvulus about a congenital band or internal hernia. Iatrogenic meconium peritonitis can result from perforation of the intestine during amniocentesis or prenatal surgery.

   A. **Inflammatory reaction** to bile and to pancreatic and intestinal enzymes causes proliferation of fibroblasts, adhesions, foreign-body granuloma formation, and calcification.

   B. The **intestinal perforation** may seal spontaneously, leaving no trace or an atretic segment.

   C. **Generalized adhesions** with **calcifications** is the most common manifestation of meconium peritonitis, with intestinal obstruction from the adhesions or at the perforation site.

   D. **Pseudocyst** formation may occur from continuing spillage of meconium. A fibrous wall forms about the affected loop of intestine and fluid collection, isolating it from the remainder of the peritoneal cavity, which is normal.

   E. **Ascites** may develop from a perforation occurring shortly before birth. Calcification may not yet be present.

   F. **Infected meconium peritonitis** results if the perforation is not sealed before birth and not recognized promptly. Bacterial colonization of the intestine leads to contamination of the peritoneal cavity.

III. **Clinical presentation**

   A. **Signs of intestinal obstruction** are the most common presenting indications of meconium peritonitis: bilious vomiting, abdominal distention, and failure to pass meconium.

   B. **Calcifications** in the abdomen or scrotum noted on abdominal film taken for intestinal obstruction may be the first clue.

   C. **Ascites**, a **scrotal mass** or calcifications, and fluid or calcification in an inguinal hernia are less common findings.

IV. **Diagnosis.** X-ray evidence of calcifications throughout the abdomen or in the scrotum are typical of meconium peritonitis. They must be differentiated from calcifications in tumors, which are localized to the mass.

V. **Indications for operation.** Not all infants with meconium peritonitis need to be operated on. Careful observation is all that is required in the asymptomatic child. Signs of sepsis, intestinal obstruction, persistent leak, free air, or an abdominal mass are indications for surgical treatment.

VI. **Operative care.** Preservation of intestine and reestablishment of intestinal continuity are the primary objectives of surgical treatment of meconium peritonitis. Calcifications and cyst walls do not need to be completely removed. Temporary ileostomy may be necessary if there is infected peritonitis with compromised bowel.

VII. **Complications.** Recurrent obstruction, cyst formation, and abscess are potential problems after surgical treatment.
VIII. **Prognosis.** Survival depends on the correctability of the underlying disease. Overall, survival is about 50–60%.

Bibliography

Birtch, A. G., Coran, A. G., and Gross, R. E. Neonatal peritonitis. *Surgery* 61:305, 1967.

Blumenthal, D. H., et al. Prenatal sonographic findings of meconium peritonitis with pathologic correlation. *J. Clin. Ultrasound* 10:350, 1982.

Boix-Ochoa, J. Meconium peritonitis. *J. Pediatr. Surg.* 3:715, 1968.

Careskey, J. M., et al. Giant cystic meconium peritonitis (GCMP): Improved management based on clinical and laboratory observations. *J. Pediatr. Surg.* 17:482, 1982.

Finkel, L. I., and Slovis, T. L. Meconium peritonitis, intraperitoneal calcifications, and cystic fibrosis. *Pediatr. Radiol.* 12:92, 1982.

Santulli, T. V. Meconium Ileus. In T. M. Holder and K. W. Ashcraft (eds.), *Pediatric Surgery*. Philadelphia: Saunders, 1980. P. 356.

Tibboel, D., Gaillard, J. L. J., and Molenaar, J. C. The "microscopic" type of meconium peritonitis. *Z. Kinderchir.* 34:9, 1981.

Wiener, E. S. Meconium Peritonitis. In K. J. Welch, et al. (eds.), *Pediatric Surgery*. Chicago: Year Book, 1986. P. 929.

Ya-Xiong, S., and Lian-Chen, S. Meconium peritonitis: Observation in 115 cases and antenatal diagnosis. *Z. Kinderchir.* 37:2, 1982.

29 Necrotizing Enterocolitis

I. **Definition.** Necrotizing enterocolitis (NEC) is a disease of complex etiology in which both the large and small intestine undergo patchy or diffuse necrosis. It is seen mostly in small premature infants, the incidence increasing with earlier birth. Approximately 7.5% of babies admitted to a neonatal intensive care unit will develop NEC.

II. **Pathophysiology**

   A. **Any part of the GI tract** may be involved, but in most patients with NEC the disease is confined to the **ileum** and **colon**. The pathologic findings vary from slight dilatation with inflammation in mild cases to frank necrosis of the entire bowel in severe affliction. Microscopically, the picture is that of **ischemia**: mucosal edema, hemorrhage, and transmural liquefaction. Frequently there is **pneumatosis**: gas bubbles in the bowel wall secondary to bacterial proliferation.

   B. **Stress** is the major etiologic factor in the development of necrotizing enterocolitis. It may occur at birth or afterward. Many of these infants have low Apgar scores at birth. **Cold** exposure, **asphyxia**, and **hypotension** are frequent antecedents. Babies with respiratory distress syndrome **(RDS), apneic spells,** severe congenital **heart disease,** and any form of **sepsis** are at increased risk of acquiring necrotizing enterocolitis.

   C. **Selective mesenteric ischemia** occurs in response to stress and results in loss of the protective mucous barrier. **Autodigestion** and **bacterial invasion** then take place. Proliferation of the bacteria leads to release of gas and bacterial toxins, which, together with the mesenteric ischemia, result in **necrosis** of the intestine.

   D. **Secondary factors** in the development of NEC are:

   1. **Prematurity.** NEC is uncommon in full-term infants.
   2. **Feeding.** Almost all babies who develop necrotizing enterocolitis have been fed. **Breast milk** offers some protection against NEC because it contains **macrophages** and **immune globulins.** Unfortunately, these elements are lost when breast milk is stored.
   3. **Bacteria.** Bacterial infection of the intestine is a constant finding in necrotizing enterocolitis, and the disease occurs in clusters, suggesting an infectious etiology. A number of organisms have been found: *Escherichia coli, Klebsiella, Aerobacter, Streptococcus, Staphylococcus,* and clostridial species.
   4. **Arterial catheters** placed through the umbilical artery may cause mesenteric ischemia, either by mechanical blockage from the catheter or a thrombus, or by inducing vasospasm.

   E. **Perforation** of the intestine results from progressive full-thickness necrosis, producing **free air** in the peritoneal cavity as seen on x-ray or an abscess palpable as an **abdominal mass.**

III. **Clinical picture**

   A. Necrotizing enterocolitis typically develops in a tiny (26–28 weeks' gestation) infant who had low Apgar scores at birth and requires ventilatory support. He has an umbilical arterial catheter in place and has been tolerating small feedings given through a nasogastric gavage tube.

B. Early signs of NEC

1. **Signs of intestinal obstruction** are usually the first abnormality noted.
   a. **Vomiting,** sometimes bilious
   b. **Delayed gastric emptying** noted by increasing gastric residuals when the stomach is aspirated before tube feeding
   c. **Abdominal distention**
2. **Reducing substances** may be noted in the stools as a result of malabsorption of carbohydrate, an early sign of NEC.
3. **Blood is found in the stools**—occult or obvious red streaking on the stools.
4. **Apneic spells** and episodes of **bradycardia** increasing in frequency may be seen early.

C. Later signs result from the systemic and local effects of the necrotic intestine and sepsis.

1. **Shock.** Poor tissue perfusion is evident by pale, gray, or mottled skin; decreased urine output; and hypotension.
2. **Acidosis.** Usually metabolic, but there may be a respiratory component, especially if abdominal distention becomes marked.
3. **DIC.** Platelets and plasma clotting factors are consumed by the necrotic process and infection.
4. **Peritonitis.** At first, peritoneal irritation is mild and generalized, but if full-thickness necrosis develops, there is localized irritation of the abdominal wall with tenderness, guarding, and eventually, erythema and edema.

IV. Diagnosis

A.
Because of its high incidence in small premature infants, NEC should be suspected if there are any abnormalities of intestinal function. **A presumptive diagnosis** of NEC is made if **two or more of the early signs (sec. III.B)** are present.

B. Physical findings, sparse initially, increase with progression of the disease.

1. Abdominal **distention** occurs early.
2. Abdominal **tenderness** is usually present during the active stage of the disease.
3. A **palpable mass** indicates severely inflamed bowel, often a necrotic segment or an abscess.
4. **Erythema and edema** of the abdominal wall signify underlying necrotic bowel.

C. Abdominal x-ray may confirm the diagnosis.

1. **Pneumatosis intestinalis**—intramural gas in either the colon or intestine (rarely the stomach)—is diagnostic of NEC (Fig. 29-1). It is seen in more than half the patients later proved to have the disease. Pneumatosis intestinalis does not indicate full-thickness necrosis, however.
2. **Portal vein gas** is also diagnostic of NEC.
3. **Free air** indicates intestinal perforation. It is best seen on a cross-table lateral or upright film.
4. **Fixed, dilated loops** of intestine are strongly suggestive of impending or actual necrosis.
5. **Ascites** and **intestinal wall edema** are sometimes detectable by x-ray.

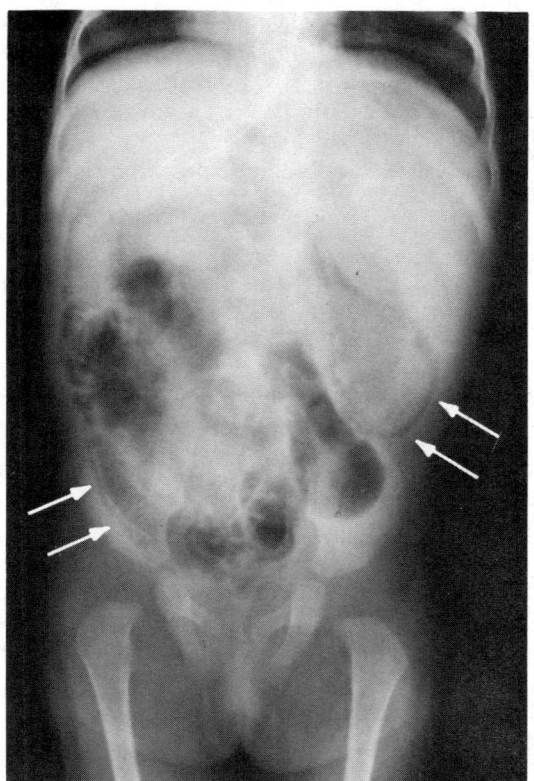

Fig. 29-1. Necrotizing enterocolitis. Pneumotosis intestinalis is evident on plain film of abdomen. (From L. L. Leape and T. M. Holder, Pediatric Surgery. In D. C. Sabiston (Ed.), *Textbook of Surgery* (12th ed.). Philadelphia: Saunders, 1981.

   6. Abscess may be seen if there has been walled-off or retroperitoneal perforation.

   7. Contrast studies are seldom indicated and contribute little.

C. Laboratory findings consistent with NEC

   1. WBC is **elevated** in most patients. A WBC below normal is an ominous sign.

   2. Thrombocytopenia is common, particularly late in the disease course.

   3. PT and PTT are elevated.

   4. Acidosis is present.

Nonoperative **treatment**

A. Nonoperative treatment is successful in a high percentage of patients with NEC if it is carried out early, before there is extensive bowel necrosis. For this reason, premature infants should be presumed to have NEC and be treated for it if any two of the diagnostic characteristics are present.

   1. Bowel rest. Feedings are stopped and a nasogastric tube is placed to evacuate the stomach and keep it empty. **Parenteral nutrition,** either peripheral or central, is required.

2. **Restoration of vascular volume.** Plasma and blood are given to replace losses caused by septic shock and intestinal edema. The volume required may be considerable.
3. **Antibiotics.** Penicillin (50,000 U/kg q6h) and gentamicin (2 mg/kg q12h) are given until antibiotic sensitivities are obtained on organisms isolated from the stool culture.
4. **Platelet transfusions** and fresh frozen **plasma** are given as needed to correct clotting deficiencies.
5. **Serial abdominal x-rays** are obtained every 6–8 hours to monitor intestinal involvement and to detect perforation.

B. **A prompt response is expected.** The infant should be much improved both clinically and according to laboratory studies within 12 hours. Lack of response usually indicates intestinal necrosis has already occurred.

C. **Intestinal rest and antibiotics** are continued for **10 days.** Feedings should be withheld for 14 days or more.

VI. Problems

A. **Rapid progression** occurs in some patients despite early and appropriate treatment. Perforation or extensive necrosis of the intestine can occur within hours.

B. **Delay in diagnosis** is a common cause of severe, progressive refractory necrotizing enterocolitis. Prolonged hypoperfusion and acidosis may result in irreversible tissue changes.

C. **Perforation** may occur without warning, even when the patient is properly treated and seems to be responding well. There may be no observed change in the infant's condition. For this reason, serial abdominal x-rays are necessary for the first 48 hours, even when treatment appears to be successful.

VII. Indications for operation

A. **Operative treatment** is necessary for the infant with necrotizing enterocolitis in whom the disease progresses to **bowel necrosis.** But it is difficult to make the diagnosis of intestinal gangrene before the development of complications. The challenge is to avoid operating on the infant with NEC who does not have necrosis, yet not delay operating on the infant who does.

B. **Absolute indications** for operation
1. **Perforation** as indicated by the presence of free air on lateral or upright abdominal x-ray
2. **Abdominal mass**
3. **Inflammation** and **edema** of the **abdominal wall**

C. **Relative indications** for operation are signs of **progressive disease.** These almost always indicate intestinal necrosis has developed. A high degree of clinical judgment and experience is required to make these distinctions.
1. **Increasing tenderness and guarding,** signs of peritoneal irritation
2. **Persistence of a fixed dilated loop** of intestine on serial abdominal x-rays, which usually indicates ischemic bowel
3. **Refractory DIC or acidosis**
4. **Clinical deterioration**
5. **Failure to improve** on medical treatment, even if the DIC or acidosis is mild

VIII. Preoperative preparation (see Chaps. 3 and 23)

A. Emergency resuscitation is necessary in most patients to prepare them for operation. Resection of the necrotic bowel must be carried out as soon as possible if the patient is to survive, leaving little time for preparation.

1. **Restore blood volume.** Transfuse plasma or blood as needed. Have blood available for use during the operation.
2. **Restore clotting factors.** Platelet transfusion and FFP are often necessary.
3. **Correct acidosis.** Give bicarbonate. Acidosis cannot be completely corrected until the dead bowel is removed.

IX. Operative care

A. The objectives of the operation are as follows:

1. **Remove all dead tissue.**
2. **Control sepsis.**
3. **Divert the fecal stream.**
4. **Preserve as much of the length of the bowel as possible.**

B. Technical considerations

1. **The entire abdominal gastrointestinal tract is examined** to determine the extent of damage and what can be saved.
2. **The peritoneal cavity is cleaned** of intestinal contents if there has been a perforation, using a copious lavage of warm saline.
3. **All obviously necrotic intestine must be removed.**
4. **Questionable segments of intestine are retained.** If the patient does not improve by the next day, a **"second look"** operation should be performed to reassess the equivocal areas.
5. **Intestinal diversion** is accomplished by creating a stoma proximal to the most cephalad area of necrosis. Continuity is restored after the intestine has healed and the patient is well—a minimum of 6 weeks later.
6. **A central venous catheter** is inserted for total parenteral nutrition. If the infant is unstable, this should be done at a later operation.

X. Postoperative care

A. Infants with necrotizing enterocolitis are among the **sickest** and **most difficult to care for** in pediatric surgery. Invariably, in small premature infants who are fragile to begin with, the massive metabolic insult of necrotic infected bowel stresses their homeostatic mechanisms to the utmost.

B. A **team** approach is essential, using the talents of the neonatologist, intensivist, cardiologist, and respiratory specialist as well as the pediatric surgeon. These babies also require the constant presence of a qualified neonatal intensive care nurse.

C. In addition to the usual monitoring and routine blood tests, these infants require:

1. **Ventilatory support** for several days after the operation.
2. **Circulatory support.** The peritoneal "burn" from peritonitis, together with edematous bowel and wound edema, constitutes a sizable "third space," which requires large amounts of fluids in the first 24 hours.
3. **Correction of DIC** may require repeated infusions of platelets and clotting factors for several days.

XI. Complications

A. Early

1. **Progressive sepsis** with shock, acidosis, and DIC is seen in patients who are operated on too late.
2. **Wound infections, disruption, and abscess formation** are more common in infants who have had massive contamination at operation.

B. Late

1. **Short bowel syndrome** develops if a long segment of intestine is removed. Long-term total parenteral nutrition is necessary.
2. **Stricture** of the intestine may develop in parts of the bowel that were ischemic without obvious necrosis. For this reason, contrast studies must be performed before the diverting stoma is closed. Stricture is also a well-recognized complication of nonoperative treatment of necrotizing enterocolitis.
3. **Malabsorption** may occur even when the length of intestine seems adequate to support enteral nutrition. Special formulas and parenteral nutrition are sometimes needed for a long time, although most infants gradually adapt.

XII. Prognosis.
Outcome in patients with NEC depends in large measure on the speed and aggressiveness of treatment. Babies who are operated on promptly after the development of intestinal necrosis usually recover. Those in whom the intestinal gangrene has progressed to the point that acidosis, shock, and DIC have occurred often do not survive.

Bibliography

Amoury, R. A. Necrotizing Enterocolitis. In T. M. Holder and K. W. Ashcraft (eds.), *Pediatric Surgery*. Philadelphia: Saunders, 1980. P. 374.

Barlow, B., et al. An experimental study of acute neonatal enterocolitis: The importance of breast milk. *J. Pediatr. Surg.* 9:587, 1974.

Book, L. S., et al. Clustering of necrotizing enterocolitis. *N. Engl. J. Med.* 297:984, 1977.

Brown, E. G., and Sweet, A. Y. (eds.). *Neonatal Necrotizing Enterocolitis*. New York: Grune & Stratton, 1980.

Dalsing, M. C., et al. Superoxide dismutase: A cellular protective enzyme in bowel ischemia. *J. Surg. Res.* 34:589, 1983.

Daneman, A., Woodward, S., and de Silva M. The radiology of neonatal necrotizing enterocolitis. *Pediatr. Radiol.* 7:70, 1978.

Ein, S. H., Marshall, D. G., and Girvan, D. Peritoneal drainage under local anesthesia for perforations from necrotizing enterocolitis. *J. Pediatr. Surg.* 12:963, 1977.

Kliegman, R. M., and Fanaroff, A. A. Necrotizing enterocolitis. *N. Engl. J. Med.* 310:1093, 1984.

Leonidas, J. C., Bhan, I., and Leape, L. L. Barium enema in suspected necrotizing enterocolitis: Is it ever indicated? *Clin. Radiol.* 31:587, 1980.

O'Neill, J. A., Jr. Neonatal necrotizing enterocolitis. *Surg. Clin. North Am.* 61:1013, 1981.

Pitt, J., Barlow, B., and Heird, W. C. Protection against experimental necrotizing enterocolitis by maternal milk. I. Role of milk leukocytes. *Pediatr. Res.* 11:906, 1977.

Rowe, M. I. Necrotizing Enterocolitis. In K. J. Welch, et al. (eds.), *Pediatric Surgery*. Chicago: Year Book, 1986. P. 944.

Schwartz, M. Z., et al. Intestinal stenosis following successful medical management of necrotizing enterocolitis. *J. Pediatr. Surg.* 15:890, 1980.

Stevenson, D. K., et al. Late morbidity among survivors of necrotizing enterocolitis. *Pediatrics* 66:925, 1980.

30 Hirschsprung's Disease

I. **Definition.** *Hirschsprung's disease* is the congenital absence of ganglion cells in the colon. The rectum is always involved, and in 90% of patients the abnormality is confined to the rectum and sigmoid. Longer segments can be affected, including the entire colon, or rarely, the entire small bowel as well. Absence of ganglion cells prevents peristalsis, resulting in functional intestinal obstruction. There is a strong hereditary factor. Up to 30% of patients have a relative with Hirschsprung's disease.

II. **Pathophysiology**
   A. **Ganglion cells are absent** both between the muscle layers of the bowel (Auerbach's plexus) and in the submucosa (Meissner's plexus). Nerve fibers are hypertrophied. Acetylcholinesterase is increased in the aganglionic segment.
   B. Failure of parasympathetic innervation results in **absence of peristalsis,** preventing propulsion of fecal contents. Colon proximal to the aperistaltic segment becomes distended and hypertrophied as it works against the obstruction.
   C. **Obstruction** may be acute and severe or chronic and indolent, depending on the extent of bowel involvement. If complete, severe fluid and electrolyte imbalance and acidosis result (see Chap. 23).
   D. **Enterocolitis** results from chronic obstruction. Ischemia of the intestinal wall from distention and mechanical trauma from fecal material result in bacterial invasion with ulceration, necrosis, pneumatosis, generalized sepsis, severe fluid loss, and sometimes, perforation.
   E. Chronic enterocolitis of a less fulminant form occurs in the older child with **hypoproteinemia** caused by protein loss from the ulcerated mucosa.

III. **Clinical presentation.** Despite the fact that Hirschsprung's disease is a congenital abnormality, present from birth, symptoms may be mild enough that the diagnosis is not initially suspected. There is great **individual variability** in symptoms.
   A. **In the newborn two major patterns of presentation are seen:** intestinal obstruction and constipation.
       1. **Acute intestinal obstruction** is the most common finding in the neonate, with the usual signs: massive distention, bilious vomiting, fluid retention in the lumen and wall of the bowel, and hypovolemia and acidosis (see Chap. 23). More than half the patients demonstrate this pattern.
       2. **Constipation** is seen in some newborns who have partial obstruction; it is intermittently relieved by spontaneous or induced bowel movements. Infrequent stools may alternate with diarrhea and distention.
       3. **Symptoms almost always begin in the first few weeks of life,** even if perceived only as constipation.
       4. **Enterocolitis** in the young infant **may occur suddenly,** with abdominal distention, watery diarrhea, vomiting, fever, and toxicity. It can be rapidly fatal.
   B. **In the older child** Hirschsprung's disease is usually perceived as typical **constipation,** but there are several **important differences.**
       1. **The urge to defecate is absent.** Since the aganglionic rectum is empty, pressure sensors are not stimulated and no "messages" are sent to the brain.

2. **Soiling (encopresis) does not occur.** The rectum is empty, not full of the large, hard stools found in typical constipation. Rarely, soiling may be seen in short-segment Hirschsprung's disease.

3. **Abdominal distention may be immense,** with muscle wasting of the extremities. **Malnutrition** results from decreased appetite because of fecal retention.

IV. **Diagnosis**

A. **Rectal biopsy** showing absence of ganglion cells definitely establishes the diagnosis of Hirschsprung's disease. Since the disease is always present from the anus up, biopsy will be positive whether the affected segment is confined to the rectum or extends throughout the colon. Blind suction or punch biopsy through the anus is usually adequate. Operative biopsy is indicated in equivocal cases.

B. **Barium enema** in the typical case is also diagnostic. It will show a narrow rectum with proximal dilated bowel and a "transition zone" of tapered bowel between them. The level of the transition zone indicates the extent of the aganglionosis.

1. Unfortunately, the **barium enema can be misleading,** failing to show the expected dilatation under certain conditions.

    a. In **the newborn,** before dilatation has had time to develop

    b. **If a colostomy has been performed** (as for unexplained perforation in the newborn)

    c. **If the "constipation" has been assiduously managed** by daily enemas, preventing fecal retention

    d. In **total-colon Hirschsprung's disease,** in which the colon may look deceptively normal

2. **Failure to evacuate the barium within 24 hours,** even in the absence of dilatation or a transition zone, is highly suggestive of Hirschsprung's disease if the infant is not septic or does not have generalized ileus for other reasons.

3. **Intestinal obstruction in the newborn** is probably caused by Hirschsprung's disease if the barium enema shows a normal or dilated colon and does not evacuate. Rectal biopsy is needed to confirm the diagnosis.

C. **Anorectal manometry** in Hirschsprung's disease shows failure of relaxation of the internal sphincter with rectal distention. Although this finding is specific, the test is more painful and time consuming than rectal biopsy, which is needed in any case for definitive diagnosis.

V. **Problems and differential diagnosis**

A. **Intestinal obstruction** (see Chap. 23)

B. **Constipation** (see Chap. 68)

VI. **Indications for operation.** Hirschsprung's disease is completely curable by resection of the affected bowel. Thus all patients with the diagnosis should undergo resection and a pull-through operation. Timing and proper staging are the critical variables.

A. **Neonates should have a colostomy.**

1. **Enterocolitis** requires rapid resuscitation and an immediate operation to prevent perforation and potentially fatal peritonitis.

2. **Intestinal obstruction,** if severe, may require emergency colostomy before a definitive diagnosis can be obtained by biopsy. Obstruction with a normal-caliber colon should be considered to be due to Hirschsprung's disease if no nonmechanical cause is found (e.g., sepsis, adrenal hemorrhage, cerebral injury).

3. **If the infant does not have enterocolitis or massive distention** and can be adequately decompressed with nasogastric and rectal intubation, colostomy can be delayed until the diagnosis is confirmed by rectal biopsy.

4. **The mildly symptomatic infant** also requires colostomy, even if he can be managed without tubes or irrigations. Although many do well, a significant number will suddenly develop fulminant enterocolitis, which can be rapidly fatal.

5. A **definitive pull-through** procedure can be done in 3 to 6 months.

B. **Older children also need a colostomy** to allow the massively dilated colon to shrink down and to permit cleansing of the colon so that a safe pull-through can be performed. Only rarely is it possible to prepare the colon adequately for pull-through without a colostomy. A **definitive pull-through** is done after the colon shrinks—about 6–12 months later.

I. Preoperative preparation (see Chaps. 3 and 23)

A. **Newborns**

1. Newborns with **enterocolitis** may require rapid resuscitation and emergency colostomy.

   a. **The colon is decompressed** by a rectal tube and gentle saline irrigations (by the physician). **Water should not be used because significant amounts may be absorbed, resulting in hyponatremia and seizures.**

   b. **Fluid resuscitation,** blood, or plasma may be needed.

   c. **Antibiotics** (gentamicin in doses of 2 mg/kg and clindamycin in doses of 10 mg/kg) are given.

2. **Uncomplicated intestinal obstruction** requires fluid resuscitation and nasogastric and rectal decompression. Operation is performed when the patient is hemodynamically stable and nearing electrolyte balance.

3. **Infants with mild symptoms** are managed with nasogastric and rectal decompression and operated on after the diagnosis has been confirmed by biopsy.

B. **The older child** is seldom as sick as the neonate with Hirschsprung's disease but benefits from evacuation of accumulated feces from the colon if this can be accomplished. Multiple irrigations rather than enemas, which cannot be evacuated, are needed.

C. Before the **pull-through** procedure is performed, the colon must be thoroughly cleansed with saline irrigations, finishing with a nonabsorbable antibiotic solution (neomycin 1 gm/liter).

Operative care

A. **Colostomy**

1. **Colostomy in the right colon** gives the greatest potential length of bowel at the time of pull-through and will not need to be taken down or redone at that time. If the patient has a transition zone above the splenic flexure, however, colostomy is performed at the end of the ganglionic segment so that the maximum length of colon is preserved for the pull-through.

2. **End colostomy** with mucous fistula or closure of the distal end is preferable to a loop colostomy since patients who have the latter are frequently plagued with recurrent prolapse.

B. **Pull-through procedure.** Removal of the aganglionic segment and anastomosis of normal ganglionic bowel to the anus are the objectives of surgical treatment. There are **three methods** of accomplishing this (Fig. 30-1).

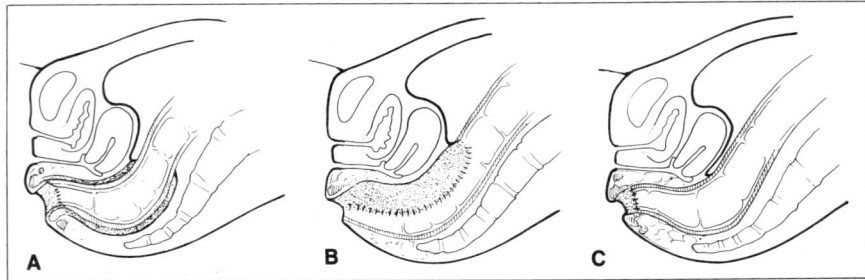

Fig. 30-1. Operations for Hirschsprung's disease. A. Soave endorectal pullthrough. The mucosa is stripped from the rectum, and ganglionic bowel is brought through the retained muscular sleeve and anastomosed to the anus. B. Duhamel procedure. Ganglionic colon is placed behind the retained aganglionic rectum and side-to-side anastomosis is performed. C. Swenson procedure. The entire rectum is removed and ganglionic colon is anastomosed at the upper end of the anal canal.

1. **Soave endorectal pull-through.** The rectum is retained, but the mucosa is removed. Aganglionic colon above the rectum is resected, and normal ganglionic colon is pulled through the rectal muscular sleeve and anastomosed above the anus. The majority of pediatric surgeons prefer this operation.
2. **Duhamel procedure.** The rectum is retained, and aganglionic colon above is resected. The ganglionic bowel is brought through the pelvis behind the retained rectum, and side-to-side anastomosis is performed as well as anastomosis to the anus. The patient is left with a double-sized rectum, half of which has ganglion cells.
3. **Swenson's procedure.** In this procedure, the original curative operation, the aganglionic segment is completely resected from just above the anus cephalad, and ganglionic colon is pulled through and anastomosed above the anus.

C. **Posterior sphincterotomy** may be performed at the time of the pull-through. Otherwise, approximately 50% of patients will have postoperative enterocolitis because of obstruction at the sphincters.

D. **Total-colon Hirschsprung's disease** may be treated by either an extended Duhamel procedure (carrying the side-to-side anastomosis to the splenic flexure) or an endorectal pull-through, anastomosing ileum to just above the anus. If the latter is used, a "training period" of 3–6 months is needed to expand the neorectum's retention capacity (see Chap. 66).

IX. Postoperative care

A. After the patient has recovered from the colostomy operation, the **distal colon is irrigated with saline** to rid it of retained feces and barium, which will otherwise become inspissated from the normal dehydrating action of the colon.

B. After the pull-through procedure, **early ambulation and feeding** are usually possible, since the bowel that was operated on is separated from the active intestinal stream.

C. In **older children or adolescents, elastic stockings** will help prevent thrombophlebitis, a common complication after an operation in which the legs are in stirrups for a prolonged period.

D. The retrorectal **drain is removed** on the second or third day, when it no longer serves any function.

E. The **anorectal anastomosis** should not be examined for 2 weeks, at which time it is gently **dilated**. It is digitally examined repeatedly every 2 weeks for at least 2 months to make sure there is no stricture formation. Daily home dilatations are carried out if stricture develops as the anastomosis heals.

F. The **colostomy is closed** after complete healing of the anastomosis has taken place and there is no evidence of stricture. This takes at least 3 months, longer if dilatations are required.

X. **Complications**

A. **Anastomotic leak** results if the anastomosis is under tension, ischemic, or infected. Prompt diagnosis and drainage will prevent cuff abscess. If the fecal stream has not been diverted, fatal peritonitis can result from an anastomotic leak, which is a major reason for doing a colostomy.

B. **Cuff abscess** after the Soave procedure is usually caused by infected hematoma. Adequate hemostasis and good drainage are the best preventive measures.

C. **Ischemic necrosis** of the pulled-through colon results if the blood supply is inadequate or under excessive tension. It is suspected if there is fever, leukocytosis, and a foul-smelling discharge at the anus. Immediate reoperation, bringing down healthy colon and a new anastomosis, is the treatment of choice. Otherwise, irremediable stricture will result and subsequent pull-through may be impossible.

D. **Thrombophlebitis** in older children results from positioning during the operation. Adequate padding and use of elastic stockings will help prevent it. Anticoagulation may be necessary treatment if there is no bleeding from the rectal cuff.

E. **Rectal stricture** results from ischemia or infection at the anastomosis. Repeated dilatations are usually adequate treatment, but on occasion repeat pull-through is necessary.

F. **Enterocolitis** occurs in some patients, sometimes as late as several years postoperatively. Sphincterotomy is usually curative; it may be preventive if done at the time of pull-through.

G. **Incontinence** of stool is a rare complication, usually the result of faulty technique with damage to both the external sphincter and the puborectalis muscle.

XI. **Prognosis.** Long-term results from pull-through procedures are excellent. Normal bowel movements are to be expected in the vast majority of instances. The only significant mortality risk is in young infants if the diagnosis is missed or colostomy is not performed.

Bibliography

Berdon, W. E., and Baker D. H. The roentgenographic diagnosis of Hirschsprung's disease in infancy. *Am. J. Roentgenol.* 93:432, 1965.

Carcassonne, M., et al. Primary corrective operation without decompression in infants less than three months of age with Hirschsprung's disease. *J. Pediatr. Surg.* 17:241, 1982.

Ehrenpreis, T. *Hirschsprung's Disease.* Chicago: Year Book, 1970.

Holzschneider, M. *Hirschsprung's Disease.* Stuttgart: Hippokrates-Verlag; New York: Thieme-Stratton, 1982.

Kleinhaus, S., et al. Hirschsprung's disease: A survey of the members of the Surgical Section of the American Academy of Pediatrics. *J. Pediatr. Surg.* 14:588, 1979.

Lefebvre, M. P., et al. Total colonic aganglionosis initially diagnosed in an adolescent. *Gastroenterology* 87:1364, 1984.

Lynn, H. B. Rectal myectomy in Hirschsprung's disease: A decade of experience. *Arch. Surg.* 1109:991, 1975.

Martin, L. W. Surgical management of total colonic aganglionosis. *Ann. Surg.* 176:343, 1972.

Martin, L. W. Hirschsprung's Disease. In T. M. Holder and K. W. Ashcraft (eds.), *Pediatric Surgery*. Philadelphia: Saunders, 1980. P. 389.

Noblett, H. R. A rectal suction biopsy tube for use in the diagnosis of Hirschsprung's disease. *J. Pediatr. Surg.* 4:406, 1969.

Sieber, W. K. Hirschsprung's disease. In K. J. Welch, et al. (eds.), *Pediatric Surgery*. Chicago: Year Book, 1986. P. 995.

Soave, F. Hirschsprung's disease: A new surgical technique. *Arch. Dis. Child.* 39:116, 1964.

Swenson, O., and Bill, A. H. Resection of rectum and rectosigmoid with preservation of the sphincter for benign spastic lesions producing megacolon: An experimental study. *Surgery* 24:212, 1948.

Swenson, O., Fisher, J. H., and Gherardi, G. Rectal biopsy in the diagnosis of Hirschsprung's disease. *Surgery* 45:690, 1959.

Swenson, O., Neuhauser, E. B. D., and Pickett L. K. New concepts of etiology, diagnosis and treatment of congenital megacolon (Hirschsprung's disease). *Pediatrics* 4:201, 1949.

Weitzman, J. J. Complications of Hirschsprung's Disease and its Management. In P. A. de Vries and S. R. Shapiro (eds.), *Complications of Pediatric Surgery*. New York: Wiley, 1982. P. 269.

Weitzman, J. J., Hanson, B. A., and Brennan, L. P. Management of Hirschsprung's disease with the Swenson procedure. *J. Pediatr. Surg.* 7:157, 1972.

31 Imperforate Anus

Definition. The term *imperforate anus* encompasses the full spectrum of obstructive anorectal malformations: anal agenesis, rectal agenesis, and rectal atresia.

A. Incidence. Major anorectal malformations occur in approximately **1 in 5000** births either as isolated findings or as part of the **VACTERL** syndrome (*v*ertebral, *a*nal, *c*ardiac, *t*racheal, *e*sophageal, *r*enal, and *l*imb anomalies).

B. Classification. Patients with imperforate anus are classified as having a "high" or "low" lesion according to whether the blind end of the rectum passes through the key muscle of continence, the **puborectalis**. If it does (a "low" defect), definitive repair by perineal operation is possible in the neonatal period. A high defect requires colostomy and a later pull-through operation. It is also important to note whether a **fistula** is present to the perineum, vagina, or urinary tract (Fig. 31-1).

1. **Low**
   a. **Anal stenosis.** "Nearly" imperforate anus
   b. **Anal agenesis.** With or without a perineal or vestibular fistula
2. **High**
   a. **Anorectal agenesis.** With or without a fistula to the vagina or urethra
   b. **Rectal atresia.** Normal anus with obstruction several cm proximal to anus

Pathophysiology. The pathologic effects of imperforate anus result from the obstruction and the fistula.

A. Low intestinal obstruction is present unless there is a large decompressing external fistula. Untreated, the patient develops abdominal distention, fluid sequestration, and vomiting.

B. A fistula may connect the blind rectum to the perineum in either sex, or the genital tract in females (most commonly the vaginal vestibule), or to the urethra in males.

1. **Hyperchloremic acidosis** may result from absorption of urine from the blind colon if there is a large fistula to the urinary tract.
2. **Recurrent urinary tract infections** may result from passage of feces into the urinary tract through a urinary fistula.

Clinical presentation

A. Physical examination reveals the diagnosis of imperforate anus in most patients. The perineum should be carefully searched for evidence of a **fistula**, which typically occurs along the median raphe in males. Most females with imperforate anus have a vestibular fistula—an opening inside the vulva but posterior to the hymen.

B. Signs of intestinal obstruction (abdominal distention, intestinal dilatation by x-ray, and vomiting) develop if the diagnosis is missed or the patient is not treated.

Diagnosis. The need for diagnostic studies depends on the physical findings.

A. If meconium is seen on the **perineum,** either at the vestibule or emerging from a perineal fistula, the patient has a **low** defect. Further studies are not necessary, and corrective anoplasty can be carried out right away.

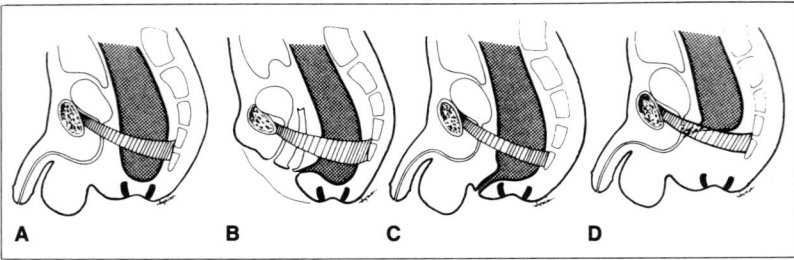

Fig. 31-1. Types of imperforate anus. A. Low defect in male without fistula. B. Low defect in female with rectovaginal fistula. C. Low defect in male with perineal fistula. D. High defect in male with rectourethral fistula. The rectum does not pass through the puborectalis muscle as it does in the low defects. (From L. L. Leape and T. M. Holder, Pediatric Surgery. In D. C. Sabiston (Ed.), *Textbook of Surgery*. Philadelphia: Saunders, 1981.)

  B. **If no fistula** can be identified, the defect may be high or low. Further studies are needed.
    1. **Urine sediment** may reveal meconium epithelial cells, confirming the presence of a fistula from a high lesion.
    2. **Retrograde urethrogram** in males may reveal a rectourethral fistula and may also demonstrate the level of the lower end of the blind rectum.
    3. **Perineal puncture contrast rectogram** is the most reliable method of demonstrating the level of the rectal pouch. The examination is safely performed under fluoroscopic control.
    4. The traditional **inverted lateral film** of the abdomen and pelvis to determine the level of the blind pouch is **unreliable** and therefore not indicated.

V. **Problems**
  A. **Associated anomalies** are present in more than 50% of patients with imperforate anus. The most common are **gastrointestinal** (esophageal atresia, intestinal atresia, malrotation), **genitourinary** (renal agenesis, hypospadias, reflux, exstrophy), **cardiac**, and **skeletal**.
  B. **Hyperchloremic acidosis** may result from urinary absorption preoperatively if operation is long delayed, or after colostomy if there is a large fistula.
  C. **Sacral anomalies** are associated with neuromuscular deficiencies in the perineum, which may result in incontinence in spite of an anatomically satisfactory repair.

VI. **Indications for operation**
  A. **High lesions** require urgent colostomy, followed by a definitive pull-through procedure at 3–12 months.
  B. **Low lesions** may be corrected by anoplasty and closure of the fistula in the neonatal period.
  C. **Anal stenosis** does not require an operation; it is treated with repeated dilatations.
  D. **Temporizing dilatations** or a simple **cutback** anoplasty of a vestibular or perineal fistula may be necessary if there are other life-threatening anomalies (including severe prematurity) that take precedence in treatment.

II. Preoperative preparation. In addition to the standard preparation for neonates (see Chap. 3), fluids and electrolytes are replaced to correct the effects of intestinal obstruction.

III. Operative care

   A. Low defect: anoplasty. The fistula is excised, the superficial external sphincter is identified, and the blind end of the rectum is brought through the sphincter and anastomosed to the anal skin.

   B. High defect: colostomy. A divided colostomy is created, separating the two ends so there is no "spillover" of fecal contents. A large urinary fistula may require closure to prevent fecal contamination or urinary absorption.

   C. A **pull-through** procedure is performed at 3–12 months. The rectum is brought through the muscles of control (puborectalis, levator ani, and external sphincters) by either the Stephens sacroabdominal-perineal approach or the Pena midsagittal perineal method. The colostomy is retained until healing is complete.

IV. Postoperative care

   A. Anoplasty. The new anus is calibrated at 2 weeks and **dilated** if necessary. Daily dilatations by the parent may be needed until healing is complete (3–6 months). Frequent (at least monthly) examinations are necessary to monitor healing.

   B. Colostomy. The infant should remain in the hospital for at least a week to make sure there is no evidence of urine absorption or infection.

   C. After the pull-through procedure, dilatations of the neorectum and anus are necessary until healing is complete and an adequate and soft anorectum is achieved. The colostomy may then be safely closed.

V. Complications

   A. Stricture of the new anus or rectum may result from devascularization or excessive tension on the pull-through segment but is common even when the operation is properly performed. Dilatations are usually adequate treatment, but operative repair is sometimes necessary.

   B. Recurrent urinary fistula results from inadequate closure, unrecognized urethral damage, or infection. Reoperation is necessary.

   C. Hyperchloremic acidosis and **urinary infections** may occur (See sec. II.B).

   D. Mucosal prolapse at the anus occurs if there is inadequate preservation of the superficial external sphincter.

   E. Constipation is common in children after repair of imperforate anus, especially high defects. Stool softening with milk of magnesia and bowel-training programs are indicated.

   F. Diarrhea most commonly results from residual obstruction at the anus or rectum. Dilatations or revision may be necessary.

VI. Prognosis. The potential for continence following repair of imperforate anus depends on the skill with which the operation is performed and on whether the child has an intact neuromuscular apparatus for control.

   A. Low defects. Almost all of these patients do well. The rectum is through the puborectalis muscle and the sensorimotor mechanisms are intact. Normal function is expected.

   B. High defects. The extent of neurologic and muscular impairment varies widely but generally parallels the severity of the rectal and urinary tract lesions and the extent of the sacral deformity.

1. **Proper placement** of the rectum within the **puborectalis** sling and preservation of all available sphincter muscles are essential. Reoperation is indicated if this has not been accomplished with the initial operation.
2. **Motivation** of the patient and intelligence of the parents are key factors in success at achieving continence when there are significant neuromuscular disabilities.
3. Many children with **severe impairment** are ultimately able to achieve satisfactory control through the use of accessory muscles and dietary regulation.
4. **Few** children with high defects **achieve continence before entering school,** when peer pressure increases motivation.
5. **Biofeedback** conditioning and muscle **sling operations** may be helpful in refractory cases.

Bibliography

de Vries, P. A. The surgery of anorectal anomalies: Its evolution, with evaluations of procedures. *Curr. Probl. Surg.* May 1984.

de Vries, P. A., and Pena, A. Posterior sagittal anorectoplasty. *J. Pediatr. Surg.* 17:638, 1982.

Khoury, M. J., et al. A population study of the VACTERL association. *Pediatrics* 71:815, 1983.

Kiesewetter, W. B. Imperforate Anus. In T. M. Holder and K. W. Ashcraft (eds.), *Pediatric Surgery.* Philadelphia: Saunders, 1980. P. 401.

Murugasu, J. J. A new method of roentgenological demonstration of anorectal anomalies. *Surgery* 68:706, 1970.

Pena, A. Posterior sagittal anorectoplasty as a secondary operation for the treatment of fecal incontinence. *J. Pediatr. Surg.* 18:762, 1983.

Pena, A., and de Vries, P. Posterior sagittal anorectoplasty: Important technical considerations and new applications. *J. Pediatr. Surg.* 17:796, 1982.

Santulli, T. V., et al. Imperforate anus: A survey from the members of the Surgical Section of the American Academy of Pediatrics. *J. Pediatr. Surg.* 6:484, 1971.

Stephens, F. D., and Smith, E. D. *Anorectal Malformations in Children.* Chicago: Year Book, 1971.

Templeton, J. M., and O'Neill, J. A., Jr. Anorectal Malformations. In K. J. Welch, et al. (eds.), *Pediatric Surgery.* Chicago: Year Book, 1986. P. 1022.

32 Gastrostomy

I. **Definition.** A gastrostomy is an opening made in the stomach and abdominal wall for the purpose of external gastric drainage or feeding. Usually there is an indwelling rubber tube, although a tubeless gastrostomy can be constructed.

II. **Indications.** Gastrostomy is performed in patients who are unable to be fed adequately by mouth and as an adjunct in the management of some surgical diseases.

   A. **Feeding problems**
   1. **Swallowing incoordination** as a result of neurologic disorders, either temporary or permanent.
   2. Difficult or time-consuming feeding in **brain-damaged** children. Gastrostomy often greatly simplifies feeding in these difficult patients.
   3. **Motility disorders** of the esophagus.
   4. **Recurrent aspiration** caused by any of the preceding.
   5. **Extreme prematurity** requiring long-term tube feedings.
   6. **Respirator-dependent** patients.

   B. **Surgical management**
   1. **Postoperative** care of neonates with **intestinal obstruction,** short bowel syndrome, or other disorder in which feeding may be long delayed. Gastrostomy also facilitates assessment of gastric emptying when feedings are initiated.
   2. **Esophageal atresia** requiring **staged** or **delayed repair.**
      a. For gastric drainage to prevent reflux aspiration in those in whom division of the tracheoesophageal fistula must be delayed
      b. For feeding in patients with isolated "long-gap" esophageal atresia while awaiting repair
   3. **Pyloroplasty,** in which adequate gastric emptying may be delayed (particularly likely in brain-damaged children undergoing fundoplication for reflux).
   4. **Esophageal stricture,** either from caustic injury or reflux esophagitis. Gastrostomy is helpful both for feeding and for retrograde esophageal dilatations.

III. **Operative technique.** The Stamm method is most commonly used. A tube is inserted via a gastrotomy within two concentric pursestring sutures, infolding a serosa-lined "cuff." The tube is brought out through a stab wound in the abdominal wall, and the stomach is sutured to the inside of the abdominal wall at the exit site. Several **technical points** deserve emphasis.

   A. **Nonabsorbable sutures** must be used. Adhesion between the stomach wall and the peritoneum is frequently imperfect and may break down if absorbable sutures are used.
   B. The stomach must be **securely sutured** to the abdominal wall to eliminate the possibility of leakage into the peritoneal cavity.
   C. A **"mushroom" (de Pezzer) catheter** must be used initially. If a balloon catheter is used and the balloon breaks, the catheter will come out. If the catheter comes out within the first 2 weeks, replacement may be impossible or cause

stomal disruption with intraperitoneal leakage. The catheter can be safely changed to a balloon catheter after 14 days.

D. Nonoperative placement of a gastrostomy tube is possible. Using a flexible fiberoptic gastroscope, the stomach and abdominal walls are punctured from within, and the tube is brought through in retrograde fashion. This method obviates the need for an abdominal incision, although not the need for anesthesia. It may or may not be safer than the operative approach.

IV. Postoperative Care

A. The catheter must be **fixed on the outside** to keep the flange snug against the stomach opening on the inside, which is necessary to prevent leakage. The problem is not that the catheter might come out, but that it may go in. A "keeper" can be fashioned of a slit piece of rubber tubing through which the gastrostomy tube is passed and the tension adjusted.

B. The tube should **not be clamped** initially but placed to gravity drainage so that acute gastric distention does not occur in the immediate postoperative period.

C. Feedings may be started with clear liquids on the first postoperative day, progressing to full-strength tube feedings as tolerated, usually within a day or two.

1. Feedings should initially be given slowly by **gravity** to mimic normal feeding. Too-rapid feeding may cause pain, bloating, vomiting, or hiccups.
2. For most patients, prepared formulas (e.g., Isocal) offer no advantage over a **regular meal blenderized** with added water.
3. The feeding is followed with clear water to rinse the tube.

D. In infants, the tube should not be clamped until the stomach is well healed to the abdominal wall—at least 10 days. It may be attached to a large syringe barrel and suspended to prevent loss of feedings.

V. Early complications.
Few simple operations are beset with as many complications as is gastrostomy. Most complications are related to improper surgical technique or **inadequate fixation** of the tube.

A. Intraperitoneal leakage. This is the most serious complication of gastrostomy and is almost always the result of a technical error. Highly irritating gastric contents cause peritonitis, which can be fatal if not promptly diagnosed and treated by immediate reoperation.

1. **Etiology**
   a. **Trauma during replacement** of a tube that has come out is particularly likely in the immediate postoperative period.
   b. **Pursestring sutures** that are **too tight** can cut through the stomach wall.
   c. **Excessive tension** on the tube can cause local necrosis of the stomach wall.
2. **Diagnosis**
   a. **Sudden deterioration** in a patient previously progressing well after the operation suggests an intraabdominal catastrophe.
   b. **Fever, abdominal distention, pain, and leukocytosis** are usually present. Tenderness is increased but may not be localized.
   c. **Upright abdominal x-ray** will usually show free intraperitoneal air.
   d. An **x-ray** study with **aqueous contrast material** introduced through the gastrostomy tube will show intraperitoneal leakage in most cases.
3. **Treatment**
   a. **Immediate emergency reoperation** is required.

b. **A new gastrostomy** is constructed at a different site in the stomach.
   c. **Copious saline lavage** of the abdominal cavity is performed to remove the gastric contents.
   d. Peritonitis is treated with **antibiotics, plasma and fluids,** and gastric decompression.
B. **Nonfunction** is most likely to result from **kinking** of the tube or **angulation** of the stomach because of improper placement of the exit site in the abdominal wall. It may also be caused by displacement of the tube end into the abdominal wall tissues because of **excessive tension.** If a functional tube suddenly stops working, it is usually because of intraluminal **plugging** with food particles.
C. **Bleeding** in the immediate postoperative period is usually due to gastric-wall blood vessels at the gastrotomy site.

Late complications. Most complications that occur in a previously properly functioning gastrostomy are the result of **inadequate fixation** of the tube.

A. **Leakage** of gastric contents around the tube occurs if the flange (de Pezzer) or balloon (Foley) is not kept snug up against the exit site of the catheter from the stomach. Lateral movement of the tube irritates and widens the skin stoma, causing irritation and leakage.
   1. **Skin breakdown** results rapidly from contact with acid-peptic gastric juice, causing erythema, seropurulent drainage, and further leakage. Infection may occur but is rare.
   2. **Granulation tissue** develops around the tube in response to chronic irritation by the gastric juice and the tube. Its presence prevents the skin from healing close to the tube.
   3. **Gastric mucosa** may prolapse or grow up at the tube exit site. Operative excision is necessary to permit healing of the skin against the tube.
   4. **Treatment of leakage**
      a. **"Snugging up" the tube** and keeping it well sealed on the inside will usually stop leakage. If the hole is enlarged, replacement with a larger tube is often effective.
      b. In refractory cases, **removal of the tube** for 4–12 hours will result in shrinkage of the stoma and a snug fit when the tube is reinserted.
      c. **Cimetidine** (10 mg/kg qid) reduces gastric acid production and may help stomal healing in difficult cases.
      d. **Granulation tissue** should be completely eradicated by vigorous treatment with **silver nitrate** sticks. Several treatments may be necessary at weekly intervals.
B. **Accidental dislodgment** may occur if the tube is caught and the child suddenly turns. Children seldom pull tubes out.
C. **Gastric obstruction** may result from pyloric occlusion by the catheter balloon if there is distal migration of an unsecured tube. Pulling the tube back corrects the problem.

Replacement of a dislodged gastrostomy tube is potentially hazardous in the immediate postoperative period or if the tube has been out a long time. A Foley (balloon) catheter should be used for replacement. A safe technique is as follows:

A. A small **Hegar dilator** (or straight sound) is passed gently into the stoma to determine the angle of entry into the stomach. It should be felt to "drop" into the gastric lumen.
B. Progressively larger dilators are introduced, following the "tract," to **stretch** it without a false passage.

C. The catheter (with keeper placed on it) is introduced after a dilator the size of the catheter has been passed. The balloon is inflated to 5 ml. If the balloon is properly positioned in the gastric lumen, it is possible to move the catheter in and out easily. The catheter is then fixed on gentle traction.

D. The catheter is **irrigated** with 10 ml of sterile saline. It should be possible to aspirate some, but not all, of the irrigant.

E. **Contrast x-ray** study is obtained to verify that the catheter is in the gastric lumen **if there is any question whatever about its position.** A positioning error is suspected if it is difficult to pass the catheter, if it does not move easily after insertion, or if it does not irrigate easily.

VIII. **Closure of gastrostomy.** The gastrostomy stoma will close spontaneously after removal of the tube at any time within the first 6–12 months. After that, operative closure is usually required under general anesthesia.

Bibliography

Bishop, H. C. Simplified closure of the long-standing gastrostomy. *J. Pediatr. Surg.* 16:571, 1981.

Campbell, J. R., and Sasaki, T. M. Gastrostomy in infants and children: An analysis of complications and techniques. *Am. Surg.* 9:505, 1974.

Ducharme, J. C., Youssef, S., and Tilkin, F. Gastrostomy closure: A quick, easy, and safe method. *J. Pediatr. Surg.* 12:729, 1977.

Gallagher, M. W., Tyson, K. R. T., and Ashcraft, K. W. Gastrostomy in pediatric patients: An analysis of complications and techniques. *Surgery* 74:556, 1973.

Gauderer, M. W. L., Ponsky, J. L., and Izant, R. J., Jr. Gastrostomy without laparotomy: A percutaneous endoscopic technique. *J. Pediatr. Surg.* 15:872, 1980.

Holder, T. M., and Gross, R. E. Temporary gastrostomy in pediatric surgery: Experience with 187 cases. *Pediatrics* 26:36, 1960.

Holder, T. M., Leape, L. L., and Ashcraft, K. W. Gastrostomy: Its use and dangers in pediatric patients. *N. Engl. J. Med.* 286:1345, 1972.

Kappel, D. A., and Leape, L. L. A method for gastrostomy fixation. *J. Pediatr. Surg.* 10:523, 1975.

Rodgers, B. M. Gastrostomy. In K. J. Welch, et al. (eds.), *Pediatric Surgery*. Chicago: Year Book, 1986. P. 808.

Sieber, W. K. The Stomach. In T. M. Holder and K. W. Ashcraft (eds.), *Pediatric Surgery*. Philadelphia: Saunders, 1980. P. 313.

33 Colostomy and Ileostomy

- **Definition.** A *colostomy* is an external opening of the colon on the abdominal wall. It is used to divert the fecal stream as an adjunct to reconstructive surgery and in the initial treatment of a variety of diseases of the colon, rectum, and anus: imperforate anus, Hirschsprung's disease, colonic atresia, necrotizing enterocolitis, and perforation of the colon from any cause. *Ileostomy* is used in a similar fashion when the colon is afflicted: NEC, ulcerative colitis, polyposis, and so on. The following discussion applies equally to both procedures.

- **Types of colostomy**

  A. **Loop colostomy** is performed by bringing the colon up through the abdominal wall as a loop in continuity and making an opening in the side wall. It is the quickest to perform but has the disadvantage that "spillover" of feces can occur into the distal limb, i.e., it does not totally divert the feces.

  B. **Divided colostomy** is created by totally dividing the colonic loop and bringing the ends out as two separated end stomas. Spillover will not occur if the appliance covers only the proximal end. This form is used for imperforate anus.

  C. **End colostomy** consists of bringing only the proximal end up to the skin. The distal end is sutured shut. This form of colostomy has no possibility of spillover and is least likely to prolapse, but it can be used only if the distal colon is open through the anus.

- **Care of a colostomy**

  A. **The stoma must be protected** from abrasion, particularly in small infants. A standard plastic bag appliance is best, but temporary petroleum jelly–impregnated gauze dressings may also be used.

  B. **Fit of the appliance** around the stoma is critical. It must not overlap the mucosa but should be close to it so little skin is exposed to intestinal contents. Use of Stomadhesive provides a good bond and prevents or treats skin breakdown.

  C. **The appliance** should be **changed** whenever it leaks but can stay on up to a week if it is functioning properly. More frequent changes are necessary at first until the stoma matures and the skin toughens.

  D. **Proper training** of the mother or other caretaker is essential before discharge from the hospital. A stomal therapist who is available to advise over the phone and see the patient when necessary improves care. It is very helpful for the child and parent to see a stoma on another child preoperatively.

  E. **Activity does not need to be limited.** The child can bathe, swim, and engage in full athletic activity with a colostomy or ileostomy and should be encouraged to do so.

- **Problems**

  A. **Bleeding** from the stoma is the most common problem. It usually results from abrasion and most commonly occurs in the first few weeks after the operation. Mucosal bleeding is easily controlled by gentle pressure—with the bag on. Bleeding in the first 24 hours is usually from a submucosal vessel and may require suture to control.

  B. **Prolapse** is eversion of the mucosa or full-thickness bowel wall. It is a common complication with loop colostomy but is rare in end colostomies. Prolapse can be reduced easily if treated promptly, before edema develops. If the prolapse is mild and occurs infrequently, no treatment is needed. Recurring severe prolapse requires operative revision of the stoma. Sometimes, narrowing the stoma by placement of a pursestring suture at the mucocutaneous junction will prevent prolapse.

C. **Stomal stricture** also is not a rare complication. The obstruction can be at the skin or at the fascial level. Sometimes it is related to progression of the underlying disease (as in NEC) and extends proximally. Higher obstruction must be excluded by contrast x-ray studies.

  1. **Frequent watery movements** or decreased frequency of stools with abdominal distention are signs of stomal stricture.
  2. **Inability to insert a small catheter** or calibration of the stoma with graduated Hegar dilators will make the diagnosis.
  3. **Dilatation** may be adequate treatment, but operative revision is frequently necessary.

D. **Fistula** usually results from a suture cutting through the bowel wall. If the fistula is below the abdominal wall, operative revision is required.

E. **Necrosis** may occur in an end colostomy if it is brought out under tension, if the blood supply is compromised, or if there is progression of NEC. If necrosis is deep to the fascia, the colostomy must be redone.

F. **Dehiscence and herniation** occur if the bowel wall is not sutured to the peritoneum and deep fascia. Small bowel will herniate through a very small space. Treatment is resuture.

G. **Intestinal obstruction** may be caused by adhesions or by an internal hernia or volvulus of a loop of intestine around the enterostomy limb. Reoperation is required.

H. **Dehydration and electrolyte imbalance** may occur if a stoma is high in the small intestine, if it is partially obstructed, or from food intolerance. Diarrhea may be profuse. Cessation of feedings and replacement with parenteral fluids or TPN is necessary. Closure or revision of the stoma may be needed.

Bibliography

Bishop, H. C. Colostomy in the newborn. *Am. J. Surg.* 101, 1961.
Bishop, H. C. Ileostomy and Colostomy. In K. J. Welch, et al. (eds.), *Pediatric Surgery*. Chicago: Year Book, 1986. P. 978.
Grosfeld, J. L., and Cooney, D. E. Care of the child with a colostomy. *Pediatrics* 59:469, 1977.
Lister, J., et al. Colostomy complications in children. *Practitioner* 227:229, 1983.
Nixon, H. H. Paediatric problems associated with stomas. *Clin. Gastroenterol.* 11:351, 1982.
Schwarz, K. B., et al. Sodium needs of infants and children with ileostomy. *J. Pediatr.* 102:509, 1983.

34 Ambiguous Genitalia

Definition. Anomalous development of the external genitalia may result in confusion in gender assignment in newborn infants. Immediate evaluation is necessary. If the baby has the adrenogenital syndrome, life-threatening adrenal insufficiency may occur. Even if there is no endocrinopathy, an infant with ambiguous genitalia is a cause of great distress to the parents to whom the first question is always, "Is it a boy or a girl?" Prompt evaluation and decision is indicated under the following circumstances:

1. **Obviously ambiguous genitalia** with a large phallus, regardless of the location of the urethral opening or the degree of fusion of the labioscrotal folds, and with or without palpable gonads
2. **A phallus with no palpable gonads,** even if the infant appears to be a male with cryptorchidism
3. **Penoscrotal or perineal hypospadias,** even if "testes" are present
4. **Unilateral cryptorchidism and hypospadias**

Pathophysiology. Intrauterine development of the genitalia depends on the presence or absence of the fetal testis.

A. **Female genital differentiation,** both internal and external, occurs autonomously and **requires no female hormones** (and thus, no ovary), but testicular hormones must not be present.

B. **Male genital differentiation requires** at least two hormones secreted by the developing **testis** as early as 6–8 weeks of fetal life.
   1. **Mullerian inhibiting substance (MIS)** induces regression of the primordial structures, which otherwise develop into the fallopian tubes, uterus, and upper vagina.
   2. **Testosterone** causes development of the vas deferens, seminal vesicles, and epididymis. **Dihydrotestosterone** (from conversion of testosterone by local tissue 5-alpha reductase) is necessary for development of the prostate, penis, and scrotum.

C. **Failure of male differentiation** occurs if there is:
   1. Absence or dysgenesis of the testis
   2. Testicular resistance to lutenizing hormone or chorionic gonadotropin
   3. Insufficient MIS or testosterone secreted by the testis
   4. Lack of 5-alpha reductase
   5. End-organ resistance to testosterone

D. **Virilization of female external genitalia** occurs if excess androgen is present from any source, such as adrenal hyperplasia, androgen-secreting tumors of mother or fetus, or maternal drugs.

Clinical presentation

A. **Incomplete virilization** is the presenting finding. It may be impossible to tell on initial examination whether the infant is a boy with severe hypospadias or a girl with clitoral hypertrophy (Fig. 34-1).
   1. **Clitoral hypertrophy** may result in a structure that appears to be a perfectly normal "penis."

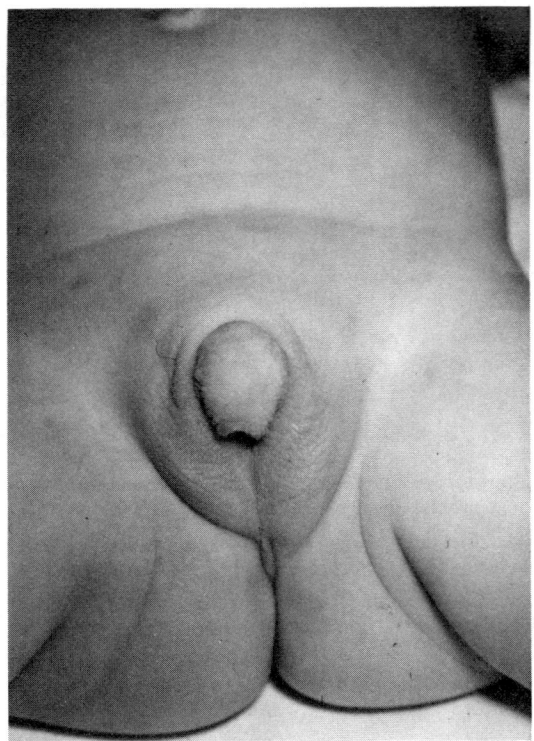

Fig. 34-1. Ambiguous genitalia. Female infant with adrenogenital syndrome and hypertrophy of the clitoris. Genitalia are similar to those of a male infant with hypospadias and undescended testes. (From L. L. Leape and T. M. Holder, Pediatric Surgery. In D. C. Sabiston (Ed.), *Textbook of Surgery*. Philadelphia: Saunders, 1981.)

      2. Fusion of the labia may mimic a scrotum, complete with rugal folds. Failure of scrotal fusion may mimic labia.

      3. Failure of separation of the urethra and vagina results in a urogenital sinus, with a single external opening. In extreme virilization, this opening may be at the end of the phallus.

      4. Severe hypospadias may result in an opening that looks like a vaginal introitus at the base of the phallus.

   B. Adrenal insufficiency is often associated with virilizing congenital adrenal hyperplasia. Collapse after a stress (such as circumcision) may be the presenting symptom.

IV. Diagnosis

   A. History. Maternal androgenic drug exposure; family history of infertility, hypospadias, or neonatal deaths.

   B. Physical examination

      1. A virilized **clitoris** may have **lateral ridges** on the ventral surface instead of the single midline raphe of the male penis.

2. **The uterus is usually palpable** by rectal examination in the virilized female. It is larger at birth than later because of stimulation by maternal hormones. Extrusion of a plug of mucus from the "urethra" during rectal examination indicates the presence of a vagina.

3. **Palpable gonads** in the labioscrotal folds or the groins are usually testes but may be dysgenetic "ovotestes."

C. **Buccal smear** is useful in demonstrating Barr bodies or Y-chromosome fluorescence. In the first few days of life, however, Barr body counts may be falsely low.

D. **Genital sinogram** will usually demonstrate the anatomy of the urogenital sinus, vagina, and sometimes the uterus, if present.

E. **Laparoscopy or laparotomy** may be necessary to determine if there is a uterus and tubes and to perform biopsy on the gonads. It is done on the first day of life if the information to be gained is essential to make the proper gender assignment. **Vaginoscopy** and **cystoscopy** can be performed at the same time.

F. **Chromosomal analysis** is performed to establish genetic sex. Unfortunately, it may take 3 to 5 days to get results, which limits its usefulness in making a decision about the emergent central question of gender assignment.

G. **Hormonal assays** (See sec. **V.C.5,** following) and serum electrolyte determinations are performed to rule out adrenal insufficiency and characterize any endocrinopathy.

Differential diagnosis of ambiguous genitalia. Because of the tremendous emotional consequences for the parents of indecision in gender assignment to their new baby, ambiguous genitalia must be treated as a **neonatal emergency.** Whatever tests and procedures are necessary to make the appropriate gender assignment are performed immediately so that the decision can be made as soon as possible.

A. **Gender assignment is based on adequacy for ultimate sexual function,** not on genetic or gonadal sex. Buccal smear and sinogram are the key tests; they should be available 24 hours a day.

B. **Positive buccal smear: Gender assignment** is female.

1. **Reconstructive surgery** can create essentially normal external genitalia regardless of the degree of virilization.

2. **Diagnostic possibilities** include:

    a. **Adrenogenital syndrome**

    b. **Maternal drug ingestion**

    c. **Masculinizing tumor** in the mother or fetus

    d. **True hermaphroditism**

3. **Hormonal assays:** serum 17-hydroxyprogesterone, androstenedione, dehydroepiandosterone, and testosterone; urine 17-ketosteroids.

4. **CT scan** or **ultrasound** of **adrenals** and **ovaries** is performed to rule out virilizing tumor.

5. **Laparotomy** with **gonadal biopsy** or gonadectomy may be necessary after hormonal analysis if true hermaphroditism is a possibility.

C. **Negative buccal smear:** Gender assignment may be **male or female** depending on functional capacity.

1. **Diagnostic possibilities**

    a. **Mixed gonadal dysgenesis**

    b. **XY gonadal dysgenesis (streak gonads)**

c. **True hermaphroditism** (very rare; 90% are XX)

d. **Anorchism**

e. **Defective testes.** Leydig-cell agenesis, block in testosterone synthesis in the testis alone or in the testis and adrenal

f. **End-organ failure.** Testosterone resistance or deficiency of 5-alpha reductase (testicular feminization)

2. **If the phallus is inadequate, a female gender assignment is given, regardless of chromosomes or gonads.** Appropriate reconstructive surgery can be performed later.

3. **If testes are not palpable,** laparotomy is performed to identify and perform biopsy on the gonads and establish the presence or absence of uterus or tubes. If the gonads are dysgenetic, they are removed and a female gender assignment is given.

4. **If the phallus could be adequate** and the testes are grossly and histologically normal, hormonal assays are needed to determine the biochemical defect and if there is response to testosterone. If there is androgen resistance, female assignment is indicated. **These are the only infants in whom an appropriate gender assignment cannot be made within 24 hours of birth.**

5. **Hormonal assays** are selected as indicated: follicle-stimulating hormone (FSH), luteinizing hormone (LH), testosterone, dihydrotestosterone, dehydroepiandosterone, androstenedione, and 17-hydroxyprogesterone; urine 17-ketosteroids.

VI. **Problems**

A. **Gender assignment is the first priority.** Ambiguous genitalia constitute a neonatal emergency. The exact hormonal abnormality can be worked out later.

B. **Gender assignment must be correct from the first.**

C. **Adrenal insufficiency** should be suspected in every virilized female baby, identified if present, and treated before it becomes symptomatic.

VII. **Treatment.** Gender assignment must precede surgical treatment. Great care must be taken in what is communicated to the parents. Casual or humorous remarks can be devastating. It is best if only one physician is responsible for the baby's care and gives all the explanations.

A. **Gender is not the same as sex,** which can be defined at four levels, only one of which concerns gender.

1. **Genetic sex** is determined by chromosomes—XX for female, XY for male. It has no direct bearing on sex-role behavior.

2. **Gonadal sex** is determined by the presence of testes or ovaries. It may not be relevant to gender assignment if the gonad is nonfunctional or dysgenetic or if there is inadequate development of the external genitalia.

3. **Genital sex** refers to the organs of procreation both internal and external. Appropriate external genitalia are necessary for sexual function and self-perception. Properly developed internal genitalia and gonads are needed for fertility.

4. **Gender refers to sexual identity,** how the individual is perceived by others and herself or himself. It is learned behavior, depending on the "messages" received from parents and the appearance of one's external genitalia. **Sex-role behavior depends on gender perception.**

B. **Functional capacity** of the external genitalia is the key factor in gender assignment. Evaluation of the infant's anatomy must be undertaken with an understanding of what reconstructive surgery is possible to permit later satisfactory

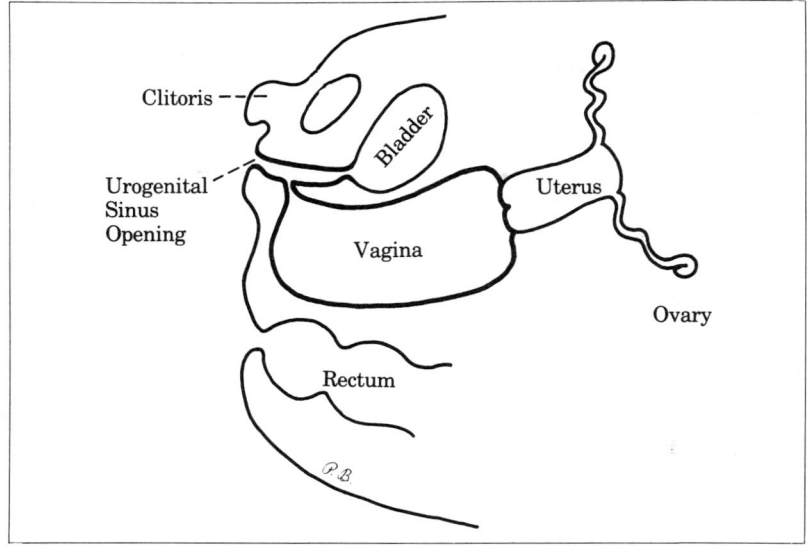

Fig. 34-2. Urogenital sinus. Typical anatomy of a urogenital sinus as seen in the adrenogenital syndrome.

sexual function. Procreative capacity, although desirable, is not essential, nor are sex-specific hormones.

C. **Female external genitalia** that are functional and acceptable in appearance **can be surgically constructed** for almost any patient, even those highly virilized.

D. **Surgical construction of a functional penis has yet to be accomplished.** A genetic male with a hypoplastic penis cannot function sexually and therefore should not be given a male gender assignment.

E. **Secondary sexual characteristics** are determined by hormones, estrogen or testosterone, which can be given exogenously as needed to develop a body habitus consonant with the gender assignment.

F. **Delay in gender assignment** leads to parental distress and, if prolonged, to ambivalent feelings toward the child, which may be detrimental to the development of appropriate sex-role behavior.

G. **Change in gender assignment** is not possible psychologically after the age of 2 years and is very difficult to accomplish after the first year of life.

I. Surgical treatment. The pediatric surgeon plays a role in both the diagnosis and the treatment of the child with ambiguous genitalia.

A. **Diagnostic**

1. **Vaginoscopy** gives information regarding the presence of a cervix and the relationship of the urethra to the urogenital sinus.

2. **Laparoscopy or laparotomy** is performed whenever it is not possible to assess the functional capacity of the genitalia with less invasive studies, particularly if there is a large phallus with a short vagina.

3. **Gonadal biopsy** is necessary in suspected true hermaphroditism and gonadal dysgenesis.

B. Therapeutic

1. **Vaginoplasty** is indicated in virilized girls with a small perineal opening of the urogenital sinus. The urethra empties into the sinus, causing pooling of urine in the vagina and recurrent urinary tract infection (Fig. 34-2). Early correction will prevent these problems.
2. **Clitoral recession** is performed to retain the clitoris while establishing a normal appearance of the external genitalia. If the operation is done in the neonatal period, the parents can consider the infant "normal" from the start.
3. **Hypospadias repair** is more likely to be successful if it is delayed until the age of 1 or 2 years.
4. **Gonadectomy** is performed if the gonads are dysgenetic or there is true hermaphroditism. It can be performed in the neonatal period.

IX. Postoperative care

A. Vaginal dilatations
are necessary for some weeks following operation for a urogenital sinus. Later reconstruction may be necessary.

B. Adrenal hormone
replacement and ACTH suppression with desoxycorticosterone acetate (DOCA) and cortisone are indicated for children with adrenal hyperplasia.

C. Estrogen or testosterone
is given at puberty to children who have undergone gonadectomy.

Bibliography

Donahoe, P. K., and Hendren, W. H. Intersex Abnormalities in the Newborn Infant. In T. M. Holder and K. W. Ashcraft (eds.), *Pediatric Surgery*. Philadelphia: Saunders, 1980. P. 858.

Donahoe, P. K., and Crawford, J. D. Ambiguous Genitalia in the Newborn. In K. J. Welch, et al. (eds.), *Pediatric Surgery*. Chicago: Year Book, 1986. P. 1363.

Federman, D. D. *Abnormal Sexual Development*. Philadelphia: Saunders, 1967.

Feldman, K. W., and Smith, E. W. Fetal phallic growth and penile standards for newborn male infants. *J. Pediatr.* 86:395, 1975.

Grumbach, M. D., and VanWyk J. J. Disorders of Sex Differentiation. In R. H. Williams (ed.), *Textbook of Endocrinology*. Philadelphia: Saunders, 1974. P. 480.

Hendren, W. H. Urogenital sinus and anorectal malformations: Experience with 22 cases. *J. Pediatr. Surg.* 15:628, 1980.

Hendren, W. H. Construction of female urethra from vaginal wall and perineal flap. *J. Urol.* 123:657, 1980.

Hendren, W. H., and Donahoe, P. K. Correction of congenital abnormalities of the vagina and perineum. *J. Pediatr. Surg.* 15:751, 1980.

Lattimer, J. K. Relocation and recession of the enlarged clitoris with preservation of the glans: An alternative to amputation. *J. Urol.* 86:113, 1961.

Shackleton, C. H., Mitchell, F. L., and Farquhar, J. W. Difficulties in the diagnosis of the adrenogenital syndrome in infancy. *Pediatrics* 49:198, 1972.

Stephens, F. D. *Congenital Malformations of the Urinary Tract*. New York: Praeger, 1983.

Wilson, J. D., George, F. W., and Griffin, J. E. The hormonal control of sexual development. *Science* 212:1278, 1982.

35   Vaginal Anomalies

Synechia vulvae. Fusion of the labia minora, partial or complete, is an affliction of girls in the first few years of life. The etiology is unknown, but low estrogen levels have been implicated. Synechia is by far the most common vulvovaginal anomaly of childhood.

- **A. Clinical picture.** Most girls are asymptomatic, but occasionally recurrent urinary tract infections or difficulty micturating occur.
- **B. Diagnosis** is obvious on inspection. The line of fusion is sometimes quite thin, even transparent. The hymen and urethra are not visible if the fusion is complete.
- **C. Treatment.** No treatment is needed if there is no obstruction to urination or infection. Daily application of estrogen cream will often result in separation. If not, direct pressure on the fusion line with a blunt instrument such as a Kelly clamp will readily separate the labia. Estrogen cream is applied to the labia bid for 2 weeks. Recurrence is not uncommon, but persistence after puberty is rare.

Imperforate hymen. Persistence of the hymenal membrane results in complete vaginal obstruction. Imperforate hymen is the most common cause of hydrometrocolpos in infants.

- **A. Pathophysiology.** High levels of maternal hormones during intrauterine life stimulate the production of copious vaginal and cervical secretions, which in turn cause **hydrometrocolpos,** massive dilatation of the obstructed vagina and uterus.
    1. Pressure from the hydrometrocolpos on neighboring organs results in **urinary obstruction** (hydronephrosis, hydroureter) and sometimes intestinal obstruction.
    2. **Leakage** of secretions retrograde through the fallopian tubes can cause peritonitis and adhesive intestinal obstruction.
- **B. Clinical picture.** Hydrometrocolpos is often the presenting finding. The infant is noted to have a large midline suprapubic mass, urinary retention, and sometimes, respiratory distress from massive abdominal distention.
- **C. Diagnosis**
    1. **Hydrometrocolpos** is usually obvious on physical examination if the physician is familiar with the entity and thinks of the diagnosis. Catheterization of the bladder does not make the mass disappear.
    2. A **bulging hymen** is evident on examination of the genitalia.
    3. **CT, MRI** or **ultrasound** will usually define the cystic midline mass, demonstrate the absence of a separate uterus, and discriminate the mass from the bladder. **Cystogram** shows anterior angulation and flattening of the bladder.
- **D. Treatment.** Hymenotomy relieves the obstruction and allows the hydrometrocolpos to evacuate and shrink. A rubber drain is left in the opening temporarily to prevent refusion. Prompt diagnosis and treatment on the first day of life will prevent ascending infection and potentially lethal peritonitis.

III. **Vaginal atresia** may be partial or complete. Complete vaginal atresia is associated with rudimentary or incomplete development of the uterus and fallopian tubes.
   A. **Clinical picture.** Distal vaginal atresia presents in the neonatal period with hydrometrocolpos. Proximal or complete vaginal atresia is seldom recognized in the neonate. It is usually diagnosed after menarche, when absence of menses leads to evaluation. Cyclic pelvic pain caused by retained menses may occur if the uterus is present.
   B. **Diagnosis.** Complete vaginal atresia, agenesis, is associated with underdeveloped labia and the absence of a vaginal opening. The external genitalia look normal in proximal partial vaginal atresia. Vaginoscopy reveals a short vagina and no cervix. Radiocontrast injection studies, cystogram, and IVP will further delineate the anatomy.
   C. **Treatment.** Vaginal reconstruction is performed by abdominoperineal pull-through. Construction of an artificial vagina is necessary for vaginal agenesis.
IV. **Septate vagina** results from either transverse or vertically oriented septa at any level and virtually any plane.
   A. **Clinical picture.** In the neonate, hydrometrocolpos, which is indistinguishable from that caused by vaginal atresia, may be the presenting finding of a transverse septum. If the septum is unrecognized in infancy, it becomes symptomatic at menarche, when the girl has amenorrhea and cyclic pelvic pain. A vertical septum may cause unilateral uterine obstruction, dyspareunia, or difficulty in delivery.
   B. **Diagnosis** is by vaginoscopy. A complete vertical septum may not be obvious until it is discovered at operation for a pelvic mass.
   C. **Treatment** is operative excision.
V. **Cloacal anomalies** are common channels composed of the gastrointestinal, urinary, and genital tracts.
   A. **Clinical picture. Obstruction** of the urinary, genital, or gastrointestinal tract is often present. **Associated anomalies** of the heart and gastrointestinal and genitourinary tracts are common, as well as anomalies of development of the vagina and uterus. Physical examination reveals a **single perineal opening** and absence of a hymen. No urethra or anus is recognized. **Hydrometrocolpos** is usually present.
   B. **Diagnosis.** Complete radiologic and endoscopic evaluation is necessary to delineate the anatomy and plan repair. This should be done promptly to prevent complications. Contrast studies of the urinary tract and injection study of the cloaca itself give the most helpful information.
   C. **Treatment.** Surgical correction is carried out in the neonatal period. It is complicated and difficult. The genital, urinary, and gastrointestinal tracts must be separated to prevent infection, the common cause of death in these infants.

Bibliography

Donahoe, P. K., and Pena, A. Abnormalities of the Female Genital Tract. In K. J. Welch, et al. (eds.), *Pediatric Surgery*. Chicago: Year Book, 1986. P. 1352.

Hendren, W. H. Reconstructive problems of the vagina and the female urethra. *Clin. Plast. Surg.* 7:207, 1980.

Hendren, W. H. Further experience in reconstructive surgery for cloacal anomalies. *J. Pediatr. Surg.* 17:695, 1982.

Hendren, W. H., and Donahoe, P. K. Correction of congenital abnormalities of the vagina and perineum. *J. Pediatr. Surg.* 15:751, 1980.

McIndoe, A. Treatment of congenital absence and obliterative conditions of the vagina. *Br. J. Plast. Surg.* 2:254, 1950.

Pratt, J., and Smith, G. Vaginal reconstruction with sigmoid loop. *Am. J. Obstet. Gynecol.* 96:31, 1966.

Ramenofsky, M. L. Vaginal Lesions. In T. M. Holder and K. W. Ashcraft (eds.), *Pediatric Surgery.* Philadelphia: Saunders, 1980. P. 891.

Ramenofsky, M. L., and Raffensperger, J. G. An abdomino-perineal-vaginal pullthrough for definitive treatment of hydrometrocolpos. *J. Pediatr. Surg.* 6:381, 1971.

36 Conjoined Twins

I. **Definition.** Incomplete separation of twins can occur at almost any locus, but the chest and upper abdomen is the site in 75% of conjoined twins. Major forms are as follows:

   A. **Thoracopagus.** Joined at the sternum, extending to the umbilicus. The livers are fused in the midline; most have a common pericardium. Seventy-five percent have conjoined hearts precluding survival of both twins after division.

   B. **Omphalopagus.** Joined from the umbilicus to the xiphoid. The livers are joined; other systems are usually separate.

   C. **Craniopagus.** Joined at the head: frontal, parietal, or occipital lobes. Rarely, the two brains are in a single skull.

   D. **Ischiopagus.** Joined at the pelvis. Lower limbs are at right angles to the body and vary in number from two to four. Intestinal or urinary obstruction, imperforate anus, and omphalocele are common. The lower urinary tract and distal bowel may be single.

   E. **Pygopagus.** Joined at the buttocks.

II. **Clinical presentation**

   A. **Antenatal diagnosis** by ultrasound is now commonplace, permitting abdominal delivery, which enhances the chances for survival.

   B. **Half** or more of conjoined twins are **stillborn**. In most of the remainder, organ systems function adequately so evaluation can be unhurried, and separation can be adequately prepared for.

III. **Diagnosis.** Preoperative evaluation is directed at clearly delineating the internal anatomy so that an assessment can be made regarding what is surgically possible and whether either or both of the twins can survive after separation. The anatomy and function of all major organ systems and the skeleton need to be evaluated. Other studies include the following:

   A. **Thoracopagus.** ECG, cardiac catheterization, and CT scan of chest and liver; isotopic biliary tract scan; contrast studies of the gastrointestinal tract.

   B. **Omphalopagus.** CT and isotopic scans of the liver and biliary tract.

   C. **Craniopagus.** Head CT scan, arteriogram, EEG.

   D. **Ischiopagus.** CT scan of abdomen and pelvis; contrast studies of gastrointestinal and urinary tracts; abdominal arteriography; genitography.

   E. **Pygopagus.** CT scan, barium enema.

IV. **Indications for operation**

   A. **Survival** of both twins after separation may not be possible even though they do well preoperatively. The anatomy may be such that only one can live if they are separated. Operative decisions require understanding and rapport between the physician and the parents. Religious convictions play an important role.

   B. **Emergency separation** of conjoined twins is required if:

      1. One twin is **stillborn** or parasitic
      2. There is a **ruptured omphalocele**

3. A correctable **life-threatening anomaly** is present (such as esophageal or intestinal atresia)
4. There is **trauma** to the connecting bridge during delivery

V. **Preoperative preparation.** Few operations in surgery require as much preoperative planning or as much teamwork in execution. In addition to the detailed anatomic and physiologic evaluations, plans for positioning, team-member responsibilities, preparation and draping, anesthetic management, and technical details of the operation must all be carefully thought out and rehearsed ahead of time. Every contingency should be anticipated and the responses rehearsed.

VI. **Operative care**
   A. **Two complete anesthetic and surgical teams** are required—one for each twin.
   B. Since no two sets are alike, the surgeons must display considerable virtuosity both in the separation of the patients and in their reconstruction.

VII. **Postoperative care.** The complexity of postoperative care is proportionate to that of the operation. Most of these patients require intensive care for a week or more postoperatively.

VIII. **Prognosis.** The outlook varies with the extent of the disease.

Bibliography

Gans, S. L., et al. Separation of conjoined twins in the newborn period. *J. Pediatr. Surg.* 3:565, 1968.

Koop, C. E. The successful separation of pygopagus twins. *Surgery* 49:271, 1961.

Luckhardt, A. B. Report of the autopsy of the Siamese twins together with other interesting information covering their life: A sketch of the life of Chang and Eng. *Surg. Gynecol. Obstet.* 72:116, 1941.

Mann, M. D., et al. The use of radionuclides in the investigation of conjoined twins. *J. Nucl. Med.* 24:479, 1983.

Simpson, J. S. Conjoined Twins. In T. M. Holder and K. W. Ashcraft (eds.), *Pediatric Surgery*. Philadelphia: Saunders, 1980. P. 1104.

Votteler, T. P. Conjoined Twins. In K. J. Welch, et al. (eds.), *Pediatric Surgery*. Chicago: Year Book, 1986. P. 771.

Surgery of the Older Child

Care of the Older Child

37 Preparation of the Child for Operation

Elective Operations

- **Definition.** An *elective operation* is one that can be performed at a time that is convenient for the patient and the physician; timing is of no significant consequence to the child's health (e.g., excision of a nevus). An *emergency operation* is one that must be performed as soon as possible to prevent serious consequences from progression of the disease (e.g., appendicitis, perforated intestine). Most pediatric surgical operations do not fit neatly into either category. An immediate operation is not required, but significant delay is inadvisable lest complications develop (e.g., hernias).

  Most children with elective surgical conditions are in good health except for the disease requiring operation; extensive preoperative preparation is unnecessary. In others, a period of preoperative hospitalization may be required to improve the patient's overall condition and nutritional status.

- **Objectives**
  - **A. Minimize operative risk** by ensuring that the diagnosis is correct, the planned operation is appropriate, and the patient is in the optimal state of health, free of correctable intercurrent disease (such as upper respiratory infection or anemia).
  - **B. Minimize psychologic trauma** by appropriate preparation of the child and parents before the operation, even before hospitalization when possible.

- **Diagnostic studies** are frequently required to confirm the clinical diagnosis or uncover related problems.
  - A. When possible, these are done on an **outpatient basis** to minimize cost and hospital utilization.
  - B. **Selection of the most useful tests** from among the many available is basic to the good practice of medicine and will be appreciated by both the patient and the insurance company. In the evaluation of an abdominal mass, for example, it is inappropriate to perform intravenous pyelography (IVP), ultrasound, and scintiscan examinations when the CT scan alone will give the necessary information.
  - C. In addition to a complete history and physical examination, all patients should have a **complete blood count** and **urinalysis** at the time of admission.
    1. No other studies should be done routinely.
    2. Specifically, "routine" preoperative **chest x-ray, ECG, and bleeding studies** have low yields in the pediatric surgical population and should not be ordered unless clinically indicated.

- **Patient evaluation** is directed toward ensuring that the child is in the optimal condition for the operation.
  - A. **Infection.** Has the child been exposed recently to a communicable disease (such as chicken pox) or does he have an upper respiratory infection or otitis?
  - B. **Nutritional status.** Is the child malnourished, and if so, is preoperative correction necessary?

C. **Pulmonary status.** If there is underlying pulmonary disease or recent infection, has that been sufficiently cleared to minimize the risk of anesthesia and postoperative atelectasis or pneumonia?

D. Is there evidence of **disease** of other systems that requires preoperative management (e.g., heart disease, seizure disorder)?

V. **Physical preparation** of the patient may require several days in the hospital preoperatively.

  A. **Bowel preparation** for intestinal surgery (pull-through operation)

  B. **Pulmonary physiotherapy** or antiasthma treatment

  C. **Nutritional buildup**—possibly **TPN**

  D. **Adjustment of medication** dosage for chronic disease

  E. **Transfusion** to correct severe anemia

VI. **Psychologic preparation** is as important as physical preparation and sometimes more difficult. Doctors and nurses frequently forget that a procedure they consider routine is the biggest event in the patient's life.

  A. **The child's ability to comprehend** depends on his age, but even the youngest patients need some preparation.

   1. **A prehospitalization program** (puppet show, video movies, games, and so on) is effective in helping young children accept or even look forward to the hospitalization.

   2. **Specific information** about the operation and the hospital routines must be tailored to the child's interest and ability to understand.

      a. **Toddlers** need only reassurance that they will not be separated from their parents.

      b. **The preschool child** is told that he will have an operation to make him better, and he is shown where the incision, or "operation," will be. Playing with stethoscopes and surgeons' masks helps to demystify these objects and allay anxiety.

      c. **The school-age child** benefits from a simple description of the operation and the details of postoperative care. It is helpful for him to know ahead of time that he will wake up with a tube in his nose and an IV line in his arm. Talking with another child who has had a similar operation is very helpful.

      d. **The teenager** often wants to know all the "gory details," and his questions should be answered in whatever detail he desires. He should participate in the decision making about whether to have the operation.

   3. **Honest answers** are essential in dealing with patients at every age. It is difficult for a child to develop a trusting relationship with his doctors and nurses if they tell him something will not hurt and it does.

   4. **Anticipation magnifies anxiety.** Painful procedures are best tolerated if they are performed without advance warning, but with a brief explanation just before an expeditious performance.

  B. **The parents' concerns** are quite different. Their anxiety may seem all out of proportion to the operation being contemplated.

   1. **Parental anxiety is universal** when a child is sick, even if the mother or father do not "show" it. There are significant ethnic differences, but even the most stoic and nonverbal individuals are frequently frightened.

   2. **Serious concerns about whether the child will survive** the operation or the anesthesia may be present and not verbalized. Similarly, there may be un-

spoken questions about whether the problem could be caused by cancer. It is helpful for the doctor to anticipate these concerns and address them even when not asked. When appropriate, it is wise to say, "And we know it couldn't possibly be cancer."

3. **Guilt is a common emotion** in parents when their children are sick. Mothers in particular often blame themselves for the child's illness, feeling that they could have prevented it, or that something they did (particularly during pregnancy) might have caused it. This, too, is frequently not expressed but should be addressed by the doctor.

4. **Misinformation is common.** It sometimes seems that every child's grandmother knows someone who had the same thing and had a bad result—10 years ago! Operations are safer than most people realize.

5. **An empathetic approach** in which the surgeon takes the time to explain what is wrong with the child, what will be done during the operation, and what can be expected goes a long way in helping worried parents cope with their child's illness and operation. Parents are quite capable of understanding even complex medical problems if the details are clearly explained. Reassurance is always necessary—it is hard to overdo it.

6. **Informed consent** means that the parents understand what is wrong, what the operation consists of, what the major risks and complications might be, and what alternatives there are for treatment. It does not mean that the surgeon merely asks them to choose among several alternatives. On the contrary, the surgeon has a clear responsibility to make a specific recommendation for therapy based on his knowledge and experience.

Preoperative checklist. The following must be completed and **recorded in the chart prior to operation** in every patient. Specific considerations are dealt with under the individual disease sections.

1. **CBC and urinalysis**
2. **Preoperative note.** Explanation of what operation is planned and what specific preparations have been completed
3. Reports of all **diagnostic studies**
4. **Blood typed** and ready for transfusion if appropriate
5. **Signed operative permit**

Emergency Operations

I. **Definition.** An *emergency operation* is one that must take place within hours (sometimes minutes) because of the severity of the disease. Either the condition is imminently life-threatening or it will worsen rapidly and increase morbidity.

II. The **objective of preparation** is the same as for elective operations: to **minimize operative risk** by having the patient in the optimal condition. However, there are **three significant differences.**
   A. **Serious physiologic imbalances** may be present because of the underlying illness (shock, acidosis, sepsis).
   B. **Correction** of the physiologic abnormalities **may be impossible** until the operative procedure removes the cause.
   C. There is **insufficient time** for complete correction. However, the patient must be **resuscitated.**

III. **Resuscitation** requires attention to the following, **in this order:**
   1. **Restoration of blood volume**
   2. **Establishment of adequate ventilation**
   3. **Correction of acidosis**
   4. **Restoration of electrolyte balance**
   5. **Replenishment of fluid deficits**
   6. **Correction of clotting deficits**
   7. **Control of sepsis**

   A. **Restore blood volume.** Inadequate perfusion inhibits function of all organs. It prevents adequate oxygenation of the tissues, increasing acidosis. Except in the rare patient who requires an immediate operation to stop exsanguinating hemorrhage, **no patient should go to the operating room until his blood volume has been restored.**
   1. **Large quantities of saline** or lactated Ringer's solution may be given **rapidly** to patients in shock caused by hypovolemia. If there has been blood or plasma loss, however, it should be replaced.
   2. **Bolus therapy** (10 ml/kg in 10–15 minutes) should be given, repeating infusions until there is clinical evidence of **return of perfusion** (decreasing pulse, rising blood pressure, improved cutaneous circulation, urine output).

   B. **Establish adequate ventilation.** Oxygenation is second only to perfusion as a primary requisite for tissue function.
   1. **An endotracheal tube** and assisted ventilation may be required.
   2. **Oxygen** should be supplied.

   C. **Correct acidosis.** Reestablishing perfusion is the most important method of combating acidosis. Adequate oxygenation is also essential. Bicarbonate should be given, but if hypoperfusion and hypoxia are not corrected, bicarbonate accomplishes little.

   D. **Restore electrolyte balance.** Complete restoration to normal is seldom possible. Intravenous fluids are tailored according to serum electrolyte determinations.

   E. **Replenish fluid deficits.** Intestinal obstruction, protracted vomiting, peritonitis, sepsis, and most injuries result in severe fluid loss. The deficit does not need to be completely corrected preoperatively, but progress should be evident.

   F. **Restore clotting mechanisms.** If there is bleeding, basic screening tests (platelet count, PT, PTT) will indicate whether correction is necessary. Disseminated intravascular coagulation (DIC) may be present. FFP or clotting factors and platelets may be needed.

- **G. Control sepsis.** In most cases, this is impossible until the operation has been performed. However, intravenous high-dose antibiotics may prevent further spread.
- **H.** Emergency resuscitation is **not** concerned with the preoperative **nutritional status** of the patient, for little can be done about that in the short time available. Similarly, little can be done about **pulmonary dysfunction** (pneumonia or chronic lung disease) in a few hours.

IV. Parents.
It is important not to neglect the family in the urgent rush to prepare the patient for the operating room.

- **A.** The responsible surgeon must explain what is wrong and what is to be done in as reassuring a manner as is realistically possible. The parental concern is often whether the child will survive. When that is not at issue, the doctor can help relieve parents' anxieties by telling them so.
- **B.** A realistic appraisal of the probable duration of the operation and clear instructions concerning where the surgeon will talk with the parents afterward are also helpful. It is worthwhile to have the patient's nurse present at this time for additional support.

V. Preoperative checklist
1. **Nasogastric tube** in place
2. **Large-bore intravenous catheters** in place
3. **Blood cross-matched**
4. **Lab studies in chart:** CBC, electrolytes, clotting factors
5. **X-rays available:** chest and others as appropriate
6. **Operative permit signed** and in chart

38 Postoperative Care

Objectives. The objective of postoperative care is to enable the patient to recover from the operation as quickly as possible with the least amount of distress, pain, and disability. The surgeon must:

A. Enhance and **assist** the body's **adaptation** to and compensation for surgical stress

B. Decrease disability by **preventing complications** and facilitating repair

C. Detect and correct **complications** promptly

D. Minimize the **psychologic effects** of trauma and hospitalization

To **realize these objectives,** it is necessary to **monitor** for evidence of physiologic instability, **maintain** fluid and electrolyte balance, **medicate** for comfort and disease, and **prevent** complications by prophylactic treatment. **Psychologic support** is necessary before and after the operation, for both the patient and the parents.

Monitoring. Careful observation by qualified pediatric nurses is essential for good postoperative care. The finest electronic gadgetry is no substitute for a nurse who knows how to take care of a sick child and recognizes problems when they develop.

A. Vital signs should include rectal temperature recordings and accurate blood pressure determinations.

B. Electronic monitoring of heart rate, blood pressure, central venous pressure, arterial gases, ventilation parameters, and so on is essential in the critically ill patient.

C. Intake and output from all sources are carefully measured, recorded, and totaled for each shift to detect changes requiring prompt corrective action.

D. Clinical assessment—whether the patient is progressing as expected—is the most important form of monitoring.

Fluids. Regardless of age, size, or disease, the basic principle of intravenous fluid therapy in the patient who is unable to use the alimentary tract is to **replace losses. Normal losses** include urine, stool, and insensible losses from the skin and lungs. Their replacement constitutes **maintenance fluids. Abnormal losses** from nasogastric tubes, wound drains, and so on are measured and replaced in kind.

A. Maintenance intravenous fluids

Solution
5% D/.25 N/S with 2 mEq KCl/100 ml
Amount
<10 kg: 100 ml/kg/day
10–20 kg: 80 ml/kg/day
20–30 kg: 70 ml/kg/day
30–40 kg: 60 ml/kg/day
>40 kg: 50 ml/kg/day

B. Replacement of gastric drainage: 0.5 N/S with 4 mEq KCl/100 ml

C. Orders for IV fluids are written for the amount to be administered **per shift.** The advantages of this method over specifying an hourly drip rate are:

1. The nurse can vary the rate as necessary to **"catch up"** when there are problems, ensuring that the total amount is given during each shift.

2. If there is an accidental rapid infusion of the entire amount, it will not be too much for an infant to tolerate.

IV. Nutrition

A. **Total parenteral nutrition** (TPN) is indicated if prolonged inability to use the intestinal route is expected.

B. **How soon** a patient can be fed after the operation depends on the patients's overall condition, whether it was an abdominal operation, and whether the intestinal tract was entered.

1. Most patients with **nonabdominal operations** who are not critically ill can rapidly resume a regular diet.

2. After **intestinal operations,** the rate at which feedings can be advanced varies considerably and depends on the nature of the operation, the prior state of the intestine, and whether or not sepsis is present.

3. Evidence of **intestinal activity** is the best guide to when to begin feedings. Decreasing volume of nasogastric drainage, disappearance of bile from the gastric drainage, passage of stools, hunger, and a flat abdomen all indicate effective peristalsis. **The presence or absence of bowel sounds is of no value whatever in this assessment.**

C. **Clear liquids** in small amounts (30 ml) are most likely to be tolerated without vomiting or diarrhea when feedings are begun.

D. Specific diet orders depend on the nature of the operation and the underlying disease. Patients with a normal intestine preoperatively can usually progress rapidly from clear liquids to full diet.

V. Analgesia.
Most major operations cause significant postoperative pain, particularly with body movement. Relief of pain is essential for patient comfort and to facilitate ambulation and pulmonary physiotherapy. Pain is a subjective response to a stimulus and is significantly affected by psychologic factors such as anxiety, parental concern, and prior experience.

A. Pain is very much **age-dependent.** Young children experience much less pain with any given operation than older children and adults.

B. The most important single factor increasing pain is **fear** of the unknown. Thus the amount of pain (and the need for analgesics) can be significantly reduced by **preoperative preparation.**

C. **Administration.** Two common errors: too **little,** too **seldom.**

1. **Analgesics are given every 3 hours (q3h), NOT prn, for the first 48 hours.** If ordered "as needed," patients will not get analgesics as often as necessary. Nurses tend to withhold narcotics for fear of side effects and addiction. With proper doses and short-term use, neither is a significant risk.

2. **Ambulation** and **pulmonary physiotherapy** should be timed to occur **after** analgesics are given to minimize discomfort.

D. **Morphine** sulfate is the narcotic of choice for serious pain relief, except in cases of biliary or ureteral colic, when meperidine should be used.

E. **Usual dose** of morphine after major abdominal or chest operations are as follows (many patients require less):

1. **Teenagers:** adult dose (10 mg)

2. **Children 6–12 years:** 0.1–0.2 mg/kg

3. **Preschoolers and infants:** 0.1 mg/kg

F. Morphine is seldom required for more than 48 hours after an operation except in unusual circumstances. Persistent need for narcotics may indicate the presence of a complication or psychologic problems.

VI. Other medications

A. Antibiotics (prophylactic or therapeutic).

B. Continuing (e.g., antiseizure medication).

C. Corticosteroids. Patients taking steroids require an increased dose for 48 hours, then return to maintenance. If appropriate, the dose may then be tapered to zero over a 6-week period.

VII. Activity.
It is a common and tenaciously persistent misconception that rest favors recovery after an operation. The evidence is all to the contrary. Inactivity leads to muscle weakness, shallow breathing, and aches and pains, while **early ambulation hastens recovery and improves the patient's sense of well-being.**

A. Wound healing is enhanced. There are few wounds that cannot tolerate the stress of movement; they are weakest on the fifth to seventh days in any case.

B. Respiratory complications are fewer in the patient who is up and about. The standing position favors diaphragmatic movement.

C. Hospital stay is shortened, since the patient does not get as weak and can resume normal activity sooner.

D. Walking, not sitting in a chair, is what is needed. Sitting requires little muscle exercise. Multiple small excursions are best, beginning the night of the operation and increasing in number and duration each day.

E. Small children, not knowing they are supposed to rest, do not. Their irrepressible activity is a major factor in their rapid recovery after major surgery.

VIII. Pulmonary physiotherapy.
Pulmonary function is compromised after any general anesthesic, especially the ability to clear secretions. **Prevention of atelectasis** is thus a primary objective in the immediate postoperative period.

A. Frequent encouragement (insistence) on **deep breathing** and **coughing** is essential—hourly at first, less often after the first 24 hours.

B. Nasopharyngeal suctioning is required if secretions are copious and poorly handled. Suctioning also stimulates coughing.

C. Pain medication should be given just before vigorous pulmonary physiotherapy to decrease discomfort and facilitate cooperation.

IX. Wounds.
Most wounds require little or no care if primary closure has been accomplished. The dressing may be removed on the first postoperative day. The incision is physiologically sealed within a few hours, and external contamination will not cause infection. Most patients are more comfortable with no dressing.

A. Examination of the incision should be performed **daily** to detect signs of poor healing or infection.

B. A **"healing ridge"** should be palpable within **3 days** if the wound is healing properly. Its absence may signify infection or dehiscence.

C. Drainage of serosanguineous fluid may indicate a dehiscence.

D. Wound **infection** should be suspected if the wound erythema worsens instead of disappearing or if there is a fever lasting for several days without another explanation.

E. Sutures may be removed at 5–7 days (except on the legs or back) in normal patients. Subcuticular sutures or Steri-strips are appreciated by patients and work equally as well as transcutaneous sutures for most wounds.

X. Psychologic support

- **A. Anxiety, fear, and lasting psychologic effects from hospitalization can be far more serious than the physical or emotional consequences of the operation itself.**
- **B. Proper preoperative preparation** of the child and parents can greatly diminish these effects and even turn the experience into a positive one for all concerned.
- **C. Daily parental visiting should be encouraged.**
- **D. Rooming-in is essential for those from 1–5 years of age,** since these children are completely dependent on the parent and view separation as a threat to life. The presence of the mother or father will make hospitalization much less traumatic for a young child. The older child is accustomed to dealing with adults and usually copes better and shows less regressive behavior if the parents are not continually present.
- **E. Frustration, guilt, and anger** sometimes lead parents to treat doctors and nurses with hostility or suspicion. They may be inordinately demanding about trivial details of the child's care or highly critical of minor mistakes. Especially if they feel responsible for the illness, it is not unusual for the internal anger and guilt to be turned outward toward those caring for the child. These feelings are seldom the result of anything the physician has done and should not be taken personally. An even temper and genuine empathy will soothe many an aggravation.

XI. Postoperative orders checklist

1. **Vital signs**
2. **Deep breathing, cough, suction**
3. **Intravenous fluids**
4. **NPO as appropriate**
5. **Nasogastric tube (gastrostomy) to gravity drainage**
6. **Medications**
   a. **Analgesics**
   b. **Antibiotics**
   c. **Continuing medications**
   d. **Corticosteroids**
7. **Ambulation**
8. **Drains and special wound care**

Bibliography

Cartwright, G. W., and Schreiner, R. L. Major complications secondary to percutaneous radial artery catheterization in the neonate. *Pediatrics* 65:139, 1980.

Committee on Hospital Care and the Pediatric Section of the Society of Critical Care Medicine. Guideline for pediatric intensive care units. *Crit. Care Med.* 11:753, 1983.

Crone, R. K. Acute circulatory failure in children. *Pediatr. Clin. North Am.* 27:525, 1980.

Driscoll, D. J., Gillette, P. C., and McNamara, D. G. The use of dopamine in children. *J. Pediatr.* 92:309, 1978.

Driscoll, D. J., Pinsky, W. W., and Entman, M. L. How to use inotropic drugs in children. *Drug Ther.* 4:39, 1979.

Fineman, A. Emotional Considerations of the Pediatric Surgical Patient. In T. M. Holder and K. W. Ashcraft (eds.), *Pediatric Surgery*. Philadelphia: Saunders, 1980. P. 84.

Hersh, S. P. Psychological Implications of Operations in Children. In K. J. Welch, et al. (eds.), *Pediatric Surgery*. Chicago: Year Book, 1986. P. 125.

Katz, R., Pollack, M., and Weibley, R. Pulmonary artery catheterization in pediatric intensive care. *Adv. Pediatr.* 30:169, 1983.

Kosloske, A. M., and Stone, H. H. Surgical Infections. In K. J. Welch, et al. (eds.), *Pediatric Surgery*. Chicago: Year Book, 1986. P. 78.

Pasnick, M., and Lucey, J. Practical uses of continuous transcutaneous oxygen monitoring. *Pediatr. in Review* 5:5, 1983.

Rowe, M. I. Fluid and Electrolyte Management. In K. J. Welch, et al. (eds.), *Pediatric Surgery*. Chicago: Year Book, 1986. P. 22.

Rowe, M. I., and Petitt, B. J. Management of the Critically Ill Patient. In K. J. Welch, et al. (eds.), *Pediatric Surgery*. Chicago: Year Book, 1986. P. 31.

IV

Head and Neck

39 Neck Masses

I. **Definition.** Children frequently develop lumps or swellings in the neck. The vast majority of these masses are benign and require no treatment. Because of the small risk of malignancy and the anxiety that it causes parents, however, accurate diagnosis and treatment are essential.

II. **Differential diagnosis.** Key factors in the diagnosis of a neck mass are its location (Fig. 39-1), its physical nature, the age of the patient, and associated symptoms.

   A. **Midline masses.** Lymphadenopathy, thyroglossal duct cyst, dermoid cyst, thyroid nodule

   B. **Anterior triangle.** Lymphadenopathy, branchial cleft cyst, salivary gland tumor or cyst

   C. **Posterior triangle.** Lymphadenopathy, metastatic tumor, bronchogenic cyst

III. **Lymphadenopathy.** An enlarged lymph node (swollen glands) is the most common mass in the neck in childhood. The swelling may vary from just detectable to several centimeters in diameter.

   A. **Lymphadenopathy may occur in any location.** The most common sites are anterior to the sternomastoid muscle just below the angle of the mandible and behind the ear.

   B. **Infection** is the usual cause of lymphadenopathy, particularly viral pharyngitis, which results in enlargement of the "tonsillar" nodes below the angle of the mandible. These nodes rarely suppurate, but the enlargement may persist for months.

   C. **Acute suppurative submandibular lymphadenitis** is due to infection by the staphylococcus or streptococcus.

      1. **Clinical findings.** Suppurative lymphadenitis is a disease of early childhood affecting children between 6 months and 3 years of age. Enlargement of the lymph node is usually preceded by pharyngitis or upper respiratory infection (URI). The child is sick, feverish, and irritable. The swelling may be dramatic, with erythema, exquisite tenderness, and surrounding cellulitis in the cheek. Fluctuation develops as the abscess forms.

      2. **Pathophysiology.** It is unknown why the submandibular glands are particularly susceptible to pyogenic infection. Prior streptococcal pharyngitis is only occasionally present.

      3. **Treatment.** Antibiotics will sometimes control the infection and allow the adenitis to subside (ampicillin, 25 mg/kg qid). In many patients the infection progresses to abscess formation. Development of fluctuance is the indication for surgical drainage. Incision and drainage requires heavy sedation but can be done without general anesthesia. The wound is packed for hemostasis and to permit healing from the inside, which takes about a week. Recurrence is rare.

   D. **Chronic lymphadenitis** is persistent enlargement of lymph nodes long after all evidence of a presumed infection has disappeared. It is very common.

      1. **Clinical findings.** "Tonsillar" nodes are most commonly affected. There may be a history of prior pharyngitis or URI with swelling of the glands, which persists after the infection is gone. The nodes are usually solitary, nontender, mobile, and soft.

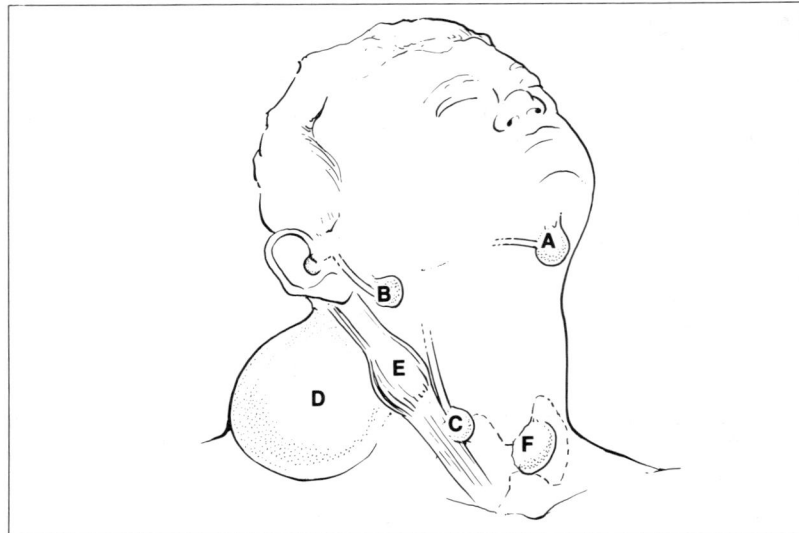

Fig. 39-1. Neck masses. A. Thyroglossal duct cyst. B. First branchial cleft cyst. C. Second branchial cleft cyst. D. Cystic hygroma. E. Congenital torticollis. F. Thyroid nodule.

  2. **Pathophysiology.** Histologic examination reveals "reactive hyperplasia" if a node is biopsied.
  3. **Treatment.** No treatment is needed if the node is less than 1 cm in diameter and is asymptomatic. Most chronically enlarged lymph nodes eventually disappear. Some require biopsy (see sec. **H** following).

E. **Mycobacterial lymphadenitis** is usually caused by the atypical mycobacteria, probably entering through the pharynx. Tuberculous adenitis is secondary to pulmonary infection, rarely seen in children in the United States.
  1. **Clinical findings.** There is no history of prior infection and no fever or leukocytosis, and the nodes are swollen but not tender or inflamed. After a few weeks, the nodes degenerate, forming a "cold" abscess. If no treatment is given, spontaneous drainage and sinus formation may occur. PPD skin test may or may not be positive.
  2. **Pathophysiology.** The granulomatous reaction of the lymph node in typical mycobacterial adenitis is indistinguishable from that caused by tuberculosis.
  3. **Treatment.** Excision of the node is curative. Antituberculous chemotherapy is of no value.

F. **Cat-scratch lymphadenitis** results from infection by the cat-scratch disease organism, probably a species of *Chlamydia*. The disease is transmitted by cats, usually kittens, who are unaffected by the disease. The injury is often not remembered by the patient.
  1. **Clinical findings.** The node is minimally tender. Fluctuance may develop, but spontaneous drainage is unusual. Skin test with cat-scratch antigen is positive.
  2. **Pathophysiology.** Swelling of the regional nodes occurs following inoculation by a scratch. Axillary adenopathy results from a scratch on the arm, cervical lymphadenopathy from a scratch on the face.

3. **Treatment.** No treatment is necessary if the diagnosis is secure (positive skin test) since the swelling will eventually subside. Antibiotics are of no value. If fluctuance develops, needle aspiration is indicated. In doubtful cases, surgical excision (not drainage) is curative.

G. **Hodgkin's disease** is rare in preschool children, but it occurs with increasing frequency in teenagers and young adults, in whom it is the most common solid tumor. Although fewer than 1 in 100 enlarged lymph nodes are malignant, this possibility is the major source of anxiety about lymphadenopathy.

1. **Clinical findings.** There are several characteristics that indicate malignant change in a lymph node.

    a. **Continuing growth** over a period of weeks.

    b. Lack of local symptoms: The node is **not tender,** red, or fluctuant.

    c. A cluster of nodes can be felt, usually **"matted"** together (although a single node can be affected).

    d. **Weight loss,** night fevers, and malaise in the absence of infection further suggest malignancy.

2. **Pathophysiology.** Hodgkin's disease may be confined to a single group of cervical nodes, but often there is bilateral or mediastinal involvement, or disease also in the abdomen.

3. **Treatment.** Chemotherapy and radiation are the primary methods of treatment of Hodgkin's disease, once the diagnosis is established by biopsy (see Chap. 87).

H. **Biopsy of chronic lymphadenitis.** Most swollen lymph nodes do not require surgical treatment. Biopsy may be necessary if the diagnosis is not clear, however. In most cases the swelling will subside within 6 weeks, and waiting that long will not compromise the chances of cure if Hodgkin's disease is present. **Excisional biopsy of an enlarged cervical lymph node is indicated if:**

1. **The node is 2 cm or more** in diameter and has been present for **6 weeks** or longer.

2. **The node is 2 cm or more** in diameter, has shown **rapid growth,** and is **continuing to enlarge,** even if it has only been noted for 2 or 3 weeks.

3. **There is a cluster** of hard, matted, nontender nodes.

Thyroglossal duct cyst

A. **Etiology.** Thyroglossal duct cyst (TGDC) results from failure of obliteration of the thyroglossal duct following descent of the thyroid in the sixth week of fetal life.

B. **Clinical findings.** Rarely evident in early infancy, the TGDC appears in early childhood as a **midline** cystic mass or as a draining sinus. It may not be apparent until infection with abscess occurs. If it is not infected, the cystic nature of the TGDC is usually apparent by palpation. The cyst is in or near the midline, usually overlying the hyoid bone, although it may be nearer the chin or the sternum. Protrusion of the tongue will cause the mass to rise.

C. **Pathophysiology.** The TGDC is connected with the oral cavity, giving bacteria ready access to cause infection. The cyst and duct are lined with stratified squamous or pseudostratified columnar epithelium and mucus-secreting glands. Ectopic thyroid tissue may be present.

D. **Treatment.** Excision is recommended both to remove the mass and to prevent recurring infections.

1. If the cyst is infected, **antibiotics** are given. It is usually possible to eradicate the infection, permitting later operation in a noninfected field.

2. Preoperative **thyroid scan** is not necessary unless the diagnosis is unclear. Thyroid tissue in a TGDC is usually dysgenetic and should be removed. Postoperative scan is obtained to assess remaining thyroid function in the rare patient who is found to have thyroid tissue in an excised TGDC.
3. The center of the **hyoid bone** must be removed, together with the cyst and a core of tissue along the duct all the way to the foramen cecum. Failure to remove the center of the hyoid bone is the most common cause of recurrence.

V. **Thyroid nodule.** A nodule in the thyroid must be considered in the differential diagnosis of a low anterior neck mass. A thyroid scan may be advisable (see Chap. 42).

VI. **Branchial cleft cyst**
  A. **Etiology.** Anomalies of closure and resorption of the primitive branchial clefts and arches are responsible for the development of cysts, sinuses, and masses.
  B. **Clinical findings**
  1. **Branchial cleft sinuses** present as cutaneous openings at the angle of the mandible (first branchial cleft) or along the anterior border of the sternomastoid muscle (second branchial cleft). Second cleft sinuses are much more common and frequently drain saliva.
  2. **Branchial cleft cysts** occur in the same locations as sinuses but may be difficult to differentiate from swollen lymph nodes or other cervical masses, particularly if they are infected. First cleft cysts are rare.
  3. **Branchial arch remnants** are small, asymptomatic subcutaneous cartilaginous masses located anywhere along the anterior border of the sternomastoid muscle or in front of the ear.
  C. **Pathophysiology.** Branchial cleft **sinuses** are embryologic remnants that are open externally, while **cysts** develop if the sinus is closed at the external end.
  1. **First branchial cleft** anomalies communicate with the external auditory canal and are intimately associated with the facial nerve.
  2. **Second branchial cleft** cysts and sinuses communicate with the tonsillar fossa, pass through the bifurcation of the carotid artery, and exit along the anterior border of the sternomastoid muscle.
  3. **Infection** results from bacteria entering from the external auditory canal or brought into the cyst by saliva from the pharynx.
  D. **Treatment.** Branchial remnants should be removed for cosmetic reasons and to prevent infection. If a cyst is infected, an attempt should be made to clear the infection with antibiotics before removal. During removal, dissection close along the sinus tract is necessary to prevent injury to neighboring nerves or vessels.

VII. **Dermoid cyst.** Inclusion cysts containing sebaceous glands and hair follicles are *dermoid cysts,* while those lacking these elements are properly termed *epidermoid cysts*. Both contain sebaceous material.
  A. **Etiology.** Dermoid and epidermoid cysts result from burial of ectodermal elements beneath the surface of the skin during embryonic fusion.
  B. **Clinical findings**
  1. Dermoid cysts are most likely to occur just above the lateral end of the eyebrow ("angular" dermoid).
  2. Epidermoid cysts are more frequently found in the midline of the neck, where they are difficult to differentiate from thyroglossal duct cysts. They can occur anywhere.
  C. **Treatment.** Cysts should be removed, since they tend to grow larger and become more unsightly. Infection is rare.

- **Salivary gland tumors.** Tumors of the salivary glands are uncommon in childhood, but an amazing variety of lesions, both benign and malignant, do occur. Infants are most likely to develop benign hemangiomas or lymphangiomas of the parotid gland, while solid neoplasms are more likely to occur in older children. Half the solid neoplasms of the salivary glands are malignant.
    - **A. Hemangioma** is the most common salivary tumor of childhood, occurring almost exclusively in infants.
        1. Typically, it is **not present at birth** but develops and enlarges rapidly in the first 3 months of life.
        2. On examination, a **fluctuant, soft, asymptomatic mass** is found in the parotid gland. There may be an overlying cutaneous capillary hemangioma.
        3. **Growth** of the lesion usually ceases by 12–18 months, and **spontaneous involution** occurs by 5 years of age.
        4. The diagnosis can usually be made on clinical grounds by an experienced physician, but biopsy is indicated if there is doubt.
        5. **Treatment.** Steroids may halt growth and hasten involution; prednisone is given, 1 mg/kg daily for 6 weeks. Radiotherapy is ineffective. Surgical excision is not indicated for this benign lesion because of its difficulty and the risk of damage to the seventh nerve. Excision of residual deformity may be indicated after spontaneous involution.
    - **B. Lymphangioma,** including cystic hygroma, of the parotid or submaxillary glands is much less common than hemangioma but is easily mistaken for it.
        1. Lymphangioma is **usually present at birth** and may show rapid growth in the first few months. Mixed hemolymphangiomas occur.
        2. Unlike hemangioma, lymphangioma **should be resected** early, before it reaches a huge size requiring a large incision and dissection. Care is taken to spare the facial nerves since this is a benign lesion.
    - **C. Mixed tumor** (pleomorphic adenoma) is the most common benign solid tumor of the salivary glands.
        1. It typically appears after the age of 7 as a hard asymptomatic mass that grows slowly.
        2. The **parotid** gland is the site of origin of 90% of mixed tumors.
        3. Treatment is wide surgical excision, taking care to spare the facial nerve. Chemotherapy and radiation are ineffective.
        4. Recurrence after resection is not unusual, especially if wide excision has not been performed.
    - **D. Other benign tumors**
        1. Hemangioendothelioma
        2. Lymphoepithelioma
        3. Cystadenoma
        4. Neuroma
        5. Lipoma
    - **E. Mucoepidermoid carcinoma,** the most common malignant tumor of salivary glands in children, is almost as common as the mixed tumor.
        1. The tumor is indistinguishable clinically from the mixed tumor.
        2. The cure rate after surgical excision is very high since this tumor rarely has distant metastases. Nodal metastases are not rare, however, and may require later excision if missed at the time of the primary operation.

F. **Other malignant tumors** include acinar cell carcinoma, anaplastic carcinoma, adenocarcinoma, and various sarcomas. Most patients with these tumors fare poorly, even after radical excision.

G. **Nonneoplastic salivary disease** may masquerade as a tumor.
   1. **Mumps.** Diffuse swelling, tenderness; patient is sick; elevated amylase.
   2. **Salivary duct stone.** Suspect if there is recurrent sialadenitis. Diagnosis: the stone is apparent on plain x-rays if calcified. Otherwise, sialography is indicated.

H. **Operative treatment is indicated** for almost all solid masses of the salivary glands. It is curative for most benign and malignant lesions. If there is any question, biopsy should be performed. If radical resection including sacrifice of the facial nerve, is required, the histologic diagnosis must be definitely established by prior biopsy and permanent section.

IX. **Miscellaneous neck masses**

A. **Cystic hygroma.** A huge, soft, cystic mass in the neck of a newborn infant is most likely to be a cystic hygroma (see Chap. 40).

B. **Bronchogenic cyst**
   1. **Etiology.** Bronchogenic cysts arise from the foregut. Although most bronchogenic cysts are found in the chest cavity, occasionally one will develop in the neck. Histologically, the cervical cyst is indistinguishable from the thoracic variety. The wall contains cartilage, mucous glands, elastic tissue, and smooth muscle.
   2. **Clinical findings.** A smooth, globular swelling in the side of the neck anterior to or deep to the sternomastoid muscle, a bronchogenic cyst can enlarge to 5 cm or larger. The mass is usually asymptomatic, but dysphagia can result from compression of the esophagus. Ultrasound or CT scan shows a thick-walled cyst.
   3. **Treatment.** Removal of the cyst is curative.

C. **Soft-tissue tumors.** Benign and malignant tumors can develop in the soft tissues of the neck and present as an asymptomatic mass. **Rhabdomyosarcoma** is the most common malignant soft-tissue tumor found in the neck (see Chap. 86). Fibroma, lipoma, neurofibroma, fibrosarcoma, liposarcoma, and neurofibrosarcoma may also occur, but these are exceedingly rare.

D. **Metastatic tumor. Neuroblastoma** is the tumor most likely to metastasize to the neck in a child. If a mass found in the posterior triangle or supraclavicular region is growing rapidly, metastatic disease should be suspected. Biopsy excision is indicated.

E. **Torticollis.** A hard mass in the sternomastoid muscle in a newborn infant is most likely to be torticollis (see Chap. 41).

Bibliography

Filston, H. C. Head and Neck: Sinuses and Masses. In T. M. Holder and K. W. Ashcraft (eds.), *Pediatric Surgery*. Philadelphia: Saunders, 1980. P. 1062.

Gray, S. W., and Skandalakis, J. E. The Pharynx and its Derivatives. In *Embryology for Surgeons: The Embryological Basis for the Treatment of Congenital Defects*. Philadelphia: Saunders, 1972.

Jaffe, B. F. Neck Masses and Malignant Tumors of the Head and Neck. In C. F. Ferguson and E. L. Kendig, Jr. (eds.), *Pediatric Otolaryngology*. Philadelphia: Saunders, 1972. Chap. 100.

Jaques, D. A., Krolls, S. O., and Chambers, R. G. Parotid tumors in children. *Am. J. Surg.* 132:469, 1976.

Kaban, L. B., Mulliken, J. B., and Murray, J. E. Sialadenitis in childhood. *Am. J. Surg.* 135:570, 1978.

Randall, P., and Royster, H. P. First branchial cleft anomalies. *Plast. Reconstr. Surg.* 31:497, 1963.

Shepard, G. H., and Rosenfeld, L. Carcinoma of thyroglossal duct remnants. *Am. J. Surg.* 116:125, 1968.

Sistrunk, W. E. The surgical treatment of cysts of the thyroglossal tract. *Ann. Surg.* 71:121, 1920.

Soper, R. T., and Pringle, K. C. Cysts and Sinuses of the Neck. In K. J. Welch, et al. (eds.), *Pediatric Surgery*. Chicago: Year Book, 1986. P. 539.

Strickland, A. L., et al. Ectopic thyroid glands simulating thyroglossal duct cysts. *J.A.M.A.* 208:307, 1969.

Welch, K. J. The Salivary Glands. In K. J. Welch, et al. (eds.), *Pediatric Surgery*. Chicago: Year Book, 1986. P. 487.

40 Cystic Hygroma

Definition. *Cystic hygroma* is a form of lymphangioma consisting of **multilocular cysts** of widely varying size. It is frequently present at birth, and all but 10% appear within the first 2 years of life. Seventy-five percent occur in the **neck** or in the **floor of the mouth.** The axilla, mediastinum, and retroperitoneum are the other major locations.

Pathophysiology

A. Pathologically, cystic hygroma may occur as an **isolated** lesion or associated with cavernous **lymphangioma** and/or **hemangioma.**

B. The typical lesion is a thin-walled multicystic mass that **insinuates** into muscle and around nerves and vessels. The individual cysts **vary tremendously in size** from a few millimeters to several centimeters. Although it "invades" the surrounding tissue, it is **not malignant** in that it does not destroy other tissues, nor does it metastasize.

C. **Symptoms** result from expansion of the cysts causing **pressure** on surrounding structures with compression or displacement of nerves, vessels, tongue, airway, or esophagus.

D. **Rapid growth** may ocur in the first 6–9 months of life. Typically, hygromas grow only slowly thereafter, but they can suddenly appear at any time during childhood. Cystic hygroma is not seen in adults.

Clinical presentation

A. An **asymptomatic mass in the neck** or under the mandible is the typical presenting finding (Fig. 40-1). It is usually **soft, mobile,** and obviously cystic, but it can be quite firm if there has been recent hemorrhage. The size may vary from just perceptible to 10 cm or larger. It will transilluminate.

B. **Hemorrhage** into a hygroma can produce sudden swelling and reddish or blue discoloration.

C. **Infected** cystic hygroma is associated with acute swelling, fever, and cellulitis with erythema and edema of the skin.

D. **Displacement of the tongue** or swelling from associated lymphangioma may prevent feeding and closure of the mouth.

E. **Respiratory distress** may result from swelling of the tongue, hygroma in the throat, or pressure on the trachea.

Diagnosis. The diagnosis is made by **physical examination.** Cystic hygroma can usually be differentiated from solid tumors or hemangioma by its appearance. A retroperitoneal cystic hygroma presents as an abdominal mass.

A. **Chest x-ray** is obtained to identify intrathoracic extension.

B. **Ultrasound or CT** imaging may help differentiate cystic hygroma from solid tumors in equivocal cases.

Problems. The **appearance** of the hygroma is the characteristic that is usually the **most distressing** for the parents. Other problems include:

1. **Respiratory distress** (stridor, cyanosis, apnea)
2. **Dysphagia**
3. **Infection**

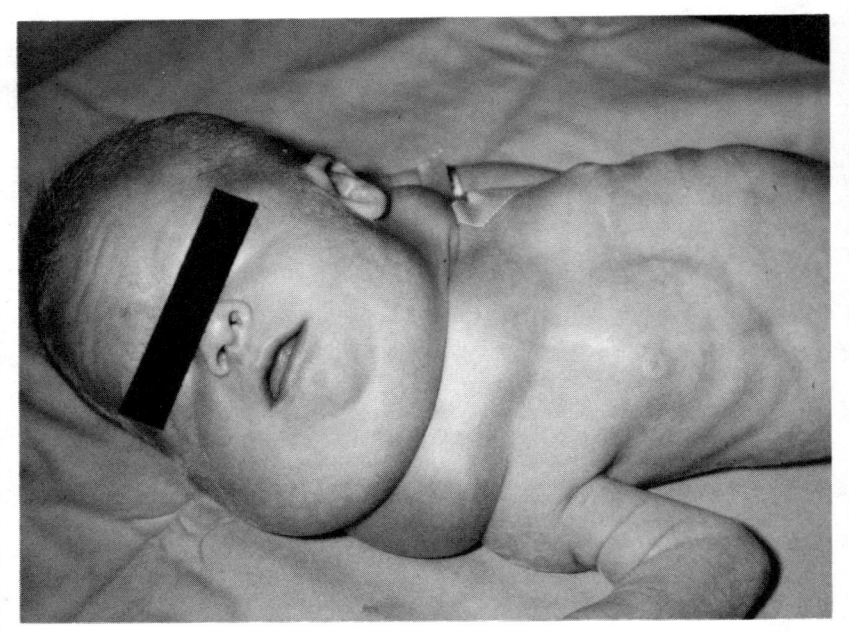

Fig. 40-1. Cystic hygroma. Typical lesion in the newborn involving neck and submandibular regions.

VI. Indications for operation

- **A. Nonoperative treatment** of cystic hygroma is **unsatisfactory.** The cysts rapidly reaccumulate if tapped. Injection of sclerosing substances is ineffective. The cysts are radioresistant. They do not spontaneously disappear.
- **B. Early operation,** soon after diagnosis, is advisable before the hygroma grows even larger and before there is compromise of respiration.
- **C. Parents** must be led to understand that complete removal is seldom possible in a large cystic hygroma because of the need to preserve vital structures.
- **D. Repeat operation** in the same site or on the opposite side may be necessary.

VII. Operative care

- **A. Removal of a huge cystic hygroma of the neck is one of the most tedious and difficult operations in surgery.** The thin-walled cysts insinuate around vessels and nerves and are removed with great difficulty. Resection is easier if the cysts can be kept unbroken.
- **B.** The major **hazard** of excision of cervical cystic hygroma is **damage to the nerves,** particularly the mandibular branch of the facial nerve and the spinal accessory. They may be markedly displaced by the cysts and hard to identify.
- **C.** It is usually **impossible to remove every trace of hygroma.** However, if gross disease is eliminated, many do not recur, and recurrences can also be resected if necessary.
- **D. Drains** are placed to remove lymph that will accumulate from divided lymphatics that supplied the hygroma.

III. Postoperative care

A. Ventilatory support may be necessary if the airway has been involved.

B. Drains are left in until no longer needed, which may be several weeks.

IX. Complications

A. Nerve injury is a serious potential complication. The mandibular branch of the facial nerve and the spinal accessory nerve are the ones at major risk.

B. Infection often occurs in cystic hygroma because of the impaired lymphatic drainage. Antibiotics are usually adequate treatment (ampicillin, 25 mg/kg, qid), but incision and drainage may be necessary.

C. Many infants get infection (possibly viral) in their hygroma whenever they have a **cold or pharyngitis.** Infections are thought to facilitate spontaneous involution of the hygroma.

X. Prognosis.
Since cystic hygroma is not a malignant lesion, the prognosis for life is excellent. Small hygromas are easily removed and rarely recur. Large cystic hygromas can defeat the best surgeon in the attempt to eradicate the disease. Multiple operations may be necessary, and results are seldom completely satisfactory to either the parent or the doctor.

XI. Lymphangioma.
Noncystic lymphangioma is much less common than cystic hygroma, although they are similar in origin.

A. Lymphangiomas consist of **multiple tiny cysts** and connecting lymphatic channels that infiltrate the surrounding tissues. They vary in size from barely detectable to huge, involving most of an extremity. Lymphangiomatous tissue may combine with hemangioma, a **hemolymphangioma.**

B. The **tongue, cheek, extremities,** trunk, and retroperitoneal tissues are most likely to be affected. Lymphangiomas are apparent at birth in 65% of children; 90% appear by age 2.

C. Most lymphangiomas are asymptomatic. Pain is rare unless the lesion becomes infected. Overgrowth of an extremity can result from the massive infiltration and vascularity of hemolymphangioma.

D. Diagnosis is by inspection. Multiple "bubbles" in the skin containing a clear fluid are distinctive.

E. Treatment of lymphangioma is excision, with skin grafting if necessary. Operation is indicated for lymphangiomas that are disfiguring or interfering with function (macroglossia).

XII. Lymphedema
is a collection of lymph in the subcutaneous space. It may be present at birth, develop during adolescence, or occur in middle age.

A. Failure of development of the lymphatics is the cause of lymphedema. Subcutaneous or subfascial lymphatics may be affected.

B. Congenital lymphedema involves the dorsum of the foot or hand but seldom the proximal extremities. Later-onset lymphedema typically involves the entire extremity and is often bilateral.

C. Treatment. Compression stockings are of considerable value in late-onset lymphedema. If lesions are disfiguring, subcutaneous excision of the fat and lymphatics is indicated.

Bibliography

Barrand, K. G., and Freeman, N. V. Massive infiltrating cystic hygroma of the neck in infancy. *Arch. Dis. Child.* 48:7, 1973.

Bill, A. H., Jr., and Sumner, D. S. A unified concept of lymphangioma and cystic hygroma. *Surg. Gynecol. Obstet.* 120:79, 1965.

Feins, N. R., et al. Surgical management of thirty-nine children with lymphedema. *J. Pediatr. Surg.* 12:471, 1977.

Fonkalsrud, E. W. Congenital lymphedema of the extremities in infants and children. *J. Pediatr. Surg.* 4:231, 1969.

Fonkalsrud, E. W. Surgical management of congenital malformations of the lymphatic system. *Am. J. Surg.* 128:152, 1974.

Fonkalsrud, E. W. Malformations of the Lymphatic System and Hemangiomas. In T. M. Holder and K. W. Ashcraft (eds.), *Pediatric Surgery*. Philadelphia: Saunders, 1980. P. 1042.

Fonkalsrud, E. W. Disorders of the Lymphatic System. In K. J. Welch et al., *Pediatric Surgery*. Chicago: Year Book, 1986. P. 1506.

Kinmonth, J. B., et al. Primary lymphoedema: Clinical and lymphangiographic studies of a series of 107 patients in which the lower limbs were affected. *Br. J. Surg.* 45:1, 1957.

Mills, N. L., and Grosfeld, J. L. One-stage operation for cervico-mediastinal cystic hygroma in infancy. *J. Thorac. Cardiovasc. Surg.* 65:4, 1973.

Ninh, T. N., and Ninh, T. X. Cystic hygroma in children: A report of 126 cases. *J. Pediatr. Surg.* 9:2, 1974.

Perkes, E. A., et al. Mediastinal cystic hygroma in infants. *Clin. Pediatr.* 18:168, 1979.

Ravitch, M. M., and Rush, B. F. Cystic Hygroma. In K. J. Welch, et al. (eds.), *Pediatric Surgery*. Chicago: Year Book, 1986. P. 533.

Seashore, J. H., Gardiner, L. J., and Ariyan, S. Management of giant cystic hygromas in infants. *Am. J. Surg.* 149:459, 1985.

Touloukian, R. J., et al. The microvascular circulation of lymphangioma: A study of xenon 133 clearance and pathology. *Pediatrics* 48:36, 1971.

Woodward, A. H., Ivins, J. E., and Soulf E. H. Lymphangiosarcoma arising in chronic lymphedematous extremities. *Cancer* 30:562, 1972.

41. Torticollis

I. **Definition.** *Torticollis* means wry neck. The infant tilts his head to one side, and there is limitation of rotation of the chin toward the affected side.

II. **Pathophysiology.** Vertebral anomalies, asymmetric muscle development, and cervical adenitis may be causes of torticollis, but the most common cause by far is **fibrosis of the sternomastoid muscle.**

   A. The **etiology** of sternomastoid fibrosis is unknown, although **trauma** before or during delivery is most likely.

   B. **Shortening of the sternomastoid muscle** causes the head tilt and the limited rotation.

   C. **Pathologic examination** of the firm mass in the sternomastoid muscle shows deposition of collagen and fibroblasts around atrophic muscle fibers.

   D. The asymmetric muscle pull of uncorrected torticollis leads to **plagiocephaly**, or asymmetry of the skull, with prominence of one side of the face and dyscoordinate ocular movements. These changes are fully reversible if the muscle imbalance is corrected early.

III. **Clinical presentation**

   A. **A hard mass** is present in the muscle in two-thirds of patients at the time of diagnosis, although a mass is almost never present at birth. Because of its hardness, the mass may be suspected of being a tumor in the muscle or an enlarged lymph node (Fig. 41-1).

   B. **Head rotation and tilting** are also seldom noted in the first week or two of life but become progressively more pronounced as the child ages. The child refuses to turn his head toward the affected side. On examination, the chin can be rotated easily to touch the acromion on the opposite side but not on the affected side.

   C. **Progressive facial asymmetry** develops if torticollis is neglected.

IV. **Diagnosis.** The diagnosis is made by physical examination. If a mass is present and there is limitation of rotation, no further studies are needed. If the diagnosis is unclear, vertebral x-rays are indicated.

V. **Nonoperative care.** Most infants with torticollis do not require an operation.

   A. **Passive stretching exercises** will elongate the sternomastoid muscle and permit full range of motion. These can be given by the infant's parent or caretaker.

   1. The infant's head is turned toward the affected side by manual pressure applied 10 times prior to each feeding.

   2. Monthly follow-up is necessary until the deformity is corrected.

   B. **The mass disappears** whether or not exercises are performed.

   C. **Facial asymmetry disappears** as the muscle lengthens.

VI. **Indications for operation.** Persistent **facial asymmetry** is the indication for operative correction. The operation must be carried out before a year of age to prevent permanent deformity. Operative division of the sternomastoid muscle is most likely to be necessary if either of the following is present:

   A. **Failure of passive stretching** to lengthen the sternomastoid muscle (persistent fibrosis)

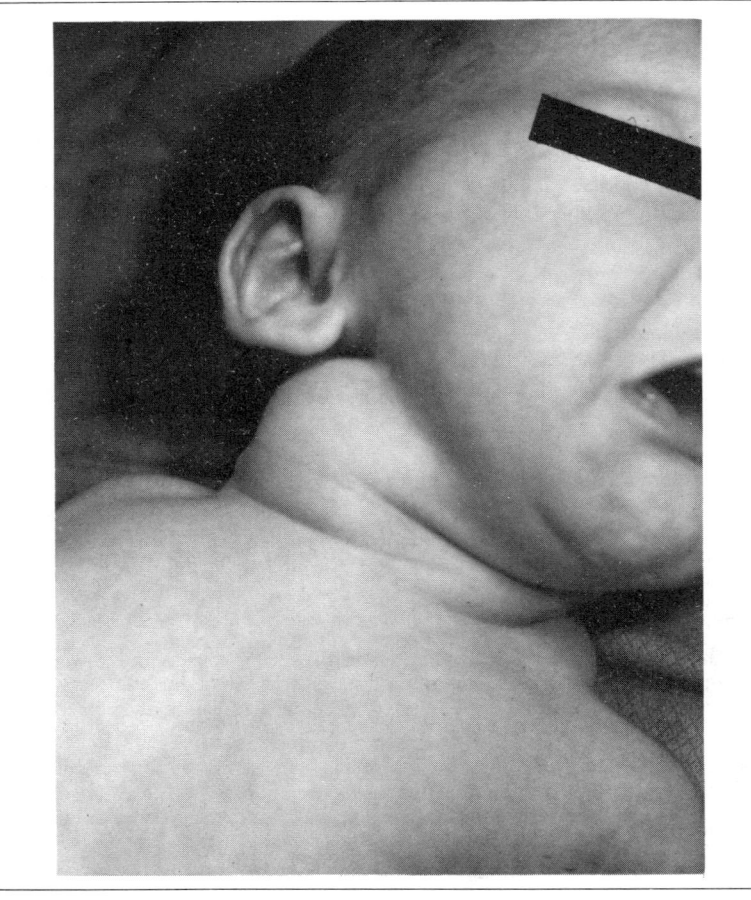

Fig. 41-1. Congenital torticollis. Hard mass in sternomastoid muscle is easily mistaken for a tumor.

    B. The child is first treated **after the age of 9 months**
VII. **Operative care.** The sternomastoid muscle is completely divided at the junction of the middle and lower thirds. The fascia colli is incised to the midline.
VIII. **Postoperative care**
    A. The neck is supported with a padded **collar** for 3 days.
    B. Active and passive rotational **exercises** begin on the third day. They are continued for 1–3 months.
IX. **Complications**
    A. **Hematoma**
    B. **Wound dehiscence**
X. **Prognosis**
    A. **Torticollis resolves** with passive stretching exercises in the vast majority of patients, never to recur.

B. Torticollis will **recur** after operation if there is inadequate physiotherapy because of poor patient or parent cooperation.

Bibliography

Armstrong, D., et al. Torticollis: An analysis of 271 cases. *Plast. Reconstr. Surg.* 35:14, 1965.

Filston, H. C. Head and neck. Sinuses and masses. In T. M. Holder and K. W. Ashcraft (eds.), *Pediatric Surgery*. Philadelphia: Saunders, 1980. P. 1062.

Jones, P. G. Torticollis. In K. J. Welch, et al. (eds.), *Pediatric Surgery*. Chicago: Year Book, 1986. P. 552.

42 Thyroid Nodules

I. **Definition.** Thyroid nodules may occur at any age but are uncommon before puberty. Nodules may represent cysts, hyperplasia, or benign or malignant neoplasm. Ionizing radiation to the head, neck, or thorax increases the risk of development of thyroid cancer. Enlargement of the entire thyroid gland occurs in thyroiditis, hyperthyroidism, and simple goiter.

II. **Pathophysiology.** Thyroid nodules develop from overgrowth of normal tissue, inflammation, or neoplasm.

   A. **Hyperplasia.** Excessive production of thyroid-stimulating hormone (TSH) by the anterior pituitary, or abnormal thyroid sensitivity to it, can give rise to thyroid hyperplasia. Administration of thyroid hormone (desiccated thyroid or thyroxine) will block production of TSH, and the hyperplasia regresses. Some hyperplastic nodules are autonomous, however, and do not respond to thyroid medication.

   B. **Thyroiditis.** Inflammation of the thyroid typically results from Hashimoto's disease (autoimmune thyroiditis), rarely from bacterial infection or other poorly understood mechanisms. Generalized swelling and tenderness of the gland is typical, but nodules may develop.

   C. **Neoplasm.** Most benign and malignant growths of the thyroid originate in the follicular cell.

   1. **Papillary carcinoma** is the most common malignant lesion and typically occurs in adolescent females. Although it may metastasize to the regional nodes, their removal is usually curative, and more distant spread is rare.

   2. **Mixed papillary-follicular** forms are occasionally seen in children and tend to behave like papillary carcinoma. Pure follicular carcinoma is rare; in addition to regional nodes, it may metastasize to lungs, liver, and bone.

   3. **Medullary carcinoma** of the thyroid **(MCT)** arises from the C cells, which produce calcitonin. Rarely seen in isolated cases, it usually occurs in the familial form, often as part of one of the syndromes of multiple endocrine adenomatosis (MEA).

      a. MEA II consists of variable associations of MCT, hyperparathyroidism, and pheochromocytoma.

      b. MEA III includes, in addition to MCT, mucosal neuromas of the lips and tongue, pheochromocytoma, and ganglioneuromas of the bowel (Sipple's syndrome).

      c. C-cell hyperplasia is the precursor of MCT, and both it and MCT secrete abnormal amounts of calcitonin.

      d. MCT and C-cell hyperplasia occur in multiple foci throughout the central sections of the thyroid gland.

   4. **Anaplastic** carcinoma is very rare in children and uniformly fatal.

   5. **Benign adenoma** may develop from follicular or stromal elements. It is indistinguishable preoperatively from malignant growths.

III. **Clinical presentation**

   A. **Most thyroid nodules are asymptomatic.** A **lump** in the neck is noted by the patient or parent. The lump moves with swallowing. It is not tender.

- **B. Thyroiditis** presents as painful swelling of the entire thyroid gland. The gland is diffusely enlarged, and may be soft, hard, or nodular. Early in the disease, it is tender.
- **C.** Symptoms of **hyperthyroidism** (heat intolerance, polyphagia, weight loss, hyperactivity, menstrual irregularities, muscle weakness, insomnia, diarrhea, irritability, and emotional instability) may precede recognition of the enlargement of the gland. Exophthalmos is common.
- **D. Dysphagia** or the feeling of a **lump in the throat** is common in any kind of thyroid disease, even when the gland is not markedly enlarged.

IV. Diagnosis

- **A. Isotope scan,** either ^{131}I or ^{99}Tc, assesses overall function and demonstrates nodular uptake of isotope. If uptake is normal or excessive (hot), malignancy is unlikely. A "cold" nodule (nonfunction) is likely to be malignant, although it can be a benign tumor or cyst.
- **B. Ultrasound** examination distinguishes solid nodules from cysts, but this is of little value in determining the need for an operation.
- **C. Thyroid function studies** are always indicated to determine if there is hypo- or hyperfunctioning. T_3 (normal: 75–220 μg/dl) and T_4 (normal: 5–12 μg/dl) are measured by radioimmunoassay.
- **D. Calcitonin-provocative testing** (pentagastrin infusion, which enhances calcitonin excretion) is diagnostic of MCT or C-cell hyperplasia if positive. The test should be carried out in all of the kindred of a patient with MCT as well as in patients with hyperparathyroidism or pheochromocytoma.
- **E. Needle biopsy** is useful in confirming the diagnosis of thyroiditis. Its role in diagnosis (or exclusion) of cancer is controversial.

V. Indications for operation

- **A.** A **cold nodule** should be removed. The risk of malignancy is high. Cysts are also "cold" on scan, but they should be removed because they may arise in a tumor.
- **B. Failure of resolution** in response to **thyroid medication** of a nodule that is normal or "hot" on isotope scan is also an indication for removal, although the statistical chances of malignancy are much lower than for a "cold" nodule.
- **C.** A positive calcitonin-provocative test.
- **D. Hyperthyroidism** (Graves' disease). Radioactive iodine (RAI) treatment is hazardous, and antithyroid drugs seldom provide long-term control.
- **E. Compression symptoms** in patients with thyroiditis may require surgical relief.

VI. Preoperative preparation

- **A.** Most patients with **isolated** thyroid nodules are otherwise well and need **no specific preoperative preparation.**
- **B. Thyrotoxicosis** must be controlled prior to operation.
    1. Suppression with **propylthiouracil** or methimazole is given for several months.
    2. **Lugol's** solution (iodine) is given for 2 weeks just prior to thyroidectomy.
    3. **Propranolol** (a beta-blocker) is given for several days preoperatively, especially if there are significant cardiac manifestations.

VII. Operative care

- **A. Hemithyroidectomy** is the operation of choice for most solitary nodules of the thyroid. The isthmus is included.

B. Total thyroidectomy is indicated in patients with bilateral disease: **MCT, thyrotoxicosis,** and **bilateral nodules** unless they are nonneoplastic (hyperplasia).
  1. There are two serious **risks related to total thyroidectomy.**
     a. Injury to the **recurrent laryngeal nerves.** (Bilateral injury produces paralysis of the vocal cords in adduction causing respiratory obstruction.)
     b. **Hypoparathyroidism,** if all four of the parathyroid glands are removed or injured.
  2. **"No-touch"** identification with sparing of the **recurrent nerve** is the first step in mobilization of the thyroid prior to division of the blood supply. Blind thyroidectomy, leaving a small rim of tissue posteriorly, is not a safe alternative.
  3. **Biopsy**-verified identification of the **parathyroid glands** is essential to their preservation. At least two should be preserved if possible. Retention of one functioning parathyroid gland will prevent hypocalcemia.
C. Frozen-section diagnosis at the time of operation is essential to confirm the preoperative diagnosis and determine whether total thyroidectomy is indicated.
D. Regional lymph nodes are removed if the nodule is malignant. Radical neck dissection is not indicated.
E. The wound is drained to prevent postoperative hematoma and compression of the trachea.
F. Later **cervical metastases** (common in patients with papillary carcinoma) are removed when and if they occur.

Postoperative care
A. Rapid recovery is the rule after thyroid operations. Pain is seldom severe or long-lasting. Complications are rare.
B. A suture set (not a tracheostomy set) is placed at the bedside to permit the incision to be opened rapidly if subcutaneous bleeding causes tracheal compression.
C. Calcium levels must be monitored after total thyroidectomy to detect possible **hypoparathyroidism.**
  1. **The Chvostek sign** is sought q4h for the first 48 hours postoperatively. Circumoral or digital paresthesias also indicate hypocalcemia. Serum calcium level is obtained immediately if any of these signs are present.
  2. **Serum calcium** level is monitored twice daily for 48 hours and daily for 1 week following total thyroidectomy.
  3. **Treatment of hypocalcemia:** intravenous calcium gluconate, 10–20 ml of 10% solution, followed by continuous infusion to maintain normal calcium levels.
D. Thyroxine or desiccated thyroid is given daily for life to patients after partial or total thyroidectomy for neoplasm, thyroiditis, or hyperthyroidism.

Complications
A. Recurrent laryngeal nerve injury is a serious and preventable complication of thyroidectomy. The "no-touch" technique of mobilization and identification prevents damage. Unilateral injury results in hoarseness; bilateral injury causes laryngeal obstruction.
B. Hypoparathyroidism results if all four parathyroid glands are removed or devascularized. Temporary insufficiency may result from operative manipulation or edema. Chronic hypoparathyroidism is treated with vitamin D, 100,000 units/day and calcium lactate, 12–24 gm per day.

C. **Superior laryngeal nerve injury** causes hoarseness and aspiration from laryngeal incoordination.

D. **Wound hematoma** may cause tracheal compression and respiratory distress in the immediate postoperative period.

X. **Prognosis**

   A. **Papillary carcinoma** recurs in regional lymph nodes in a significant percentage of patients. Mortality is low, however, since these can be removed and distant metastasis is rare.

   B. **Medullary carcinoma** is cured by thyroidectomy in most patients. If metastasis has occurred, the prognosis is poor.

   C. **Other malignancies** have a poor prognosis. Fortunately, they are very rare.

   D. **Nonmalignant thyroid disease** usually responds well to chronic thyroid suppression.

Bibliography

Altman, R. P. *Thyroid-Parathyroid.* In T. M. Holder and K. W. Ashcraft (eds.), *Pediatric Surgery.* Philadelphia: Saunders, 1980. P. 1088.

Andrassy, R. J., Buckingham, B. A., and Weitzman, J. J. Thyroidectomy for hyperthyroidism in children. *J. Pediatr. Surg.* 15:501, 1980.

Block, M. A. Surgery of thyroid nodules and malignancy. *Curr. Probl. Surg.* 20:137, 1983.

Bradley, E. L., and Liechty, R. D. Modified subtotal thyroidectomy for Graves' disease: Two-institution study. *Surgery* 94:955, 1983.

Buckwalter, J. A., Thomas, C. G., and Freeman, J. B. Is childhood thyroid cancer a lethal disease? *Ann. Surg.* 181:632, 1975.

Cooper, D. S. Antithyroid drugs. *N. Engl. J. Med.* 311:1353, 1984.

Hayek, A., Chapman, E. M., and Crawford, J. D. Long-term results of treatment of thyrotoxicosis in children and adolescents with radioactive iodine. *N. Engl. J. Med.* 283:949, 1970.

Leape, L. L., et al. Total thyroidectomy for occult familial medullary carcinoma of the thyroid in children. *J. Pediatr. Surg.* 11:831, 1976.

Lee, T. C., et al. Propranolol and thyroidectomy in the treatment of thyrotoxicosis. *Ann. Surg.* 195:766, 1982.

Thompson, N. W. Thyroid and Parathyroid. In K. J. Welch, et al. (eds.), *Pediatric Surgery.* Chicago: Year Book, 1986. P. 522.

Thompson, N. W., et al. Surgical treatment of thyrotoxicosis in children and adolescents. *J. Pediatr. Surg.* 12:1009, 1977.

43 Hemangioma

1. **Definition.** *Hemangiomas* are benign hamartomas developing from vascular tissue. There is no agreed on terminology or classification, but the following differentiation is clinically useful:
    A. **Intradermal capillary hemangioma.** A flat discoloration of the skin. These lesions do not regress spontaneously.
        1. **"Salmon patch."** A pale intradermal discoloration in the distribution of the trigeminal nerve.
        2. **"Port wine stain."** A deep purple discoloration, also in the distribution of the trigeminal nerve.
    B. **Capillary hemangioma,** also called **"strawberry birth mark."** A cutaneous lesion 2 mm–4 cm in diameter that can occur anywhere but occurs predominantly on the head, neck, and upper extremities. These are very common lesions that are, fortunately, harmless. Spontaneous involution is the rule.
    C. **Cavernous hemangioma.** A subcutaneous collection of dilated veins that feels like a **"bag of worms"** and has a blue discoloration. Found predominantly on the extremities, it involutes only partially if at all.
    D. **Mixed capillary-cavernous hemangioma,** cutaneous and subcutaneous components. This is blue with a red surface in parts. It can occur anywhere but is most commonly seen on the face and extremities. It can show both **rapid growth** and significant involution.
    E. **A-V fistula.** An arteriovenous malformation that tends to occur in the extremities in the subcutaneous tissue, muscle, or bone, causing **gigantism,** and occasionally, **heart failure.** It usually is associated with cavernous hemangioma and may also occur in the **liver** as part of a mixed capillary-cavernous type. It does not involute.
    F. **Hemangioendothelioma.** A solid tumor arising from endothelial cells, particularly in the airway and mediastinum. It does not involute.
    G. **Hemolymphangioma.** A mixture of cavernous hemangioma and lymphangioma that predominantly occurs on the extremities or trunk, involving the skin and subcutaneous tissue and sometimes muscle and bone. It may cause gigantism; it does not involute.
    H. **Syndromes** involving hemangioma
        1. **Osler.** Hereditary multiple telangiectasias of skin and mucous membranes
        2. **von Hippel–Lindau.** Angiomas of retina, CNS, and viscera
        3. **Sturge-Weber.** Angiomas of skin and CNS
        4. **Malfucci.** Angiomas of skin and enchondroma of bone
        5. **Jaffe.** Angiomas of skin and viscera

Pathophysiology

A. **Natural history**
    1. Except for intradermal capillary lesions, most hemangiomas are **not obvious at birth** but become clinically evident in the first few weeks of life.

2. **Significant growth** occurs in the first 6 months, followed by a period of no relative growth, after which involution, if it is to take place, slowly occurs. If involution takes place, it is complete by age 5 years in 80% of patients.
3. **Cutaneous capillary hemangiomas are by far the most common** type of hemangioma. They typically **involute completely,** leaving only some irregularity of the skin.
4. **Mixed capillary-cavernous hemangiomas** also are capable of significant regression, but other types of hemangioma show little involution.

B. **Growth** of a hemangioma can result in local **tissue destruction** (particularly notable on the **face** where the nose or eyelids can be destroyed), **compression** of adjacent structures, or **obstruction** of the airway by an intrinsic or extrinsic lesion (subglottic hemangioma).

C. **Increased blood flow** through an arteriovenous fistula may cause **heart failure** (especially in hepatic hemangiomas) or local **gigantism**—unsightly overgrowth of part or all of an extremity or the jaw.

D. **Rapid growth** or thrombosis results in **necrosis** in some cutaneous-capillary or mixed hemangiomas. **Ulceration** with bleeding or infection may result, but involution is hastened by its healing. Ulceration of an intestinal or bronchial hemangioma is a cause of **occult gastrointestinal or pulmonary bleeding.**

E. Large mixed or cavernous hemangiomas may cause a **consumptive coagulopathy** as intravascular clotting utilizes platelets and clotting proteins **(platelet-trapping hemangioma).**

III. **Clinical presentation**

A. **Cutaneous hemangioma.** Capillary hemangiomas begin as flat or slightly raised bright red lesions that expand and become slightly elevated above the skin surface.

B. **Cavernous hemangioma.** A soft or "squishy" subcutaneous mass, typically on the extremities, face, or neck. If near the surface, there is a blue coloration. If an **A-V fistula** is present, a bruit may be heard. Differential enlargement of the extremity may not be evident for several years.

C. **Mixed hemangioma.** Characteristics of both capillary and cavernous hemangiomas are a red surface and a spongy mass beneath.

D. **Hepatic hemangioma.** Diffuse enlargement of the liver in a neonate or young infant. A bruit may be heard. **Heart failure** may be the presenting symptom. **Ecchymoses** may result from a platelet-trapping hemangioma.

E. **Subglottic hemangioma.** The presenting symptom is **stridor** that is not present from birth but develops at 1–3 months of age. There may be cutaneous capillary hemangiomas in the face, neck, or chest.

F. **Other sites.** Hemangioma can occur **anywhere** in the body: gastrointestinal tract, bronchi, bone, brain, and so on. **Parotid hemangioma** develops in early infancy as a soft mass in the paratoid gland, often with a blue coloration that distinguishes it from cystic hygroma.

IV. **Diagnosis**

A. **The typical** cutaneous or subcutaneous **hemangioma is obvious on examination.** Aspiration or biopsy can be performed in equivocal cases, but this is rarely necessary.

B. **CT scan** with enhancement is the most accurate method of diagnosing hepatic hemangiomas at present. Angiography is equally satisfactory but invasive.

C. **Intestinal hemangiomas** are difficult to diagnose. **Angiography** will demonstrate a bleeding lesion if the blood loss is 1 ml/min or if there is a sizable A-V fistula.

D. **Peripheral A-V fistulas** are best demonstrated by arteriography.
E. **Subglottic and bronchial hemangiomas** are diagnosed by bronchoscopy. Biopsy is not recommended since life-threatening hemorrhage can result, which is difficult to control through the infant bronchoscope.

V. Indications for treatment

A. **Capillary hemangioma.** Most need **no treatment.** Surgical treatment is limited to excision of residual deformed skin after maximal involution has occurred—age 5 or later.
B. **Mixed capillary-cavernous hemangioma.** Rapid growth, particularly if disfiguring, is an indication for treatment.
   1. **Prednisone,** 1 mg/kg daily, is given for 6 weeks. If given during the active proliferative phase, dramatic shrinkage may occur.
   2. Rarely is surgical excision warranted in infants. It may be difficult and hazardous.
C. **A-V fistula and hemolymphangioma.** Repeated excisions and skin grafting are necessary for cosmetic improvement and to correct surface bleeding and irritation.
D. **Hepatic hemangioma.** Intractable heart failure or coagulopathy require treatment. Prednisone, 1 mg/kg, is tried first. Surgical treatment is reserved for medical failures.
E. **Subglottic hemangioma.** Respiratory obstruction is the indication for both diagnosis and treatment.
F. **Parotid hemangioma.** Biopsy is sometimes needed for diagnosis. Treatment is seldom required, but prednisone is used if rapid growth occurs. Most parotid hemangiomas ultimately involute.

VI. Preoperative preparation

A. **Coagulation studies,** particularly a platelet count, are necessary prior to operation on any patient with a hemangioma.
B. **Adequate blood** must be available for transfusion. Excision may result in significant blood loss.

VII. Operative care

A. **Small mixed or cavernous hemangiomas** in older children are removed by direct excision. The major large feeding vessels are identified and ligated early if possible. If the lesion is on an extremity, use of a tourniquet greatly decreases blood loss.
B. **Large cavernous hemangiomas and hemolymphangiomas** are resected in stages, limiting the operation to several hours. The skin and subcutaneous tissue must be completely removed and the wound closed with skin flaps or grafts.
C. **Hepatic hemangioma** can be resected if localized. Otherwise, embolization of the hepatic arterial branch or direct ligation of the hepatic artery is employed.
D. **Subglottic hemangioma** usually requires tracheostomy and systemic steroids. If there is no response, laser coagulation is useful; however, it cannot be done in the young infant. Fortunately, most subglottic hemangiomas involute spontaneously, after which the tracheostomy can be removed.
E. **Intradermal capillary hemangioma** is best treated by laser coagulation or excision and skin grafting. Alternatively, covering with makeup may be satisfactory if the lesion is small. Treatment should take place in early childhood to spare the child psychologic trauma.

VIII. Postoperative care. Individual variations in disease and the required operation entail individualized treatment. See Chap. 89 for details of postoperative care after liver resection.

IX. Complications

    A. Bleeding is the most common complication after removal of a large hemangioma because of the difficulty of securing all feeding vessels. Suturing is usually necessary for control.

    B. Complications of liver resection are detailed in Chap. 89.

    C. Recurrence of cavernous hemangioma frequently occurs after resection because of new growth from remaining feeding vessels. Repeat resection may be necessary.

X. Prognosis. Death from hemangioma is rare. Permanent disfigurement is not, especially in patients with huge mixed lesions of the extremities or face. For these unfortunate patients, we still have no completely satisfactory treatment.

Bibliography

Apfelberg, D. B., et al. Results of argon laser exposure of capillary hemangiomas of infancy—preliminary report. *Plast. Reconstr. Surg.* 67:188, 1981.

Brown, S. H., Neerhout, R. C., and Fonkalsrud, E. W. Prednisone therapy in the management of large hemangiomas of infants and children. *Surgery* 71:168, 1972.

Edgerton, M. T. Vascular hamartomas and hemangiomas: Classification and treatment. *South. Med. J.* 75:1541, 1982.

Edgerton, M. T., and Hiebert, J. M. Vascular and lymphatic tumors in infancy, childhood and adulthood: Challenge of diagnosis and treatment. *Curr. Probl. Cancer* 2:2, 1978.

Edgerton, M. T., and Morgan, R. F. Hemangiomas: Congenital Hamartomas. In K. J. Welch, et al. (eds.), *Pediatric Surgery*. Chicago: Year Book, 1986. P. 1511.

Fonkalsrud, E. W. Malformations of the Lymphatic System, and Hemangiomas. In T. M. Holder and K. W. Ashcraft (eds.), *Pediatric Surgery*. Philadelphia: Saunders, 1980. P. 1042.

Fosh, N. C., and Esterly N. B. Successful treatment of juvenile hemangiomas with prednisone. *J. Pediatr.* 72:351, 1968.

Li, F. P., Cassady, J. R., and Barnett, E. Cancer mortality following irradiation in infancy for hemangioma. *Radiology* 113:177, 1974.

Lofgren, E. P., and Lofgren, K. A. Surgical treatment of cavernous hemangioma. *Surgery* 97:474, 1985.

Mulliken, J. B., and Glowacki, J. Hemangiomas and vascular malformations in infants and children: A classification based on endothelial characteristics. *Plast. Reconstr. Surg.* 69:412, 1982.

Olcutt, C., et al. Intra-arterial embolization in the management of arteriovenous malformations. *Surgery* 79:3, 1976.

44 Tracheostomy

Definition. *Tracheostomy* is the insertion of a tube into the trachea by means of a surgical opening in the neck.

Advantages. Tracheostomy is an alternative to endotracheal intubation. It has several advantages.

A. **A larger and shorter tube** can be used, facilitating ventilation and removal of secretions. It is easier to clean and less likely to plug than an endotracheal tube.

B. **No foreign body** passes through the larynx. The risk of laryngeal or subglottic scarring is eliminated.

C. The tracheostomy tube is **easy to remove and reinsert,** making it possible for a parent to care for the child at home and greatly **decreasing the risk associated with emergency replacement** of the tube after accidental dislodgment.

D. Tracheostomy is much **more comfortable** for the patient than either nasotracheal or orotracheal intubation.

E. A tracheostomy tube is **more secure** than a naso- or orotracheal tube. It can be tied in. Movement of the tube—in or out—is much less. The end will not accidentally slip into the bronchus. **Accidental dislodgment occurs much less frequently than with endotracheal tubes.**

Disadvantages

A. An **operation** is required to insert a tracheostomy tube. The risk is small, but the procedure does leave a scar in the neck.

B. **Development of the larynx is inhibited** in the neonate. There is some evidence that active breathing is essential for the development of the infant larynx. Inadequate growth of the larynx can complicate removal of the tube.

C. **Decannulation** is **not** more difficult than removal of an endotracheal tube, as commonly supposed. It is easier.

Indications for tracheostomy. There are three indications for airway intubation: airway obstruction, impaired ventilation, and difficulty removing secretions.

A. **Airway obstruction.** Congenital anomalies of the larynx, oropharynx, or trachea, such as subglottic stenosis, tracheomalacia, and Pierre Robin syndrome; burns; tumor, hemangioma or cystic hygroma

B. **Inadequate ventilation.** Head injury or encephalopathy; prematurity; severe illness of any kind; pneumonia and empyema; diaphragmatic paralysis

C. **Retention of secretions.** Neurologic diseases, muscle weakness, severe illness, and a variety of lung disorders associated with the inability to mobilize secretions.

Timing of tracheostomy. Tracheostomy is a substitute for endotracheal intubation to be employed when **long-term intubation** will be required. It should be a planned procedure.

A. **Endotracheal tubes are well tolerated by infants** and can be left in place for weeks or months if necessary.

B. In **older children,** tracheostomy is performed **earlier** because of the discomfort and psychologic effects of naso- or orotracheal intubation.

C. **Tracheostomy is a poor method of emergency intubation,** fraught with hazard, especially when performed by a novice under adverse conditions (such as at the bedside). Endotracheal intubation should precede tracheostomy unless the airway is totally obstructed (trauma, burns, tumor).

VI. Operative care

A. Tracheostomy is performed **in the operating room** under general anesthesia with a full team, good lighting, and proper instruments.

B. **Transverse skin incision** gives the best later cosmetic result, midline fascial dissection causes the least bleeding, and vertical incision (not excision) of rings 3–5 of the trachea causes the least permanent damage. Retention sutures are placed in the cartilage to facilitate reinsertion of the tube if it accidentally comes out in the immediately postoperative period.

VII. Care of tracheostomy. Tracheostomy is an intrinsically hazardous form of management. Obstruction of the tube or its accidental dislodgement can be rapidly fatal. Expert care is essential.

A. **Continuous monitoring** is required. The child should never be out of sight of someone familiar with and competent in tracheostomy management. **Electronic devices are no substitute for a competent caretaker.**

B. **Humidification** of inspired air is essential since tracheostomy bypasses the normal physiologic humidification mechanism of the nose and pharynx. Adding moisture prevents drying of secretions and plugging of the tube.

C. **Suction aspiration** of secretions is needed since the normal cough mechanism is rendered ineffective by the tube. It is done hourly at first, later at 2- or 3-hour intervals, as well as prn, using sterile technique.

D. The **tube is changed** immediately if it becomes obstructed. It is changed routinely at 10 days, when the wound tract is well established, and at weekly intervals thereafter.

VIII. Complications. A simple operation, tracheostomy is uniquely susceptible to complications, several of which are potentially fatal.

A. **Operative.** Bleeding and improper location of the incision in the trachea are preventable complications clearly related to experience.

B. **Occlusion** of the small tubes used in neonates by secretions occurs readily. Adequate humidification, frequent suctioning, and prompt replacement of the tube when it is partially occluded prevent this complication.

C. **Accidental dislodgment** occurs if the tube is not securely tied in place. Partial extubation is more hazardous than complete extubation because it results in complete airway occlusion, which may be rapidly fatal.

D. **Infection** of the tracheobronchial tree occurs more readily with a tracheostomy since the normal protective mechanisms are bypassed. Meticulous attention to sterile technique in suctioning is essential. Cultures of tracheal secretions should be obtained frequently, followed by prompt treatment of infection when it develops.

E. **Granulation tissue** may develop at the tracheal stoma or at the end of the tube, requiring bronchoscopic removal. **Granulomas** sometimes occur as epithelialization takes place.

F. **Erosion** of the tracheal mucosa may be caused by the end of the tube if it is malpositioned, too long, or curved improperly.

G. **Stricture** may result from use of a cuffed tube in an older child if the cuff pressure is not carefully regulated.

H. **Skin irritation** readily occurs in infants from the pressure and moisture around the retaining tape. Use of a foam pad or Stomahesive is preventive.

K. **Decannulation.** Removal of a tracheostomy tube from an infant is significantly more difficult than from an older child or adult because the infant is not motivated toward removal and finds breathing through the nose and pharynx more difficult than through the tube. Two methods have been used.

A. **A one-way valve** is attached to a fenestrated or smaller tube, permitting inspiration through the tracheostomy but requiring expiration through the glottis. The infant learns to accommodate the resistance. The valve is then progressively occluded until both phases of respiration occur through the normal nasal passage. The tube is then removed.

B. **Progressively smaller tracheostomy tubes** can also be used, increasing the resistance and leading to breathing around the tube. The tube is then occluded and later removed when breathing is normal.

C. **Closure** of the cutaneous stoma occurs spontaneously if the tracheostomy has not been in place more than 6 months. Otherwise, surgical closure is performed a month or two after the tube has been removed.

Bibliography

Aberdeen, E., and Downes, J. J. Artificial airways in children. *Surg. Clin. North Am.* 54:1155, 1974.

Ashcraft, K. W., and Holder, T. Airway Malformations and Obstructions. In T. M. Holder and K. W. Ashcraft (eds.), *Pediatric Surgery*. Philadelphia: Saunders, 1980. P. 183.

Ashcraft, K. W., and Leape, L. L. The use of a one-way valve to aid in tracheostomy decannulation. *J. Thorac. Cardiovasc. Surg.* 64:161, 1972.

Johnson, D. G. Lesions of the Larynx and Trachea: Tracheostomy. In K. J. Welch, et al. (eds.), *Pediatric Surgery*. Chicago: Year Book, 1986. P. 622.

Rodgers, B. M., Rooks, J. J., and Talber, J. L. Pediatric tracheostomy: Long-term evaluation. *J. Pediatr. Surg.* 14:258, 1979.

Tepas, J. J., et al. Tracheostomy in neonates and small infants: Problems and pitfalls. *Surgery* 89:635, 1981.

V Chest

45 Endoscopy

Bronchoscopy

Definition. Visual examination of the airway below the vocal cords, accomplished by means of a rigid-tube ventilating bronchoscope with telescopic insert or a flexible fiberoptic instrument.

A. The rigid tube method has several advantages.
 1. **The bronchoscope** serves as an **airway,** permitting optimal ventilation.
 2. **Anesthetic** gases may be administered through the tube while the procedure is being carried out.
 3. **The telescope** is much better optically, with a sharp, clear, bright, magnified image.
 4. **Biopsy, or excision of masses, and removal of foreign bodies** are much easier through the large inside lumen of the bronchoscope than through the suction or instrument channel of the fiberoptic device.
 5. **Tiny bronchoscopes** are available that permit examination of segmental bronchi in the smallest infants while maintaining a secure airway.

B. The flexible fiberoptic bronchoscope has found less use in pediatric care than in adult practice because of the difficulty of maintaining adequate ventilation through a small airway with the endoscope in place. In the older child, this instrument offers the advantage of examination without the need for anesthesia.

Indications

A. Airway obstruction is the primary indication for bronchoscopy in children. In infants, congenital anomalies of the larynx or trachea are most likely. In older children, aspiration of a foreign body is the first consideration. **Bronchoscopy should be performed in any infant or child with unexplained stridor, dyspnea, or wheezing.**

B. Foreign bodies of the airway, known or suspected.

C. Persistent atelectasis or pneumonia localized to a lobe or segment.

D. Hemoptysis.

E. Suspected "H"-type tracheoesophageal fistula is more reliably diagnosed by bronchoscopy than by radiologic examinations.

F. Mediastinal mass.

Technique

A. General anesthesia is required for elective bronchoscopy.
 1. **Unanesthetized infants will not cooperate** and hold still for the examination, greatly increasing the risk of injury from the procedure.
 2. **The examination is terrifying for older children,** who must be cruelly held down or strapped.
 3. **The examiner is more relaxed** and can perform an unhurried, careful study, taking time to recognize and evaluate subtle changes that would otherwise be overlooked.

4. **A qualified pediatric anesthesiologist** is as essential as a qualified endoscopist for safe bronchoscopy.

B. **Dexamethasone,** 1 mg per year of age, is given prior to instrumentation to inhibit tracheal and laryngeal edema formation. It is continued q4h for 24 hours postoperatively.

C. **Experienced assistance** is essential—someone in addition to the endoscopist who is familiar with the complicated instruments and their use.

D. **Experience** counts for more in endoscopy than in most areas of surgery. Properly performed, bronchoscopy should be nontraumatic and expeditious, although unhurried.

E. **Close cooperation** between the anesthetist and the surgeon is essential to safe bronchoscopy.

IV. **Complications.** Diagnostic bronchoscopy in an older child is a safe and simple procedure. Bronchoscopic removal of a foreign body in a toddler in respiratory distress or management of a congenital obstructing lesion of the airway in an infant can be one of the most risky procedures in pediatric surgery.

A. **Hypoxia** from inadequate ventilation may result from an obstructing lesion of the airway or from insufficient ventilatory pressure.

B. **Cardiac arrest** can occur from inadequate ventilation—because of either an obstructed airway or too light anesthesia resulting in the patient resisting ventilation.

C. **Bleeding,** from either bronchoscopic trauma or an intrinsic lesion, immensely complicates the process, making visualization impossible and ventilation difficult.

D. **Perforation** of the airway can occur, particularly in tiny infants, if the operator is inexperienced or the patient is not kept motionless by anesthesia.

E. **Laryngeal edema** is the most common complication of bronchoscopy, particularly in small infants.

1. **A millimeter of edema** can make a big difference in the cross-sectional area of an airway whose normal diameter is only 7 mm.
2. **Dexamethasone,** given **before** instrumentation, helps diminish edema formation.
3. **Retention of an endotracheal tube** for a day or two after the procedure will be necessary in some infants.

F. **Pneumothorax** may result from excessive ventilatory pressures by an inexperienced anesthetist or under conditions of duress. Less commonly, it can result from perforation of the trachea.

V. **Aftercare**

A. **Humidified air** facilitates mobilization of secretions in the immediate postoperative period.

B. **Pulmonary physiotherapy** will improve ventilation and clearing of secretions if there have been previously obstructed segments.

C. **Endotracheal intubation** may be required for several days in a small infant with an obstructing airway lesion.

Esophagoscopy

I. Definition. Examination of the interior of the esophagus, performed by a rigid tube with telescopic insert or a flexible fiberoptic instrument.

- **A. The rigid esophagoscope** permits use of larger instruments and is preferred if dilatations or removal of a large or impacted foreign body is necessary.
- **B. The flexible instrument** has the advantage of permitting **gastroscopy** at the same time and is therefore preferable if evaluation of the stomach is indicated (as in undiagnosed upper gastrointestinal hemorrhage or pain).

Indications

- **A. Dysphagia.** Any patient who has food sticking in the esophagus should undergo esophagoscopy. The differential diagnosis includes, in order of frequency:
    1. **Reflux esophagitis or stricture**
    2. **Anastomotic stricture** (following repair of atresia)
    3. **Foreign body**
    4. **Vascular ring**
    5. **Achalasia**
    6. **Congenital web or stenosis** (rare)
- **B. Lye ingestion**
- **C. Upper GI bleeding**
- **D. Foreign body**
- **E. Dilatation of strictures**
- **F. Esophagitis**

Technique

- **A. General anesthesia** is preferred for the same reasons it is used in bronchoscopy. Although esophagoscopy can be performed under sedation, the examination is frequently unsatisfactory and often distressing to the child.
- **B.** An **endotracheal tube** ensures adequate ventilation.
- **C.** Esophagoscopy is an appropriate **ambulatory** surgical procedure.

Complications. Perforation of the esophagus is the major hazard. It is prevented by:

- **A. Adequate anesthesia** so that the patient doesn't move
- **B. Proper positioning** of the patient
- **C. Advancing** the instrument only when the **lumen can be seen**
- **D. Care in dilatation** of strictures, avoiding overdilatation
- **E. Experience**

Aftercare

- **A. Observation for several hours** is indicated to detect possible **perforation**. Fever, mediastinal pain, and crepitus are indications for a chest x-ray or possibly an esophagogram.
- **B. Oral intake** does not need to be restricted after the observation period.

Laparoscopy

I. **Definition.** Laparoscopy is the examination of the peritoneal cavity and its contents by means of a telescope introduced through a small incision in the umbilicus.

II. **Indications.** Laparoscopy is a substitute for laparotomy. It is indicated for diagnosis when noninvasive modalities are inadequate and laparotomy would otherwise be performed. Simple disorders such as ovarian cysts or painful adhesions can often be treated laparoscopically as well. Some of the uses of laparoscopy are:

  A. **Recurrent or chronic abdominal pain.**

  B. **Liver biopsy,** when it is hazardous or not possible by the blind percutaneous route.

  C. **Possible appendicitis** in atypical cases, particularly if there are complicating factors such as immunosuppression or steroid medication.

  D. **Fever of unknown etiology.**

  E. **Equivocal inflammatory bowel disease.**

  F. **Cholestatic jaundice**—to perform cholangiogram and obtain liver biopsy.

  G. **Ambiguous genitalia.**

  H. **Precocious puberty.**

  I. **Gynecologic disorders:** amenorrhea, dysmenorrhea, pelvic pain, gonadal dysplasia, pelvic inflammatory disease, endometriosis, ovarian cyst, pelvic or adnexal mass.

  J. **Removal** of a malfunctioning **ventriculo-peritoneal shunt.**

  K. **Laparoscopy is contraindicated** if there is massive intestinal distention, peritonitis, shock, or extensive adhesions.

III. **Technique**

  A. Laparoscopy is performed in an operating room under hyperventilation **general anesthesia.** Instruments and personnel must be available for laparotomy if needed.

  B. **Pneumoperitoneum** is created by insufflation of carbon dioxide gas through a special atraumatic needle after creation of an intraumbilical stab wound.

  C. A **trocar** is then introduced followed by the examining telescope.

  D. A **probe** may be inserted through a second stab wound to manipulate the viscera to permit adequate visualization.

  E. Pelvic organs, the appendix, the gallbladder, the liver, the spleen, and most of the intestine are easily visualized unless there are adhesions or inflammation.

  F. If a condition requiring **operative treatment** (such as acute appendicitis) is discovered, laparotomy should be performed under the same anesthesia.

IV. **Complications.** In experienced hands, operative complications are quite rare. The most likely are:

  A. **Bleeding** from the stab wound or from injured viscera.

  B. **Perforation** of the bowel when the trocar is introduced.

  C. **Cardiac arrest** may occur if anesthesia is inadequate and there is overdistention of the abdomen. Increased intraabdominal pressure can cause respiratory insufficiency and diminished venous return. Accumulation of carbon dioxide contributes to cardiac depression.

V. **Aftercare.** Routine. Laparoscopy may be performed as an ambulatory procedure.

Bibliography

Fitzpatrick S. B., et al. Indications for flexible fiberoptic bronchoscopy in pediatric patients. *Am. J. Dis. Child.* 137:595–597, 1983.
Gans, S. L., and Austin, E. Foreign Bodies. In T. M. Holder, and K. W. Ashcraft (eds.), *Pediatric Surgery.* Philadelphia: Saunders, 1980. P. 116.
Gans, S. L. *Pediatric Endoscopy.* New York: Grune & Stratton, 1983.
Johnson, D. G. Bronchoscopy. In K. J. Welch, et al. (eds.), *Pediatric Surgery.* Chicago: Year Book, 1986. P. 619.
Johnson, D. G. Esophagoscopy. In K. J. Welch, et al. (eds.), *Pediatric Surgery.* Chicago: Year Book, 1986. P. 667.
Leape, L. L., and Ramenofsky, M. L. Laparoscopy in children. *Pediatrics* 66:215–220, 1980.
Leape, L. L., and Ramenofsky, M. L. Laparoscopy for questionable appendicitis: Can it reduce the negative appendectomy rate? *Ann. Surg.* 191:410–413, 1980.
Schapiro, M. Flexible Fiberoptic Esophagoscopy. In G. Berci (ed.), *Endoscopy.* New York: Appleton-Century-Crofts, 1976.
Sharp, R. J. Esophageal Foreign Bodies. In K. W. Ashcraft, and T. M. Holder (eds.), *Pediatric Esophageal Surgery.* Orlando, FL: Grune & Stratton, 1986. P. 137.

46. Foreign Bodies of the Airway

Definition. Aspiration of foreign bodies is most likely to occur in the **second and third years of life,** when children are mobile and able to put things in their mouths but not wise enough not to.

Peanuts and popcorn are the most commonly inhaled objects that require bronchoscopic removal. Many parents are unaware of this hazard. Parts of toys, plastic, and virtually any small household object may be aspirated.

Pathophysiology

A. **Laryngeal obstruction** produces sudden, severe dyspnea and rapid demise unless the object is coughed out. Objects small enough to obstruct the larynx incompletely pass through unless they are sharp.

B. **Tracheal foreign bodies** either lodge in a main bronchus or are coughed out in most cases.

C. **The main bronchus** is the most common site of foreign-body obstruction.

D. **Complete obstruction of a bronchus** leads to atelectasis of the affected segment as the air is absorbed. This takes several days or longer.
   1. **Infection** may develop behind an obstruction if it is prolonged.
   2. **Local irritation** causes an inflammatory reaction in the bronchial mucosa.

E. **Partial obstruction** frequently results in a "ball-valve" effect with **air trapping** in the affected segment, causing overinflation of the lobe or lung.

Clinical picture

A. **A history of choking** while eating peanuts or popcorn is highly suggestive. However, in 50 percent of cases, the aspiration incident is not observed.

B. **Non-specific symptoms** often bring the patient to the doctor.
   1. **Chronic or recurrent cough**
   2. **Wheezing.** The child may be treated for **asthma.**
   3. **Recurrent fevers**
   4. **Recurrent or nonclearing pneumonia** in one lobe.
   5. **Dyspnea** or significant respiratory distress is unusual in bronchial obstruction.

C. **Physical examination**
   1. **Unilateral wheezing.** (May be absent if there is complete bronchial occlusion.)
   2. **Diminished air entry** on the affected side.
   3. **Hyperinflation** and **mediastinal shift.**
   4. **Cyanosis** and **tachypnea** are not common.

Diagnosis. The diagnosis can usually be made by **chest x-ray.**

A. **Inspiratory and expiratory films** usually reveal **air trapping** on the obstructed side with mediastinal shift away from the obstruction on expiration (Fig. 46-1). This finding is diagnostic.

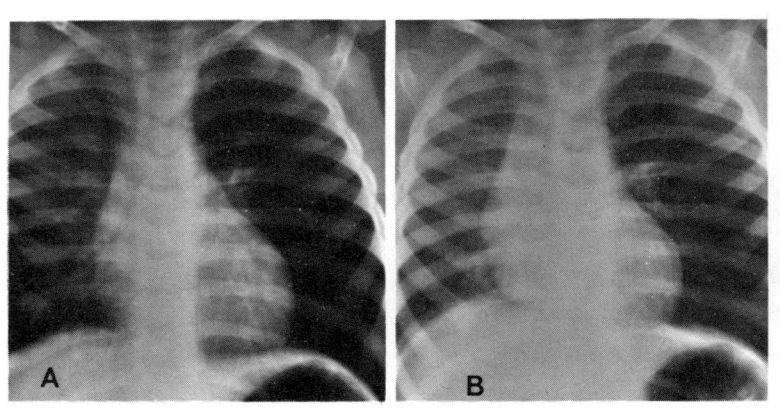

Fig. 46-1. Foreign body in the airway. X-rays of a child with a peanut impacted in the left main stem bronchus. A. Inspiratory film is unremarkable. B. Expiratory film shows air trapping on the affected side with mediastinal shift away from the obstruction. (From L. L. Leape, Thoracic Surgical Problems in Infants and Children. In F. H. Ellis (Ed.), *Thoracic Surgery*. Philadelphia: Lippincott/Harper & Row, 1983.)

- B. **Persistent atelectasis** of a lobe or segment may be the only sign.
- C. **Nonclearing pneumonia** may be the only clue to foreign-body obstruction.
- D. Occasionally the foreign body is **radiopaque** and can be seen on the chest x-ray.

V. **Indications for bronchoscopy**
- A. **A history of** an episode of **choking** with subsequent persistent **wheezing**, regardless of x-ray findings
- B. **Mediastinal shift** and **air trapping** on inspiratory/expiratory chest x-rays
- C. **Unilateral wheezing**
- D. **Nonclearing pneumonia or atelectasis**
- E. **Demonstration** of an **opaque foreign body** on the **chest x-ray**
- F. **Unexplained dyspnea**

VI. **Preoperative preparation** is nonspecific. Unless the patient is in significant respiratory distress, bronchoscopy should be performed as an urgent, but not emergency procedure under optimal conditions, with the child fasting.

VII. **Bronchoscopic technique**
- A. Bronchoscopy for removal of a foreign body from the airway is **one of the most demanding procedures** in pediatric surgery, requiring technical skill and cooperation of the surgeon and the anesthesiologist.
- B. **Anesthetic management is difficult.**
    1. **Ventilation is impaired** since only one lung is available for air exchange.
    2. **Absorption of anesthetic gases is slower** for the same reason.
    3. **The airway is irritable** because of the local inflammatory reaction.
    4. **Anesthesia and ventilation** must be administered via the bronchoscope **while the surgeon is working** through it.

C. **Removal** of the foreign body can be **technically quite challenging** for the surgeon.
   1. **A wide variety of instruments** have been devised for this purpose and should be available.
   2. **The safest and least traumatic method is to use a Fogarty catheter.** The catheter is inserted beyond the obstructing object, the balloon is inflated, and the catheter is withdrawn, dislodging the foreign body into the bronschoscope.
   3. **The first attempt is the easiest.** Multiple manipulations lead to bleeding from the inflamed mucosa, which obscures vision and makes ventilation more hazardous. **Experience** of the operator is a major factor in the success, safety, and speed of bronchoscopic removal of foreign bodies.
   4. **Removal of nonvisible peripheral bronchial foreign bodies** may sometimes be accomplished by use of the **fluoroscope** to guide the grasping forceps passed through the bronchoscope.
   5. **Complete bronchoscopic examination** of all the segmental bronchi is necessary after removal of the foreign body to make sure there is not a second one or a fragment that has broken off and lodged in another bronchus.
D. Some foreign bodies require operative removal by thoracotomy and bronchotomy. This is most likely to happen if the object is lodged in a peripheral bronchus or if delay in diagnosis has led to an extreme inflammatory reaction which makes extraction of the foreign body impossible.

II. Postoperative care

A. **Ventilation is improved** by removal of the obstruction, so most patients are improved postoperatively.
B. **Humidified air** helps with mobilization of secretions.
C. **Pulmonary physiotherapy** assists in reexpanding atelectatic areas of lung and in mobilizing secretions.
D. **Antibiotics are not indicated** unless there is evidence of infection (pneumonia or pus in the bronchus behind the foreign body).
E. **Discharge** from the hospital is possible as soon as the patient is asymptomatic and the chest x-ray shows clearing. Follow-up chest x-rays are indicated at weekly intervals until they are normal.

X. Complications

A. **Partial retention** of a foreign body may occur if it fragments during removal. Nuts and popcorn are particularly likely to do this. Failure of the patient to recover completely both symptomatically and according to chest x-ray suggests residual foreign body and is an indication for repeat bronchoscopy.
B. Sometimes it is **impossible to remove** a visible foreign body at the time of bronchoscopy. Bronchoscopy is repeated after 48 hours. Operative removal is rarely required.
C. **Bronchial stricture** may develop after removal of a foreign body that was in place for a long time. Partial lung resection may be necessary.

Bibliography

Aytac, A., et al. Inhalation of foreign bodies in children. *J. Thorac. Cardiovasc. Surg.* 74:145, 1977.
Blazer, S., Naveh, Y., and Friedman, A. Foreign body in the airway. *Am. J. Dis. Child.* 134:68, 1980.
Gans, S. L. *Pediatric Endoscopy.* New York: Grune & Stratton, 1983.

Gans, S. L., and Austin, E. Foreign *bodies*. In T. M. Holder and K. W. Ashcraft (eds.), *Pediatric Surgery*. Philadelphia: Saunders, 1980. P. 116.

O'Neill, J. A., Holcomb, G. W., and Neblett, W. W. Management of tracheobronchial and esophageal foreign bodies in childhood. *J. Pediatr. Surg.* 18:475, 1983.

Saw, H. S., Ganendran, A., and Somasundaram, K. Fogarty catheter extraction of foreign bodies from tracheobronchial trees of small children. *J. Thorac. Cardiovasc. Surg.* 77:240, 1979.

47 Pectus Excavatum

Definition. *Pectus excavatum,* or funnel chest, is a depression of the sternum resulting from a malformation of the costal cartilages. The cause is unknown, but the condition is often familial. The degree of deformity varies considerably.

Pathophysiology. The vast majority of patients have no symptoms. Cardiac and respiratory impairment may occur if the defect is severe.

A. **Cardiac abnormalities** are related to compression and displacement of the heart by the depressed sternum.
   1. **Decreased cardiac output** and reduced stroke volume
   2. **Inability to increase cardiac output with exercise**
   3. **Systolic heart murmur** with split S1-S2
   4. **ECG abnormalities.** right axis deviation, depressed ST segments, tall P waves
   5. **Prolapse** of the posterior leaflet of the **mitral valve**

B. **Pulmonary abnormalities** are those of a **restrictive defect. Ventilation and perfusion** scans sometimes show a **difference** between the two sides.

Clinical picture

A. **Most patients are asymptomatic.** They come to the doctor's attention because of concern about the **appearance** of their chest, not because of physical limitations.

B. **Symptoms in patients with severe defects** include decreased exercise tolerance, dyspnea on exertion, chronic cough, chest pain, and recurrent upper respiratory infections or pneumonia.

C. **Marfan's syndrome** is occasionally seen in pectus excavatum.

D. **Scoliosis** often accompanies severe pectus deformities.

E. **Psychologically,** a significant pectus deformity can have a profound effect on the child's self-image, particularly in boys.
   1. Young children are seldom bothered by the defect, but adolescent boys may shun athletics and beach activities, during which the abnormality is apparent and they are exposed to ridicule by peers.
   2. Girls have similar problems, but if there is adequate breast development, the defect is less noticeable.

F. **Spontaneous improvement** frequently occurs in infancy but is rare after the age of 3 years. **Worsening** of the defect may occur in the early years but is unusual after the age of 6.

Diagnosis. The presence of pectus excavatum is obvious on inspection of the chest. Few studies are necessary unless the patient has a severe defect with symptoms.

A. **Chest x-ray with true lateral view** is obtained to document the severity of the deformity and to detect pulmonary or additional chest-wall abnormalities, particularly scoliosis.

B. **Measurements of the defect** further document its severity. Complicated formulas, contour maps, and so on are unnecessary. The deformity can be characterized as mild, moderate, or severe, with the last category reserved for those with significant asymmetry or maximum depression of 2 cm or more.

C. **Cardiac and pulmonary function studies** are indicated in patients with symptoms.

V. **Indications for operation.** Few conditions in pediatrics produce as much disagreement regarding the indications for surgical treatment as **asymptomatic** pectus excavatum. Most of the disagreement is about whether an operation is appropriate for a body-image problem.

   A. **Symptomatic patients** require operative correction. These are a tiny fraction of those with pectus deformities and are usually older children. Infants and toddlers are rarely symptomatic.

   B. **Asymptomatic patients** are candidates for repair according to their age and the severity of the appearance of the deformity.

      1. **Correction** is indicated at an **early age** if the patient has a **severe** defect that will predictably cause either symptoms or body-image problems later on.

      2. The **ideal age** for repair is **2 years.** The possibility of spontaneous improvement has passed, and the operation is simpler than in an older child.

      3. **Moderate-sized defects should be repaired** if they cause the child to be ridiculed or limit full activity for psychologic reasons. Typically, patients request correction as teenagers. A parent who has lived with an uncorrected pectus excavatum himself often will bring a child in early for the operation.

VI. **Preoperative preparation.** Cardiopulmonary evaluation is indicated in symptomatic patients, as indicated in sec. **IV.** Otherwise, no special preparation is necessary. All patients should have:

   A. **Preoperative chest x-ray**

   B. **Blood available for transfusion**

VII. **Operative care**

   A. **A transverse inframammary incision** provides a far better cosmetic result than a vertical incision.

   B. **All of the deformed cartilage must be removed**—usually four or five cartilages on each side.

   C. **Internal fixation** using a Rehbein stainless steel **strut** stabilizes the chest, maintains position of the sternum during cartilage regeneration, and protects against injury during the early postoperative period. The strut is **removed after 3–6 months.**

   D. **Suction drainage** facilitates adherence of the skin and muscle flaps, as does a pressure dressing.

VIII. **Postoperative care**

   A. **Chest x-ray** is obtained in the recovery room to identify an unsuspected **pneumothorax,** which is treated by aspiration if greater than 20%.

   B. **Ambulation** and meals are resumed as tolerated.

   C. **Suction drains** are removed when no longer needed—2–4 days.

   D. The patient is **discharged** from the hospital once the drains are out and may resume full activities other than contact sports, which should be avoided for 6–8 weeks.

IX. **Complications**

   A. **Pneumothorax** may result from accidental entry of the pleura.

   B. **Atelectasis,** particularly of the lower lobes, is not uncommon postoperatively. Early ambulation and pulmonary physiotherapy may prevent it.

C. Seroma formation under the flaps is seen after removal of the suction drains in 10% of patients. It is treated by needle aspiration at 2- to 3-day intervals.

D. Wound infection may require opening of the incision and removal of the strut.

E. Migration of the strut may necessitate its removal earlier than planned.

K. Prognosis. Following repair of pectus excavatum, a significant improvement in the patient's sense of well-being, energy, and activity is typically seen. Even those who preoperatively deny any symptoms often report they are "better" afterward and have increased exercised tolerance.

Recurrence is rare—fewer than 5% if the operation is properly done. Reoperation can be performed if necessary.

Bibliography

Allen, R. G., and Douglas, M. Cosmetic improvement of thoracic wall defects using a rapid setting Silastic mold. *J. Pediatr. Surg.* 14:745, 1979.

Beiser, G. D., et al. Impairment of cardiac function in patients with pectus excavatum, with improvement after operative correction. *N. Engl. J. Med.* 287:267, 1972.

Brown, A. L., and Cook, O. Cardiorespiratory studies in pre- and post-operative funnel chest (pectus excavatum). *Dis. Chest* 20:378, 1951.

Humphreys, G. H., Jr., and Jaretzki, A. Pectus excavatum: Late results with and without operation. *J. Thorac. Cardiovasc. Surg.* 80:686, 1980.

Pickard, L. R., et al. Pectus carinatum: Results of surgical therapy. *J. Pediatr. Surg.* 14:228, 1979.

Ravitch, M. M. The operative correction of pectus carinatum (pigeon breast). *Ann. Surg.* 151:705, 1960.

Ravitch, M. M. *Congenital Defects of the Chest Wall and Their Operative Correction.* Philadelphia: Saunders, 1977.

Ravitch, M. M. The Chest Wall. In K. J. Welch, et al. (eds.), *Pediatric Surgery.* Chicago: Year Book, 1986. P. 563.

Rehbein, F., and Wernicke H. M. The operative treatment of the funnel chest. *Arch. Dis. Child.* 32:5, 1957.

Robicsek, R., et al. Pectus carinatum. *J. Thorac. Cardiovasc. Surg.* 78:52, 1979.

Welch, K. J. Chest Wall Deformities. In T. M. Holder and K. W. Ashcraft (eds.), *Pediatric Surgery.* Philadelphia: Saunders, 1980. P. 162.

Welch, K., and Vos. A. Surgical correction of pectus carinatum (pigeon breast). *J. Pediatr. Surg.* 8:659, 1973.

48 Breast Disease

I. **Definition.** A variety of conditions may afflict the breast, most of little seriousness but frequently of great concern to parent and child. Few require surgical treatment. Tumors of the breast are uncommon in children, and malignancy is exceedingly rare.

II. **Pathophysiology.** Breast tissue enlarges in response to estrogen and prolactin at any age. Stimulation may occur from endogenous production of female sex hormones (puberty), maternal hormones crossing the placenta (neonatal hypertrophy), or hormones abnormally produced by an adrenal or ovarian tumor or intracranial lesion.

III. **Abnormal enlargement**

   A. **Neonatal hypertrophy** is seen in the majority of infants, male and female, in the first week of life because of stimulation by maternal hormones. "Milk" secretion is sometimes noted. Swelling and secretions subside spontaneously within several weeks. No treatment is indicated.

   B. *Premature thelarche,* enlargement of one or both breasts before the age of 8 years, may occur in boys or girls. It is the most common lesion of the breast and is harmless.

   1. Typically there is a firm 2- to 4-cm **disk-shaped subareolar mass,** which is nontender.
   2. Failure of enlargement of the nipple and areola distinguishes this lesion from precocious puberty. The location differentiates it from fibroadenoma. No diagnostic tests or treatments are necessary.
   3. **Spontaneous disappearance** usually occurs, but in some children the enlargement persists until pubertal development.
   4. **These "lumps" must not be surgically removed or biopsied. To do so destroys the normal breast tissue.**

   C. *Precocious puberty* is defined as maturation of the breast, including the nipple, in a girl before the age of 8 years. It is usually idiopathic, but endocrine evaluation is necessary to exclude tumor or hyperfunction of the adrenal, ovary, or pituitary. No treatment of the breast itself is indicated.

   D. *Virginal hypertrophy* is the rapid enlargement of one or both breasts soon after the onset of puberty. The breasts may grow to an enormous size, causing embarrassment and pain. The cause is presumably an abnormal sensitivity of the breast tissue to estrogen. Surgical reduction is appropriate.

   E. *Gynecomastia,* breast enlargement in males, usually occurs at puberty and is thought to result from hormonal imbalance, particularly testicular estradiol production. Spontaneous regression can be anticipated, but in extreme cases surgical resection may be indicated. Gynecomastia in a prepubertal boy is an indication for endocrine evaluation for the same reasons as is precocious puberty in girls.

IV. **Congenital anomalies**

   A. **Absence of the breast** (amastia) or hypoplasia is rare but may occur in association with lack of development of the pectoralis muscle (Poland's syndrome), rib cage, or shoulder girdle. Augmentation mammoplasty is indicated after full development of the other breast.

B. **Supernumerary breasts, nipples, or areolae** are common lesions, occurring along the anterior axillary line anywhere from the axilla to the groin. They are more common in girls and are bilateral in about half of patients. Excision may be indicated for cosmetic reasons.

V. **Infections. Breast abscess** may occur at any age but is most common in the neonatal period, probably as a complication of neonatal hypertrophy and secretion. *Staphylococcus* is most commonly found to be the responsible organism. If antibiotic therapy in the initial phase of cellulitis is ineffective, circumareolar incision and drainage should be performed as soon as fluctuation is present to prevent destruction of breast tissue.

VI. **Tumors**

A. **Fibroadenoma,** the only tumor of the breast seen with any great frequency in childhood, usually occurs at puberty. The tumor may be small or huge and is sometimes mistaken for unilateral hypertrophy of the breast. These tumors may grow rapidly but are usually asymptomatic. Even with giant tumors, excision can be performed through a nondisfiguring circumareolar incision.

B. **Carcinoma of the breast** is exceedingly rare under the age of 18; fewer than 40 cases have been reported in the literature. For this reason, the physician should reassure parents of a child with a breast lesion that malignancy is not a concern.

Bibliography

August, G. P., Chandra, R., Hung, W. Prepubertal male gynecomastia. *J. Pediatr.* 80:259, 1972.
Boley, S. J. Lesions of the Breast. In T. M. Holder and K. W. Ashcraft (eds.), *Pediatric Surgery.* Philadelphia: Saunders, 1980. P. 1080.
Bower, R., Bell, M. J., and Ternberg, J. L. Management of breast lesions in children and adolescents. *J. Pediatr. Surg.* 11:337, 1975.
Farrow, J. H., and Ashikari, H. Breast lesions in young girls. *Surg. Clin. North Am.* 49:261, 1969.
Gogas, J., Sechas, M., and Skalkeas, G. Surgical management of diseases of the adolescent breast. *Am. J. Surg.* 137:634, 1979.
Iverson, R. E., and Hegg, S. I. Cystosarcoma phyllodes presenting as massive unilateral breast hypertrophy in an adolescent. *Ann. Plast. Surg.* 4:315, 1980.
Rudoy, R. C., and Nelson, J. D. Breast abscess during the neonatal period. *Am. J. Dis. Child.* 129:1031, 1975.
Seashore, J. H. Breast enlargements in infants and children. *Pediatr. Ann.* 4:7, 1975.
Seashore, J. H. Disorders of the Breast. In K. J. Welch, et al. (eds.), *Pediatric Surgery.* Chicago: Year Book, 1986. P. 559.
Stone, A. M., Shenker, I. R., and McCarthy, K. Adolescent breast masses. *Am. J. Surg.* 134:275, 1975.

49 Mediastinal Masses

Definition. A wide variety of tumors and cysts, benign and malignant, may develop in the mediastinum. The mass is often discovered on a chest x-ray taken for nonrelated symptoms. Surgical removal is almost always necessary and is usually curative.

Clinical picture. The effects of a mediastinal cyst or tumor depend on its location, its size, and whether or not it is malignant.

A. **Malignant tumors make up more than half** of all mediastinal masses: Neuroblastoma, lymphoma, and teratoma are the most common.

B. **Masses of the mediastinum sometimes grow to a large size** before causing symptoms.

C. **A majority of patients are asymptomatic.** The presence of a mass is unsuspected until the chest x-ray is taken.

D. **Symptoms**

   1. **Stridor or dyspnea** may result from compression of the airway.

   2. **Dysphagia** may result from esophageal compression.

   3. **Pain** rarely occurs. It may result from nerve root compression or from pressure within the mediastinum.

   4. **Fever and weight loss suggest tumor** but are also seen in chronic infections (such as tuberculosis and histoplasmosis).

Diagnosis. Operative removal is required in almost all mediastinal masses. Although precise diagnosis beforehand is frequently impossible, several tests may help.

A. **Chest x-ray** should be repeated if not of top quality. Lateral and oblique views aid in localization of the mass.

B. **Barium swallow esophagogram** will demonstrate impingement of the esophagus.

C. **Skin tests** for tuberculosis, histoplasmosis, and other infections are indicated if the mass appears on x-ray to be enlarged hilar lymph nodes.

D. **CT scan** is the study most likely to give valuable information preoperatively. It will often demonstrate that a structure is cystic (almost always benign) or solid, give a clue to the organ of origin, and demonstrate calcification. Most important, it will usually show the extent of involvement of adjacent tissues (such as the ribs or spine in neuroblastoma) and thereby help determine resectability.

E. **Myelogram** is indicated to assess the extent of intraspinal extension in neuroblastoma if spinal involvement is noted.

F. **Bronchoscopy** is useful if the mass is central or if there is evidence of airway compression or middle lobe syndrome. It is performed immediately prior to thoracotomy unless it is likely that bronchoscopic findings would permit nonoperative treatment.

G. **Urine measurement of vanillylmandelic acid (VMA), homovanillic acid (HVA),** and other catecholamine breakdown products is indicated for posterior masses when neuroblastoma is a possibility.

H. **Arterial blood gases** may be indicated to assess the severity of respiratory compromise, although this is usually quite evident clinically.

IV. **Differential diagnosis.** The location in the mediastinum is the primary diagnostic clue. The mediastinum is clinically divided into three compartments: anterior, middle, and posterior.

  A. **Anterior mediastinum**
  1. Anterior mediastinal masses are **frequently asymptomatic** but may cause airway compression. **Teratoma, undifferentiated sarcoma, and tumors and cysts of the thymus** are most common. **Pericardial cysts and cystic hygroma** are other possibilities.
  2. **The major problem** in evaluating anterior masses in children is in differentiating on chest x-ray neoplasms from the **thymus,** which may be quite large. The "sail sign" and bilateral symmetry are encouraging features.
  3. **Sarcomas** are usually solid: **teratomas** may be either solid or cystic or both and may demonstrate some calcification.
  4. **Cysts** are usually benign.

  B. **Middle mediastinum**
  1. Middle mediastinal masses are **most likely to be symptomatic,** causing airway or esophageal compression. At times, the vena cava may be occluded, causing edema and cyanosis of the head and neck.
  2. **Lymph node disease** is responsible for the majority of middle mediastinal lesions: lymphosarcoma, Hodgkin's disease, and inflammatory lymphadenopathy (tuberculosis, histoplasmosis).
  3. **Positive skin tests** may establish a diagnosis of tuberculosis or histoplasmosis, but an operation may be necessary for proof.
  4. **Middle lobe syndrome** may result from compression of the middle lobe bronchus by granulomatous enlargement of mediastinal lymph nodes.
  5. **Enlarged lymph nodes in the neck or axilla** are suggestive of lymphoma or Hodgkin's disease. The various forms cannot be differentiated without biopsy.
  6. **A huge, round, smooth tumor practically filling the chest** and causing respiratory distress is almost certainly a **lymphosarcoma.** It may cause the **superior mediastinal syndrome:** caval obstruction with edema and cyanosis of the head and neck. The patient **can deteriorate within hours** as the tumor rapidly grows.

  C. **Posterior mediastinum**
  1. Posterior masses are **usually asymptomatic** until they grow large enough to compress the esophagus or cause nerve root irritation.
  2. **Neurogenic tumors** make up the bulk of posterior masses: **neuroblastoma, ganglioneuroma,** and **neurofibroma,** as well as **undifferentiated sarcomas** and **foregut cysts** (e.g., bronchogenic cysts, esophageal duplications).
  3. **Neuroblastoma** has a much higher cure rate when it arises in the mediastinum than elsewhere, particularly in infants (Fig. 49-1). Often the tumor is found to be mixed—**ganglioneuroblastoma**—which behaves like a benign tumor.
  4. **Widening of the vertebral foramen** and erosion of the adjacent rib is almost diagnostic of **neuroblastoma** but is also seen in ganglioneuroma.
  5. **Urinary catecholamine** breakdown products are elevated in 50% of patients with neuroblastoma.

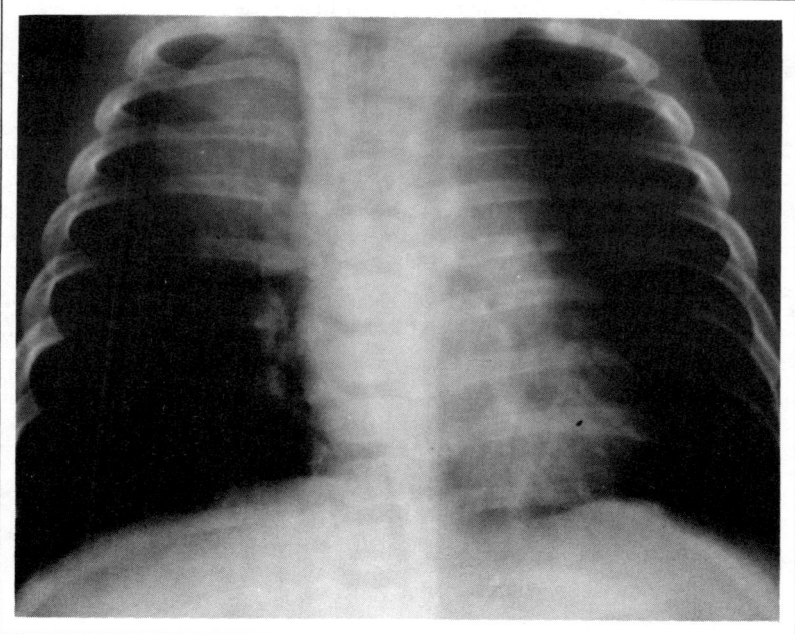

Fig. 49-1. Mediastinal neuroblastoma in an asymptomatic two-year-old child who is alive and free of disease ten years following resection. (From L. L. Leape, Thoracic Surgical Problems in Infants and Children. In S. H. Ellis (Ed.), *Thoracic Surgery*. Philadelphia: Lippincott/Harper & Row, 1983.)

    6. **Neurofibroma** should be suspected if there are other stigmata of **von Recklinghausen's disease** (café au lait spots, subcutaneous nodules, family history).

V. **Indications for operation.** Unless a nonsurgical diagnosis can be unequivocally established by other means, surgical exploration is required in all patients with a mediastinal mass.

VI. **Preoperative preparation**

  A. **Giant lymphosarcoma with the superior mediastinal syndrome requires emergency treatment.** If the patient is **in extremis,** treatment is necessary before biopsy.

    1. **Intubation and ventilatory assistance** may be necessary.

    2. **Intravenous prednisone** (1 mg/kg bid) and **radiation therapy** can produce dramatic relief of symptoms within hours (see Fig. 88-1).

    3. **Allopurinol, alkalinization of the urine,** and intravenous **hyperhydration** are used to prevent the formation of **kidney stones** from the hyperuricemia that results from rapid destruction of tumor cells.

  B. **Nonemergent cases** usually require little in the way of special preparation preoperatively other than availability of adequate blood for transfusion if necessary.

VII. **Operative care**

  A. **A standard posterolateral thoracotomy** is appropriate for most mediastinal tumors. A sternal splitting incision is occasionally indicated for anterior tumors that appear bilateral. The thymus and its tumors can be resected through a lateral thoracotomy.

- B. **Most mediastinal masses are completely resectable.** Since even malignant tumors are frequently curable in children if they can be resected, an aggressive approach is indicated.
- C. **Complete resection of neuroblastoma,** although desirable, **is not essential for cure;** therefore, damage to vital structures should be avoided.
- D. **Spinal exploration is indicated for** neuroblastoma that is causing **spinal cord compression.** If there are signs of progressive neurologic damage, this should be done urgently before thoracotomy. Otherwise, the operations can be combined.
- E. **Antibiotics are seldom indicated** but are given prophylactically if the airway is entered or therapeutically if the mass is infective in origin.

VIII. Postoperative care
- A. **Standard postthoracotomy care** is appropriate for most of these patients. Careful attention is given to:
  1. **Full expansion of the lung** and sealing of air leaks
  2. **Evacuation of blood or serum** from the pleural cavity with replacement as necessary
  3. **Aggressive pulmonary physiotherapy**
  4. **Early ambulation** and resumption of normal diet
  5. **Analgesics** as necessary
- B. **Bone-marrow aspirate,** skeletal survey or isotope scan, and other studies may be indicated in patients with **tumor** to determine if there is evidence of spread outside the chest.
- C. **Specific therapy** is given as indicated for the **underlying lesion** if resection is not curative.
- D. **Most patients recover promptly** and are able to be discharged from the hospital in 5–7 days.

IX. Complications
- A. **Air leak** from damage to the lung or airway is treated with chest-tube suction. Bronchopleural fistula may require reoperation.
- B. **Bleeding** can usually be controlled by chest-tube evacuation and replacement. Reoperation is rarely required.
- C. **Paralysis** may result from spinal-cord damage caused by tumor or its removal.
- D. **Scoliosis** is a late complication sometimes seen in patients with asymmetric spinal column involvement or following spinal irradiation. Spinal fusion may be indicated at the time of thoracotomy. Alternatively, the patient must be carefully followed so that fusion can be carried out before severe curvature of the spine develops.

X. **Prognosis** is that of the underlying lesion. Most patients are cured by the operation and require no further therapy.

Bibliography

Beiger, R. C., and McAdams, A. J. Thymic cysts. *Arch. Pathol.* 82:535, 1966.
Emmens, R. W., et al. Thymic cyst causing dysphagia. *Am. J. Dis. Child.* 133:219, 1979.

Filler, R. M., et al. Favorable outlook for children with mediastinal neuroblastoma. *J. Pediatr. Surg.* 7:136, 1972.

Haller, J. A., Mazur, D. O., and Morgan W. W., Jr. Diagnosis and management of mediastinal masses in children. *J. Thorac. Cardiovasc. Surg.* 68:385, 1969.

King, R. M., et al. Primary mediastinal tumors in children. *J. Pediatr. Surg.* 17:512, 1982.

Pokorny, W. J., and Goldstein, I. R. Enteric thoracoabdominal duplications in children. *J. Thorac. Cardiovasc. Surg.* 87:821, 1984.

Pokorny, W. J., and Sherman, J. O. Mediastinal Tumors. In T. M. Holder and K. W. Ashcraft (eds.), *Pediatric Surgery*. Philadelphia: Saunders, 1980. P. 241.

Ramenofsky, M. L., and Leape, L. L. Bronchogenic cyst: Myths and realities. *J. Pediatr. Surg.* 14:219, 1979.

Ravitch, M. M. Mediastinal Cysts and Tumors. In K. J. Welch, et al. (eds.), *Pediatric Surgery*. Chicago: Year Book, 1986. P. 602.

Saade, M., et al. Posterior mediastinal accessory thymus. *J. Pediatr.* 1:71, 1976.

Whittaker, L. D., and Lynn H. B. Mediastinal tumors and cysts in the pediatric patient. *Surg. Clin. North Am.* 53:893, 1973.

Young, D. G. Thoracic neuroblastoma/ganglioneuroma. *J. Pediatr. Surg.* 18:37, 1983.

50 Empyema

I. **Definition.** *Empyema* is the term for pus in the pleural space. Causes include pneumonia, esophageal perforation, spinal osteomyelitis, subphrenic abscess, trauma, and postoperative complications such as esophageal leak, bronchopleural fistula, or infected lung resection.

II. **Pathophysiology.** Contamination of the pleural space by bacteria results in a predictable sequence of events caused by the progressive tissue response to infection.

   A. **Exudative phase.** Pleural effusion with a thin fluid containing few cells and bacteria. The fluid is easily removed with tube drainage, and the lung readily reexpands.

   B. **Fibrinopurulent phase.** Accumulation of white cells and fibrin occurs over several days, producing loculation of the fluid and fixation of the lung. This fluid is more difficult to remove, and lung reexpansion is incomplete.

   C. **Organization phase.** Fibroblasts infiltrate the purulent coagulum resulting in the development of a tough inelastic "peel," which restricts lung expansion. Persistence and contraction of the fibrous "envelope" results in **fibrothorax** and **scoliosis.**

III. **Clinical presentation**

   A. **Pleural effusion** on chest x-ray following treatment of pneumonia is the most common finding suggesting empyema. There is frequently no noticeable change in the patient's course.

   B. **Massive empyema** is associated with **respiratory distress** and high fever, sometimes with **septic shock.**

   C. **Postoperaive empyema** is heralded by fever and the appearance of purulent drainage from the chest tube. Other symptoms may predominate (e.g., mediastinitis if there is esophageal leak).

IV. **Diagnosis**

   A. **Chest x-ray** reveals a pleural effusion.

   B. **Thoracentesis** yields purulent fluid from which the responsible organism often may be recovered by culture.

   C. **The pleural fluid may be sterile** if the patient has received effective antibiotic treatment for an antecedent pneumonia.

   D. The most **common organisms** responsible for the development of empyema nowadays are *Staphylococcus, Escherichia coli, Pseudomonas,* and *Klebsiella.* Sterile empyema occurring after pulmonary infection is most likely caused by *Haemophilus influenzae* or *Streptococcus pneumoniae.*

V. **Treatment**

   A. **Early drainage** is essential for effective treatment of empyema. The fluid can be easily and completely drained during the exudative phase, difficult to get out during the fibrinopurulent phase, and impossible to remove without an operation in the organization phase.

   B. **A chest tube must be inserted.** Repeated needle thoracentesis is inadequate because fluid reaccumulates, perpetuating the pleural abscess. If the purulent fluid is continuously drained, lung reexpansion obliterates the pleural space. Healing will then occur quickly.

C. **Loculated or organized empyema usually requires operative treatment.** However, if the patient is afebrile and cultures from the fluid are negative, healing and resolution of the empyema may take place over a period of several weeks to months with prolonged antibiotic treatment alone. If nonoperative treatment is chosen, the patient is monitored by weekly chest x-rays to ensure that there is resolution, not progressive fibrosis.

VI. Problems

A. **Delay in treatment** is the most common error in the management of empyema. If a chest tube is not inserted during the exudative phase, the fluid becomes organized and removal is difficult or impossible to accomplish without an operation.

B. **Inadequate drainage** is not uncommon, even when the tube is inserted early. Insertion of a second tube may be necessary to achieve complete evacuation of the pleural space.

VII. Indications for operation

A. **Inadequately drained empyema in a symptomatic patient** (fever, dyspnea, pain)

B. **Organized empyema in a symptomatic patient**

C. **Organized empyema in an asymptomatic patient** if there is lack of resolution within several weeks or if there is progressive lung constriction by **fibrosis** despite clearing of inflammatory changes

VIII. Preoperative preparation

A. **Appropriate antibiotic** treatment of the underlying infection

B. **Correction of malnutrition** with total parenteral nutrition (TPN) if the patient is cachectic after a prolonged septic course

IX. Operative care

A. **Loculated empyema requires partial rib resection** for drainage.

B. **Organized empyema requires decortication**—surgical removal of the fibrous peel from the surface of the lung and the inside of the thoracic cavity. A **complete** visceral and parietal pleurectomy must be carried out to free the lung.

X. Postoperative care

A. **Complete reexpansion of the lung** is the primary objective after decortication.

   1. **Adequate chest-tube suction** (two tubes are often required) is necessary to evacuate air from lung leaks and serous exudate from the pleurectomy.
   2. **Pulmonary physiotherapy** facilitates lung expansion and clearing of secretions.
   3. **Early ambulation** improves ventilation.

B. **Antibiotics** are given to prevent flare-up of previously treated infection.

XI. Complications

A. **Recurrent empyema** may occur if drainage is inadequate.

B. **Persistent air leak** results from lung damage from the decortication.

C. **Fibrothorax** can occur if decortication is inadequate.

XII. Prognosis

A. Prompt and effective drainage of empyema results in rapid recovery.

B. Organized empyema will often heal without the need for decortication if infection can be completely eliminated. Several months may be required.

C. Decortication results in recovery within 2 weeks in most patients.

Bibliography

Altemeier, W. A., and Lewis, S. A. Cyclic variations in emerging phage types and antibiotic resistance of *Staphylococcus aureus*. *Surgery* 84:534, 1978.

Bartlett, J. G., et al. Bacteriology of empyema. *Lancet* 1:338, 1974.

Bechamps, G. J., Lynn, H. B., and Wenzl, J. E. Empyema in children: Review of Mayo Clinic experience. *Mayo Clin. Proc.* 45:43, 1970.

Kosloske, A. M. Infections of the lungs, pleura, and mediastinum. In K. J. Welch, et al. (eds.), *Pediatric Surgery*. Chicago: Year Book, 1986. P. 657.

Kosloske, A. M., Cushing, A. H., and Shuck, J. M. Early decortication for anaerobic empyema in children. *J. Pediatr. Surg.* 15:422, 1980.

Mayo, P., Saha, S. P., and McElvein, R. B. Acute empyema in children treated by open thoracotomy and decortication. *Ann. Thorac. Surg.* 34:401, 1982.

Murphy, D., Lockhart, C. H., and Todd, J. K. Pneumococcal empyema. *Am. J. Dis. Child.* 134:659, 1980.

Telander, R. L. Acquired Lesions of the Lung and Pleura. In T. M. Holder and K. W. Ashcraft (eds.), *Pediatric Surgery*. Philadelphia: Saunders, 1980. P. 209.

51 Chylothorax

Definition. *Chylothorax* is the accumulation of lymph in the pleural space, caused by leakage from the **thoracic duct.** In the neonate, chylothorax may result from congenital malformations of the thoracic duct, birth injury, or unknown causes. In the older child, malignant tumors and operative injury to the thoracic duct are the most common causes, but trauma, lymphangioma, or violent coughing may be responsible.

Pathophysiology

A. The thoracic duct travels upward on the right side in the lower portion of the chest, crossing over to the left side at the level of T5. Leakage from the duct can thus produce either a left- or a right-sided collection depending on the level of the injury.

B. The volume of chyle and the rate of flow in the thoracic duct are related to diet, particularly the fat content. Fat content can be as high as 4 gm/dl, and protein can be as high as 6 gm/dl. Lymphocytes are also present in abundance.

C. Fluid accumulation in the pleural space **compresses the lung and displaces the mediastinum.** The neonate's flexible mediastinum permits compression of the opposite lung as well, resulting in significant respiratory compromise.

D. Continued leakage of chyle causes **depletion of fat and protein** and significant malnutrition. Depletion of lymphocytes also occurs. The bacteriostatic qualities of chyle prevent infection in most children with chylothorax.

Clinical presentation

A. Newborns are almost always symptomatic in the first week of life, sometimes within hours after birth.

B. Respiratory distress is the common symptom, and it is usually progressive and severe. Breath sounds are absent, and there is flatness to percussion. The mediastinum is shifted away from the fluid collection.

C. Malignant chylothorax is usually a **late complication** of advanced disease: lymphoma, neuroblastoma, or metastatic tumor.

D. Leakage of chyle may be impressive: several hundred milliliters per day in a young infant and **over 1000 ml/day** in an older child. Untreated, nutritional depletion rapidly ensues.

Diagnosis

A. Chest x-ray shows a pleural effusion that to the experienced eye is more radiolucent than the usual effusion (because of the fat content).

B. Thoracentesis yields milky fluid. In the newborn infant who has not been fed, the fluid will initially be serous.

Treatment

A. Total parenteral nutrition with complete intestinal rest is the preferred method to stop the flow of chyle. Healing of a leak in the thoracic duct will usually take place once the flow of chyle has been eliminated. A trial of feeding is given once a week to assess results. Treatment may be required for several weeks.

B. A chest tube is placed to reexpand the lung and evacuate the fluid from the chest. It should be left in until the patient can take a regular diet without fluid leakage.

C. **Plasma** infusion may be needed in the neonate if leakage is significant in spite of TPN.

D. **In mild cases,** use of medium-chain triglycerides **(MCT)** in a nonfat formula may sufficiently diminish chyle flow to permit healing without the use of TPN. The process is usually faster with TPN, however.

VI. **Indications for operation**

   A. **Operative ligation** of the thoracic duct is a **difficult** operation not to be undertaken lightly. It is indicated if the site of injury is known and if the average daily chyle loss exceeds 100 ml in a newborn or 100 ml/year of age in the older child.

   B. If the cause of the chylothorax is unknown, **TPN with bowel rest** is carried out for at least **2 weeks**—longer if the flow is diminishing.

   C. Operative treatment is ineffective and **not indicated** in patients with **malignant chylothorax.**

VII. **Operative care.** Operative detection of the chyle leak can be difficult and frustrating. A fatty meal fed after the induction of anesthesia, dyed with a fat stain, may make recognition of the leak site easier. The opening in the duct is oversewn with nonabsorbable suture. Because leaks may be multiple, care is taken to identify all of them.

VIII. **Prognosis.** In most patients, the leak will stop spontaneously, never to recur.

Bibliography

Austin, E. H., and Flye, M. W. The treatment of recurrent malignant pleural effusion. *Ann. Thorac. Surg.* 28:90, 1979.

Glenn, W. W. L. The lymphatic system: Some surgical considerations. *Arch. Surg.* 116:989, 1981.

Kosloske, A. M., Martin, L. W., and Schubert, W. K. Management of chylothorax in children by thoracentesis and medium-chain triglyceride feedings. *J. Pediatr. Surg.* 9:365, 1974.

Randolph, J. G. Chylothorax. In K. J. Welch, et al. (eds.), *Pediatric Surgery*. Chicago: Year Book, 1986. P. 654.

Selle, J. G., Snyder, W. H., and Schreiber, J. T. Chylothorax: Indications for surgery. *Ann. Surg.* 177:245, 1973.

Telander, R. L. Acquired Lesions of the Lung and Pleura. In T. M. Holder and K. W. Ashcraft (eds.), *Pediatric Surgery*. Philadelphia: Saunders, 1980. P. 209.

Vain, N. E., Swarner, O. W., and Cha, C. C. Neonatal chylothorax. *J. Pediatr. Surg.* 15:261, 1980.

52 Gastroesophageal Reflux

I. **Definition.** *Reflux* means reverse flow. *Gastroesophageal reflux* (GER) refers to reverse flow of gastric contents up the esophagus. GER is common is early infancy but rare in older children. *Hiatal hernia* refers to displacement of part of the stomach into the chest through the esophageal hiatus. Most patients with hiatal hernia have GER, but most children with GER do not have a hiatal hernia.

I. **Pathophysiology.** It is unclear what the normal mechanism of gastroesophageal competence is, but the lower esophageal sphincter (not a true sphincter) and the intraabdominal segment of esophagus (exposed to the higher abdominal pressure) are thought to be the key factors in preventing GER. There are several consequences of reflux.

  A. **Vomiting** is the most common result of GER. When severe, it can lead to inadequate intake and **growth retardation**.

  B. **Esophagitis** results from acid-peptic irritation of the lower esophagus. It may result in **pain, bleeding, esophageal spasm, ulceration,** and if prolonged, **esophageal stricture.**

  C. **Aspiration** may occur if refluxed gastric contents spill over into the airway. **Protective reflexes** may be deficient in patients with GER who aspirate, since most patients with reflux do not have this problem. The **upper esophageal sphincter** normally protects against aspiration. **Laryngospasm** secondary to acid irritation may result in apnea in young infants.

. **Clinical presentation.** Gastroesophageal reflux is a great masquerader. It is the cause of a wide variety of disease states and symptoms that may at times appear to be from other causes.

  A. **Vomiting** is the most common symptom in infants, and may be either regurgitant or projectile. The differential diagnosis includes overfeeding, formula intolerance, and pyloric stenosis.

   1. **Failure to thrive** may result if caloric intake is inadequate.

   2. **Gagging, gulping,** and **regurgitation** are frequently present. The parent may hear the reflux.

   3. **Rumination** is caused by GER. Although it is a behavioral disorder, it only occurs in the presence of GER.

   4. In the **older child,** vomiting is socially unacceptable even if it is no nutritional threat.

  B. **Esophagitis** occurs to some degree in all patients with GER, but is often asymptomatic.

   1. **Pain** is the most common symptom of esophagitis. It is typically substernal or epigastric.

     a. **In the infant,** the pain may be interpreted as "**colic**" or noted as general "**fussiness.**" Usually it is most severe after feedings, although it can occur at any time.

     b. In the **older child,** the pain may be **substernal** or **epigastric** in location. Esophagitis may be a cause of **chronic or recurrent abdominal pain.**

   2. **Gastrointestinal bleeding,** usually occult but occasionally frank hematemesis or melena, can result from esophagitis. It may be the cause of unexplained iron-deficiency **anemia.**

3. **Ulceration** of the esophagus can result in pain, bleeding, or rarely, **perforation** of the esophagus with acute mediastinitis.
4. **Spasm** of the esophagus results in **dysphagia**.
5. **Stricture** results from long-standing acid irritation of the esophagus. Patients in whom stricture develops often have no prior history of pain.
6. **Sandifer's syndrome,** spasmodic torticollis associated with GER, may be secondary to esophagitis.

C. **Aspiration syndromes** are common complications of GER.
   1. **An apneic spell** is clearly the most serious complication of GER. **Infants** under the age of 6 months are at greatest risk. Most do not have vomiting.
      a. The spell may result from **laryngospasm** due to acid irritation or may be a **vagal** response to acid irritation of the esophagus.
      b. The infant **struggles** to breathe but is unable to pass air. He has a **startled** and **frightened** look, turns **red**, and **then turns pale and cyanotic** as he becomes **limp** from inadequate oxygenation.
      c. Apneic spells may be **life-threatening** but can almost always be "broken" by vigorous stimulation or mouth-to-mouth resuscitation.
      d. GER may be a cause of the **sudden infant death syndrome (SIDS).** The clinical and epidemiologic characteristics of infants with reflux apneic spells are identical to those of infants with aborted SIDS.
   2. **Recurrent pneumonia** is the most common serious complication of GER.
      a. A **migratory** pattern, **diffuse** involvement, **inconsistent bacterial flora,** and **poor response to antibiotic therapy** are clues that the episodes are caused by recurrent aspiration rather than infection. Any type of parenchymal consolidation may be seen, however.
      b. **GER is probably the major cause of recurrent pneumonia in infancy.**
   3. **Recurring bronchitis** due to GER has a similar pattern: no characteristic flora and poor response to antibiotic therapy.
   4. **Coughing, choking, congestion, and wheezing** are other symptoms of recurrent aspiration.
   5. **Asthma** may result from GER, which should be suspected if the wheezing is noted in the night or on arising in the morning.

IV. **Diagnosis**

A. **The history should suggest the diagnosis** of GER, especially if several symptoms are present simultaneously. **Physical examination is usually unremarkable.** There are no characteristic physical findings of GER, only of its complications.

B. **Laboratory studies**
   1. The **upper gastrointestinal series** (UGIS) radiogram will establish the diagnosis of GER in most patients (Fig. 52-1). It also demonstrates other abnormalities that could be responsible for the symptoms.
   2. A **12-hour pH probe study** is the most reliable method of evaluating reflux. It is indicated if the UGIS fails to demonstrate suspected reflux and for more complete evaluation of reflux in the complicated patient.
   3. **Scintiscan** evaluation of GER using technetium 99m may demonstrate GER when the UGIS fails to do so.
   4. **Esophagoscopy and biopsy** will confirm the diagnosis of esophagitis, and thus of reflux, when other studies fail.

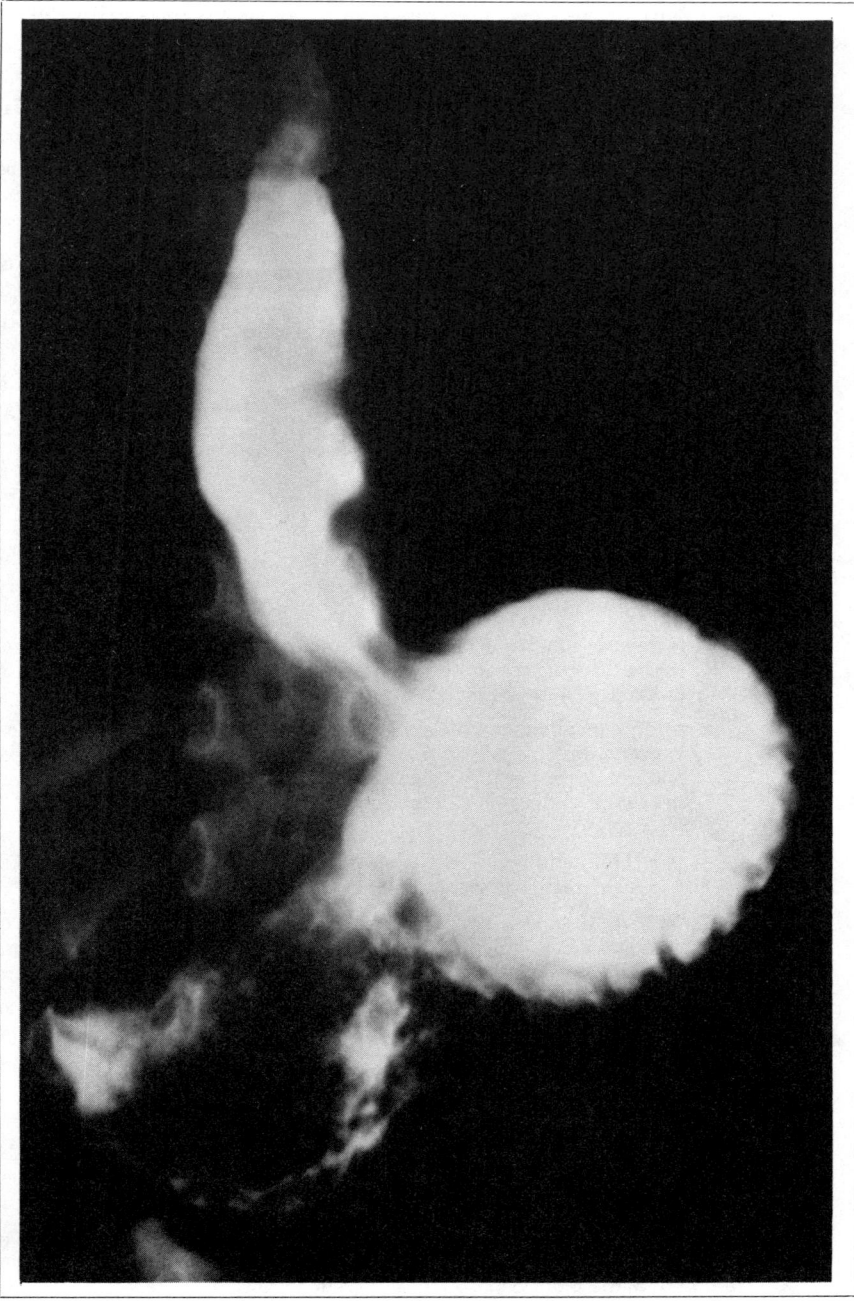

Fig. 52-1. Gastroesophageal reflux. With adequate filling of the stomach with barium, there is free reflux up the esophagus. (From L. L. Leape, Thoracic Surgical Problems in Infants and Children. In F. H. Ellis (Ed.), *Thoracic Surgery*. Philadelphia: Lippincott/Harper & Row, 1983.)

C. Patients with **recurrent pneumonia** require further evaluation to eliminate other causes such as **cystic fibrosis, immune deficiency, anatomic abnormalities** of the airway, and **allergies.**

D. **Apneic spells** cannot be attributed to GER unless its presence is documented and other causes of apnea are eliminated. **Seizures, arrhythmias, and periodic apnea** due to **immaturity** of the respiratory center must be considered. Complete cardiologic and neurologic evaluations are indicated, including ECG and EEG as well as 24-hour pneumogram.

V. **Medical treatment**
   A. **Natural history**
      1. **Infants "grow out" of reflux** as the lower esophageal sphincter matures and they assume the upright posture. Ninety percent of symptomatic infants will be **well by 15 months** of age. **Treatment** is aimed at controlling symptoms until they spontaneously disappear.
      2. **In older children,** spontaneous disappearance rarely occurs. Surgical treatment is necessary if symptoms are serious or there are significant complications. A trial of nonoperative therapy is indicated in most patients.
   B. **Treatment of infants**
      1. **Dietary and positional therapy** will usually control symptoms.
         a. **Thickened feedings** reduce reflux by increasing viscosity. **Cereal** is added to the formula, **1 tablespoon/oz. No** unthickened liquids are given.
         b. **Reduced volume** of feedings is equally important. A good "rule of thumb" is to give 1 oz of thickened feeding every 3 hours for each month of life (e.g., 4 oz q3h for a 4-month-old).
         c. **Upright positioning** prevents reflux by use of gravity. The ideal position is **prone at 45** degrees, but sitting in an infant **car seat** usually works and is much easier to arrange. If symptoms are severe, the infant is kept in the upright position **24 hours a day.**
         d. Dietary and positional therapy is **successful** in controlling symptoms in **90% of infants** with GER. The usual course of treatment is **6 weeks,** although treatment sometimes must be continued for many months.
      2. **Cimetidine, 10 mg/kg qid** 30 minutes before meals, is given if symptoms of **esophagitis** persist in spite of dietary and positional therapy. Aluminum hydroxide antacid preparations may also be required (1 tablespoon 20 minutes after each feeding).
      3. **Metoclopramide, 0.1 mg/kg qid,** may control GER in patients whose symptoms are refractory to dietary therapy.
      4. **Surgical treatment is not necessary** in infants unless medical therapy is unsuccessful and the baby's health or life is threatened by continuing complications, such as recurrent pneumonia, failure to grow, and refractory pain.
      5. **Infants with apneic spells** caused by GER require operative treatment if the spells are life-threatening. A home monitoring program is an alternative, but it is riskier and also psychologically taxing.
   C. **Treatment of the older child.** Medical therapy is much less likely to be successful in older children.
      1. Dietary and positional therapy is of no value since the child is already taking solid food and is upright most of the time. **Elevation of the head of the bed** at night is seldom effective.

2. **Esophagitis** usually will respond to **cimetidine** (10 mg/kg qid to a maximum of 300 mg qid) for 6 weeks.
   a. **Aluminum hydroxide antacids** may also be necessary to bring complete relief of pain (15–60 ml, 20 minutes after meals and at bedtime).
   b. **In refractory cases, metoclopramide,** 0.1 mg/kg qid to a maximum of 20 mg/day, may help.
3. **Aspiration syndromes (recurrent pneumonia, bronchitis, asthma, chronic cough)** may respond to long-term treatment with cimetidine. Long-term **metoclopramide** therapy has not been evaluated.

Indications for operation

A. **Stricture.** There is no nonoperative treatment for stricture. The stricture must be dilated, and the acid reflux must be eliminated to prevent further scarring. Long-term administration of cimetidine has not been effective treatment.

B. **Life-threatening apneic spells.** An antireflux operation is the surest method of preventing recurrence of apnea caused by GER. Operative risk is less than that of nonoperative therapy with an apnea-monitoring program.

C. **Failure of medical therapy** is the indication for surgical therapy in all other patients with gastroesophageal reflux.

D. **Brain-damaged children** have an increased incidence of serious complications from GER that require surgical treatment.

Preoperative preparation

A. Severe **malnutrition** is treated by a 2- to 3-week course of **parenteral nutrition.**

B. **Pulmonary complications** are controlled by intensive in-hospital physiotherapy, antibiotics, and bronchodilators. It may be necessary to stop feedings and give parenteral nutrition. **It may be impossible to clear the lungs until the reflux is eliminated.**

Operative care

A. **The abdominal approach** provides the opportunity to note and correct any other abdominal abnormalities and perform gastrostomy or pyloroplasty if indicated.

B. **The Nissen fundoplication** is the operation of choice. It is a complete (360-degree) wrap of the fundus of the stomach around the mobilized intraabdominal esophagus.

C. **A large bougie in the esophagus** at the time of fundoplication will ensure that the wrap is not too tight (size 30F in an infant, 50F in an adult).

D. **Pyloroplasty** is necessary in brain-damaged patients or others with delayed gastric emptying.

E. **Gastrostomy** is indicated if there is a feeding problem, but not otherwise.

Postoperative care

A. **Nasogastric tube** decompression is necessary to prevent acute gastric distention and possible tearing of the sutures in the immediate postoperative period.

B. **Liquid feedings** may be begun after a day or two.

C. **A blenderized diet** is necessary for **2 weeks** after fundoplication until the postoperative swelling subsides.

D. **Discharge from the hospital** is possible in 4–7 days.

E. **Follow-up UGIS** is obtained after 6 weeks, when the postoperative swelling has disappeared, to assess whether GER has been completely eliminated.

F. **Dilatations of esophageal strictures** are performed under anesthesia at 10- to

14-day intervals. A minimum of three dilatations is necessary, many more in some patients.

X. Complications

A. Early complications

1. **Perforation of the esophagus** from a suture is a rare but potentially fatal complication that must be considered if the child does not recover promptly and has a fever or persistent abdominal pain.

    a. Diagnosis: contrast esophagogram

    b. Treatment: prompt operative closure and drainage

2. **Delayed gastric emptying** is more common in infants but is also seen in brain-damaged children if pyloroplasty has not been performed.

    a. **Simethicone** (0.5–1.0 ml ac) is usually effective in mild cases of "gas bloat."

    b. **Metoclopramide** (0.1 mg/kg qid) is used in refractory or very symptomatic cases.

    c. **Pyloroplasty** may be necessary in severe cases that do not respond to medical management.

3. **Retching and hiccuping,** occasionally seen in the immediate postoperative period, are due to diaphragmatic irritation and distention of the stomach. Antiemetics, simethicone, and the passage of time usually bring relief.

B. Late complications

1. **Gas bloat.** Gastric distention, particularly after feeding, is seen in 5–15% of patients after fundoplication. It is more common in infants. It usually resolves spontaneously as the gastric capacity increases. Simethicone with feedings (0.5–1.0 ml) may be helpful.

2. **Inability to vomit** occurs in 50% of patients who undergo Nissen fundoplication. This percentage may decrease with time. Although distressing in prospect, this limitation is not harmful to the patient.

3. Dysphagia may result from a **tight fundoplication.** Esophageal dilatation is usually curative.

4. **Symptomatic recurrent GER** occurs in 2–5% of patients after a standard Nissen fundoplication. If symptoms persist, reoperation is indicated. **Radiologic reflux** without symptoms is seen in 5–10% of patients. In the absence of symptoms, no treatment is needed.

5. **Herniation of the fundoplication** into the chest occurs in 1–2% of patients and requires operative correction if symptomatic.

6. **Intestinal obstruction secondary to adhesions** occurs in about 5% of patients, most within the first 2 months after the operation.

7. **Refractory stricture** is not a postoperative complication, but the effect of long-standing preoperative scarring. If there is no response to repeated dilatations after the reflux has been eliminated, segmental resection of the esophagus may be necessary.

XI. Prognosis

A. **Overall, 90% or more** of patients with GER **are cured by operation** and have no adverse effects.

B. **Failures are of two kinds.**

1. **Operative failures.** Improper technique, suture disruption, tissue abnormalities, and so on: 2–5%

2. **Selection failures** (misdiagnosis). Almost entirely patients with pulmonary symptoms not caused by GER or that have advanced beyond reversibility: 5%

Bibliography

Ashcraft, K. W., Holder, T. M., and Amoury, R. A. Treatment of gastroesophageal reflux in children by Thal fundoplication. *J. Thorac. Cardiovasc. Surg.* 82:706, 1981.

Boix-Ochoa, J. Gastroesophageal Reflux. In K. J. Welch, et al. (eds.), *Pediatric Surgery*. Chicago: Year Book, 1986. P. 712.

Boix-Ochoa, J., and Canals, J. Maturation of the lower esophageal sphincter. *J. Pediatr. Surg.* 11:749, 1976.

Carre, I. J. Natural history of partial thoracic stomach ("hiatus hernia") in children. *Arch. Dis. Child.* 34:344, 1959.

Darling, D. B., et al. Gastroesophageal reflux in infants and children: Correlation of radiological severity and pulmonary pathology. *Radiology* 127:735, 1978.

Darling, D. B., et al. The child with peptic esophagitis: A correlation of radiological signs with esophageal pathology. *Radiology* 145:673, 1982.

DeMeester, T. R., et al. Clinical and in vitro analysis of determinants of gastroesophageal competence: A study of principles of antireflux surgery. *Am. J. Surg.* 137:39, 1979.

Herbst, J. J. Gastroesophageal reflux and pulmonary disease. *Pediatrics* 68:132, 1981.

Johnson, D. G., et al. Evaluation of gastroesophageal reflux surgery in children. *Pediatrics* 59:62, 1977.

Leape, L. L. Surgical Treatment of Asthma. In B. Berman (ed.), *Differential Diagnosis of Childhood Allergies*. Boston: Little, Brown, 1981. P. 117.

Leape, L. L. Gastroesophageal Reflux. In T. M. Holder and K. W. Ashcraft (eds.), *Pediatric Surgery*. Philadelphia: Saunders, 1980. P. 292.

Leape, L. L., Bhan, I., and Ramenofsky, M. L. Esophageal biopsy in the diagnosis of reflux esophagitis. *J. Pediatr. Surg.* 16:379, 1981.

Leape, L. L., and Ramenofsky, M. L. The surgical treatment of gastroesophageal reflux in children: Results of Nissen fundoplication in 100 children. *Am. J. Dis. Child.* 134:935, 1980.

Leape, L. L., et al. Respiratory arrest in infants secondary to gastroesophageal reflux. *Pediatrics* 60:924, 1977.

Little, A. G., et al. Abnormal gastric emptying in patients with gastroesophageal reflux. *Surg. Forum* 28:347, 1977.

Nissen, R. Gastropexy and fundoplication in surgical treatment of hiatus hernia. *Am. J. Dig. Dis.* 6:954, 1961.

Ramenofsky, M. L., and Leape, L. L. Continuous upper esophageal pH monitoring in infants and children with gastroesophageal reflux, pneumonia and apneic spells. *J. Pediatr. Surg.* 16:374, 1981.

53 Achalasia

I. **Definition.** *Achalasia* is an obstructive abnormality caused by failure of relaxation of the lower esophagus. It is also known as *cardiospasm*. The etiology is unknown, although an abnormality of the ganglion cells has been incriminated.
II. **Clinical presentation.** Achalasia may develop at any age but is rare in young children. **Difficulty swallowing** is the usual presenting symptom, but slow feeding or complications of aspiration may be the first evidence in some patients.
III. **Diagnosis**
   A. **Barium swallow** reveals the diagnostic changes in the esophagus.
      1. **Dilatation** of the esophagus with food retention
      2. **Distal narrowing**
      3. **Markedly delayed emptying**
      4. **Altered motility**
   B. **Motility studies** are helpful in equivocal cases and show absence of primary peristalsis with disordered tertiary waves.
IV. **Treatment.** Modified **Heller myotomy** of the lower esophagus is the treatment of choice. Dilations have high failure and perforation rates and are not recommended. No special preoperative preparation is needed.
V. **Complications. Esophageal leak** with mediastinitis resulting from unrecognized operative perforation is the most serious complication. Adequate drainage usually results in satisfactory spontaneous closure, although it may take several weeks.
VI. **Prognosis.** Most patients are cured by the operation, but some have recurrent symptoms. **Reflux** esophagitis or stricture may occur if the myotomy is extended too far onto the stomach. If reflux symptoms are severe, an antireflux operation may be required.

Bibliography

Berquist, W. E., et al. Achalasia: Diagnosis, management, and clinical course in 16 children. *Pediatrics* 71:798, 1983.

Boyle, J. T., Cohen, S., and Watkins J. B. Successful treatment of achalasia in childhood by pneumatic dilatation. *J. Pediatr.* 99:35, 1981.

Ellis, F. H., Jr., Gibb, S. P., and Crozier, R. E. Esophagomyotomy for achalasia of the esophagus. *Ann. Surg.* 192:157, 1980.

Fonkalsrud, E. W. The Role of Surgery in the Treatment of Gastroesophageal Reflux and Gastric Dysmotility Disorders in Children. In K. W. Ashcraft and T. M. Holder (eds.), *Pediatric Esophageal Surgery*. Orlando, FL: Grune & Stratton, 1986. P. 217.

Friesen, D. L., Henderson, R. D., and Hanna, W. Ultrastructure of the esophageal muscle in achalasia and diffuse esophageal spasm. *Am. J. Clin. Pathol.* 79:319, 1983.

Hill, J. L. Neuromotor Esophageal Disorders. In K. J. Welch, et al. (eds.), *Pediatric Surgery*. Chicago: Year Book, 1986. P. 720.

Othersen, H. B., Jr. Esophageal Lesions. In T. M. Holder and K. W. Ashcraft (eds.), *Pediatric Surgery*. Philadelphia: Saunders, 1980. P. 253.

Tachovsky, T. J., Lynn, H. B., and Ellis, F. H., Jr. The surgical approach to esophageal achalasia in children. *J. Pediatr. Surg.* 3:226, 1968.

54 Caustic Ingestion

I. **Definition.** Ingestion of caustic substances, whether predominantly alkaline (lye) or acid, may result in serious injury to the esophagus, oropharynx, and stomach.
   A. **Drain cleaners** are the most commonly ingested strong caustics. **Sodium and potassium hydroxide** are the key corrosive ingredients, either in liquid or granular form.
   B. **Mild caustics,** such as **bleach** (sodium hypochlorite), **ammonia,** and **dishwasher and laundry detergents,** must be ingested in large amounts to be harmful.
   C. **Clinitest tablets** contain concentrated lye, which can be very damaging to the esophagus if accidentally swallowed.
   D. **Acid ingestion** is rarely seen in children in the United States. Battery acid and industrial products are the common sources.

II. **Epidemiology.** Lye ingestion in older children and adults almost always results from a **suicide attempt.** Lye ingestion in young children is usually **accidental,** as is ingestion of other poisons.
   A. **Social stress** is a major factor in "accidental" poisonings, for they frequently occur in situations of family upset.
   B. **Educational programs** temporarily decrease the incidence of poisonings, but they do not seem to be of lasting value in prevention.
   C. Use of **child-proof containers** and the elimination from the home of seriously hazardous products seem to be the only realistic means of preventing caustic ingestion.

Pathophysiology
   A. **Lye injury** results from penetration of the tissues and denaturation of intracellular proteins by hydroxyl radicals. There is an intense inflammatory reaction and small vessel thrombosis. Transmural penetration can occur rapidly if the caustic is in liquid form.
      1. **The esophagus** is most likely to be injured, although if large quantities of lye are consumed, extensive burns to the stomach and intestine can also occur.
      2. **In severe burns** the necrotic tissue sloughs with healing by granulation and scar tissue formation. If the burn is full-thickness and circumferential, **stricture** develops.
      3. **The extent of the injury** depends on the **concentration of the caustic,** the **quantity ingested,** and the **duration of contact** with the tissues.
      4. **Granular lye** goes into solution slowly, so burns are usually localized and not severe. The burning sensation in the mouth leads to expectoration. Serious burns of the esophagus occur in only about 5% of patients.
      5. **Liquid lye** produces far more serious injuries than granular forms because it penetrates the tissues almost instantaneously and because a large amount can be swallowed before the child realizes what he has done. Most patients have a serious esophageal burn.
      6. **Antidotes are of no value** in liquid lye ingestion, for the rapid penetration can cause full-thickness injury within seconds.

B. **Acid ingestion** causes a coagulative necrosis on the surface, which limits the degree of injury unless large quantities are consumed. In large ingestions, full-thickness necrosis and perforation may occur rapidly, or later, when the necrotic eschar sloughs. **Gastric destruction** is most common in acid injury, with either early perforation or late antral scar formation.

IV. **Clinical picture.** The severity of the symptoms varies considerably according to the nature of the ingested caustic and the amount ingested.

   A. **Lye ingestion in large quantities** usually results from a **suicide attempt** by an older child or the accidental ingestion of **concentrated liquid lye** by a toddler. The patient is obviously ill and may be in shock. Emergency treatment is necessary.

   1. **Vascular collapse (shock)** may occur from the outpouring of fluid into the burned tissues.
   2. **Toxicity and fever** result from the absorption of necrotic cellular breakdown products.
   3. **Chest or back pain** suggests that mediastinitis has resulted from perforation or necrosis of the esophagus.
   4. **Bloody vomitus** may be present.
   5. **Peritonitis** may result from gastric perforation or intestinal necrosis, causing abdominal pain and rigidity.
   6. **Dyspnea, stridor, and hoarseness** are symptoms of laryngeal injury. Progressive respiratory compromise may occur over a period of hours, necessitating intubation.
   7. **Overwhelming sepsis** may rapidly ensue.

   B. **Ingestion of smaller quantities of lye** is more commonly seen and is less serious.

   1. **The history of ingestion may be inadequate.** Frequently the event is not witnessed, so the physician must rely on inferential evidence.
   2. **Oral burns** are evidence that ingestion has occurred. Unfortunately, they do not give a clue to the quantity (and thus the severity) of the ingestion.
      a. **Severe esophageal burns** can occur in the absence of significant oral burns. This is most likely when concentrated liquid lye is swallowed.
      b. **Severe oral burns** may occur without any esophageal injury if the child spits the caustic out before swallowing any. This is most likely when granular lye is taken.
   3. **Drooling, edema, and erythema** of the lips and tongue are seen. The child may be **unable to swallow.**
   4. **Fever and leukocytosis** suggest a moderately severe amount of tissue injury.

   C. **Acid ingestion** typically results in abdominal symptoms: pain, bloody vomiting, and if large quantities are ingested, shock.

V. **Diagnosis.** In the typical case of lye ingestion, there are three questions that must be answered: Did the ingestion in fact occur? What was the substance? Is there damage to the esophagus?

   A. **Did ingestion occur?** If it was witnessed or if there are obvious oral burns, the question is answered. If there are no burns and the parent is unsure, further investigation is indicated if the substance suspected is strong lye.

   B. **What was it?** Since bleach, ammonia, and a wide variety of detergents and cleaning agents are relatively harmless and seldom require treatment for ingestion, positive identification of the substance, preferably through examination of the container, is highly desirable. The local poison control center can give information regarding ingredients and treatment.

C. **Is there esophageal damage?** Damage to the esophagus can only be determined by **esophagoscopy,** which should be performed in every patient in whom the ingestion of concentrated lye is reasonably possible.

   1. **Signs and symptoms are unreliable** in determining whether there is esophageal injury.

   2. **Radiologic examination is also unreliable,** except in the rare instance in which there is perforation, marked atony, or ulceration from ingestion of a large quantity of caustic.

D. **Esophagoscopy should be performed 12–24 hours after injury,** after there has been time for the stomach to empty, but before the risk of perforation increases.

   1. **The purpose of esophagoscopy is to determine whether there is a burn of the esophagus, not to determine its extent.**

   2. **If there is no burn,** no further treatment is indicated, and the patient is not at risk of late stricture formation. Seventy-five percent **of patients have no esophageal burn.**

   3. **If esophageal burn is detected, the examination is stopped.** Attempts to examine the entire esophagus increase the risk of perforation.

   4. **The depth of burn cannot be evaluated** by esophagoscopy, so it is impossible to tell if there will be full-thickness scar formation. However, if there is **circumferential** burn, it is more severe and the possibility of stricture formation exists.

Treatment

A. **Mild or moderate injury**

   1. **Admission to the hospital** overnight is essential for every patient with suspected or actual caustic ingestion because of the risk of airway injury, which may take hours to develop.

   2. **Nothing is given by mouth** because of the tendency to vomit, which would further increase the injury.

   3. **Local treatment of the mouth burns** with emollients and local analgesics may be necessary.

   4. **Intravenous fluids** are given as indicated.

   5. **Ampicillin, 250 mg qid,** is given as prophylaxis for infection of the burned tissues.

   6. **Prednisone, 0.5 mg/kg qid,** is given to decrease scar formation and later esophageal stricture.

   7. **Esophagoscopy** is performed the next day.

B. **If there is no esophageal burn,** treatment with steroids and antibiotics is stopped, and the patient may be sent home.

C. **If there is an esophageal burn,** administration of antibiotics should be continued for 10 days and of prednisone for 3 weeks.

   1. **Feeding** may begin when the patient is able to swallow—usually within a day or two of injury.

   2. **Gastrostomy** may be necessary if the esophageal injury is severe.

   3. **Discharge from the hospital** is appropriate once the patient is comfortable and able to eat without difficulty.

4. **Barium swallow** examination of the esophagus should be obtained at 3 weeks, earlier if there is dysphagia.
5. **Esophageal dilatations** are necessary if stricture develops.

D. **Severe injury**
1. **Plasma or blood** is required to resuscitate the patient if shock or sepsis is present.
2. **Antibiotics** are given, but steroids are withheld because they increase the risk of perforation and sepsis and are ineffective treatment of necrotic tissue.
3. **Early laparotomy or thoracotomy** may be necessary as a lifesaving measure if there are signs of extensive necrosis (peritonitis or mediastinitis).
4. **Gastrectomy or esophagectomy** is performed as an emergency measure if either or both of these organs are destroyed by the lye.

E. **Acid ingestion**
1. **A nasogastric tube** is passed and residual acid in the stomach evacuated to decrease further injury.
2. **Antacids (aluminum hydroxide)** are administered to neutralize any remaining acid in the stomach.
3. **Nothing is given by mouth** until the extent of gastric injury is defined and there are no signs of toxicity.
4. **Peritoneal signs** result from extensive organ damage and are an indication for immediate laparotomy to evaluate the extent of necrosis.
5. **Gastrectomy,** partial or complete, may be necessary, as well as resection of the **esophagus** if it is also destroyed.
6. **Less severe injuries** are treated symptomatically.
7. **Antral scarring** is a late consequence of acid gastric injury. It should be sought by barium study at 3 weeks or earlier if there is evidence of gastric dysfunction.

VII. **Complications**

A. **Esophageal stricture** occurs in 5–10% of granular lye ingestions and 50–100% of concentrated liquid lye ingestions (Fig. 54-1).
1. **Diagnosis** of stricture is made by routine barium swallow examination at 3 weeks, or later if dysphagia develops.
2. **Esophageal dilatations** are effective treatment for all but the most severe strictures.
   a. **Early dilatation** is desirable, before the scar tissue is mature and has contracted extensively.
   b. **Frequent dilatations** (at 7- to 10-day intervals) are more likely to be successful. If treatments are delayed each time until the patient is symptomatic, strictures are more difficult to dilate and the process drags on for many months.
   c. **General anesthesia** should always be used. Although it is possible to perform dilatations without anesthesia, the procedure is terrifying to the patient. Esophageal dilatation is a safe and simple **day-surgery** procedure.
3. **Ninety percent** of esophageal strictures caused by granular lye will respond to dilatations.
4. **Only 10–20% of strictures** caused by concentrated liquid lye will respond to

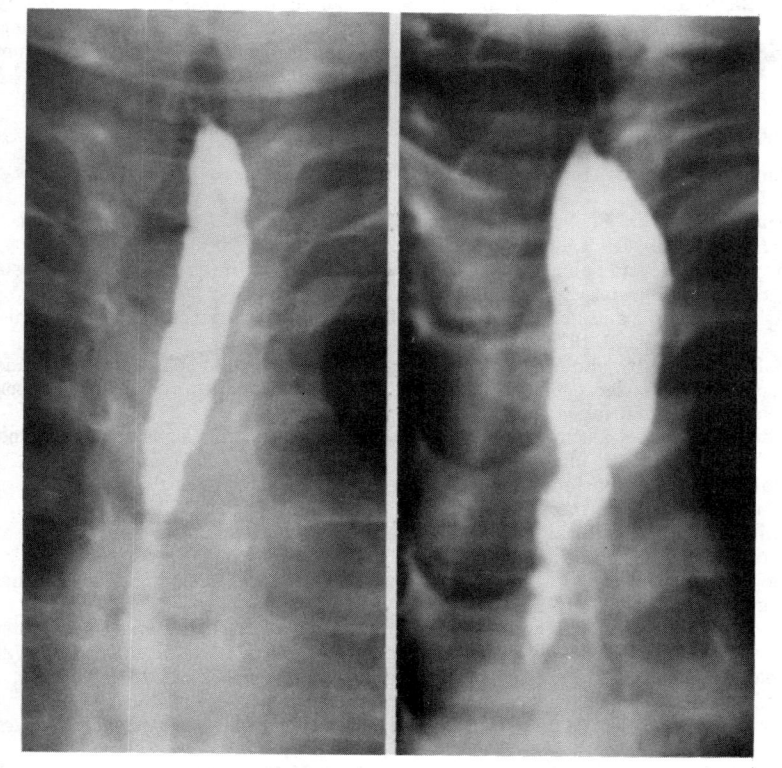

Fig. 54-1. Lye ingestion. Esophogram two weeks after ingestion of a small quantity of liquid lye (left). At two months stricture is worse despite repeated dilatations (right).

dilatations. Most of these patients require an esophageal substitution operation. If the injury is obviously severe, repeated dilatations will be futile.

B. **Laryngeal and tracheal strictures** are rare but difficult to treat when present. Segmental tracheal resection may be necessary. **Tracheostomy** is almost always required.

C. **Tracheoesophageal fistula** results from perforation of a severe lye injury from the esophagus into the trachea. These patients are usually quite ill.

   1. **Severe esophageal injury** is always present; emergency esophagectomy may be required.
   2. **Cough or expectoration of gastric or esophageal contents** is a typical symptom.
   3. **Contrast esophagogram** using bronchographic medium will usually demonstrate the fistula.
   4. **Bronchoscopy** may be necessary to establish the diagnosis.
   5. **Repair is difficult.** The tissues are very friable and heal poorly. **Esophageal exclusion** with cervical esophagostomy and gastrostomy may allow the fistula to close. Esophageal substitution is performed later on.

D. Carcinoma of the esophagus has been reported in patients with long-standing esophageal stricture, occurring 40 years or more after injury. Because the mortality risk of prophylactic esophagectomy appears to be higher than that from later cancer development, the procedure is not advised.

Bibliography

Amoury, R., et al. Tracheoesophageal fistula after lye ingestion. *J. Pediatr. Surg.* 10:273, 1975.

Anderson, K. D. Replacement of the Esophagus. In K. J. Welch, et al. (eds.), *Pediatric Surgery*. Chicago: Year Book, 1986. P. 704.

Appelqvist, P., and Salmo, M. Lye corrosion carcinoma of the esophagus: A review of 63 cases. *Cancer* 45:2655, 1980.

Ashcraft, K. W., and Padula, R. T. The effect of dilute corrosives on the esophagus. *Pediatrics* 53:226, 1974.

Baltimore, C., Jr., and Meyer, R. J. A study of storage, child behavioral traits and mother's knowledge of toxicology in 52 poisoned families and 52 comparison families. *Pediatrics* 44 [Suppl. 5]:816, 1969.

Gaudreault, P., et al. Predictability of esophageal injury from signs and symptoms: A study of caustic ingestion in 378 children. *Pediatrics* 71:767, 1983.

Haller, J. A., and Bachman, K. The comparative effect of current therapy on experimental caustic burns of the esophagus. *J.A.M.A.* 186:262, 1963.

Hill, J. L., et al. Clinical technique and success of the esophageal stent to prevent corrosive strictures. *J. Pediatr. Surg.* 11:443, 1976.

Hopkins, R. A., and Postlethwait, R. W. Caustic burns and carcinoma of the esophagus. *Ann. Surg.* 194:146, 1981.

Leape, L. L. Chemical Injury of the Esophagus. In K. W. Ashcraft and T. M. Holder (eds.), *Pediatric Esophageal Surgery*. Orlando, FL: Grune & Stratton, 1986. P. 73.

Leape, L. L., et al. Hazard to health: Liquid lye. *N. Engl. J. Med.* 284:578, 1971.

Leape, L. L., et al. Tracheal resection for lye stricture. *Surgery* 72:357, 1972.

Maull, K. I., et al. Surgical implications of acid ingestion. *Surg. Gynecol Obstet.* 148:895, 1979.

Othersen, H. B., Jr. Esophageal Lesions. In T. M. Holder and K. W. Ashcraft (eds.), *Pediatric Surgery*. Philadelphia: Saunders, 1980. P. 253.

Sobel, R. The psychiatric implications of accidental poisoning in childhood. *Pediatr. Clin. North Am.* 17:653, 1970.

Tunell, W. P. Corrosive Strictures of the Esophagus. In K. J. Welch, et al. (eds.), *Pediatric Surgery*. Chicago: Year Book, 1986. P. 698.

United States Department of Health, Education and Welfare, Public Health Service, Food and Drug Administration. *Bulletin, National Clearinghouse for Poison Control Centers*, 1982.

Votteler, T. P., et al. The hazard of ingested alkaline disk batteries in children. *J.A.M.A.* 249:2504, 1983.

VI Abdomen

55 Foreign Bodies

- **Definition.** A *foreign body* is any ingested object that is neither food nor medication, or any object that enters the body through a route other than the gastrointestinal tract (Also see Chap. 46 Foreign Bodies of the Airway).
- **Gastrointestinal foreign bodies.** Virtually every imaginable object may be ingested by young children—particularly between the ages of 1 and 3 when children are mobile but unwise! Fortunately, most objects pass through without causing trouble.
  A. **Esophagus.** Foreign bodies of the esophagus may result from a witnessed ingestion or may be totally unsuspected by the parent, who notes only that the child has suddenly developed dysphagia or is drooling and spitting up food.
     1. Esophageal foreign bodies are most likely to stick at the cricopharyngeus, at the crossing of the left mainstem bronchus, and at the gastroesophageal junction. If the child has had prior esophageal surgery, the anastomotic site is the typical point of obstruction.
     2. **Diagnosis** is by chest x-ray if the foreign body is radiopaque or by barium swallow if it is not.
     3. Because **perforation** occurs more readily in the esophagus than elsewhere, even from smooth foreign bodies, prompt removal is indicated. If there is complete obstruction, aspiration of saliva is also a hazard.
     4. **Removal** of a smooth foreign body (such as a coin) that has been ingested recently often can be accomplished by use of a Foley catheter under fluoroscopic control with the child in the head-down position. For all other objects, endoscopic removal under general anesthesia is required (see Chap. 45).
  B. **Stomach.** Gastric foreign bodies are seldom symptomatic and are often unrecognized unless the ingestion has been witnessed.
     1. Gastric foreign bodies, having navigated the narrow places of the esophagus, will pass the rest of the way through the gastrointestinal tract in 95% of cases. Round and smooth objects, such as coins, seldom perforate or cause symptoms, but even sharp objects usually pass without difficulty.
     2. Long objects are more likely to get caught in the duodenum or terminal ileum. Perforation may occur if the object is sharp or becomes stuck in one part of the intestine for a prolonged period.
     3. **Diagnosis** is by plain abdominal x-ray if the object is opaque, by contrast study if it is not.
     4. **Treatment.** Watchful waiting will result in recovery of most objects within a few days.
        a. All **stools are strained** for the foreign body. Cheesecloth is placed under the toilet seat prior to defecation, and hot water is poured over the stool to cause it to disintegrate and reveal the foreign body.
        b. If the object is not recovered, **x-rays** are taken **weekly** to determine whether it has left the stomach and is progressing satisfactorily. If the foreign body is still in the stomach at **4 weeks**, endoscopic removal is performed.
        c. If a **long or sharp object** leaves the stomach but remains in one place in the intestine for a week, operative removal is carried out. Earlier removal is indicated if the child develops pain, vomiting, bleeding, or fever.

C. **Alkaline batteries** from calculators, cameras, and hearing aids are easily ingested by a toddler and constitute a special hazard. They may leak concentrated KCl, which can cause local necrosis. Their prompt passage or removal must be ensured.

1. If a battery lodges in the **esophagus,** endoscopic removal is carried out immediately with careful examination for evidence of lye injury. If lye injury is found, barium swallow is obtained 2 weeks later in search of stricture.

2. If the battery is in the **stomach** or **intestine,** accelerated passage is encouraged by the administration of magnesium citrate. Stool is strained, and daily x-rays are obtained. Once the battery reaches the colon, enemas are given to evacuate it.

3. If the battery does not leave the stomach within 24 hours, endoscopic removal is performed.

4. Prompt operative removal of a battery in the intestine is indicated if the child develops pain, fever, or symptoms of obstruction; if the battery case is broken; or if the battery fails to progress along the intestine each day.

D. **Bezoars** are collections of foreign material in the stomach, usually either vegetable matter (phytobezoar) or hair (trichobezoar). The latter usually result from the child eating her own hair (90% are girls). Trichophagy may or may not indicate an emotional disorder.

1. **Symptoms** are often subtle and gradual in onset, with progressive decrease in appetite, weight loss, heavy feeling in the stomach, and vomiting. Physical examination in these thin girls usually easily reveals a midepigastric mobile mass.

2. **Diagnosis** is by barium x-ray, although some bezoars are clearly evident on plain x-rays of the abdomen.

3. **Treatment** is operative removal and psychotherapy if appropriate.

III. **Orifices.** Young children may insert objects into any orifice of their own or their siblings' bodies as part of normal exploratory play. Symptoms result from local erosion, bleeding, or infection.

A. **Ear or nose.** Pain, discharge, and bleeding are the usual symptoms that bring the patient to the physician. The object is usually evident on examination. Impacted foreign bodies are best treated by an otorhinolaryngologist.

B. **Vagina.** Vaginal discharge is the common symptom of a foreign body of the vagina, often foul-smelling and refractory to treatment. Vaginoscopy is indicated for diagnosis and treatment. Unfortunately, vaginal foreign bodies are suspected as a cause of vaginal discharge far more often than they are found. Bleeding is a rare complication.

C. **Rectum.** Pain and bleeding are the usual symptoms, but foreign bodies of the rectum are rarely seen in children.

IV. **Soft tissues.** Foreign bodies of the soft tissues result from trauma, which may range from trivial (wood splinter) to tragic (gunshot wound) and may affect any tissue in the body.

A. **Superficial foreign bodies** under the skin are typically known to the patient or result from incomplete removal at the time of treatment of an impalement.

1. **Symptoms.** A hard lump, recurrent infections, failure to heal, or continued drainage from a wound.

2. **Treatment.** If a foreign body can be seen or felt, its removal under direct vision is easily accomplished. If it cannot be seen or felt, exploration under local analgesia in the emergency room should be limited to 5 or 10 minutes since success is unlikely. The child should be taken to the operating room

where removal can be accomplished with the assistance of fluoroscopy or a foreign body finder. A broken-off needle in the foot is particularly hard to find and almost always requires a trip to the operating room.

B. **Foreign bodies in muscle** are harder to diagnose. A hard lump or persistent pain is the presenting symptom. Failure of a wound to heal suggests a foreign body. Operative treatment is required.

C. Foreign bodies of **internal organs** are usually best left in place except in the unusual situation in which they are symptomatic. Treatment of each case must be individualized, but removal of an asymptomatic foreign body may cause more damage than its retention.

Bibliography

Alexander, W. J., Kadish, J. A., and Dunbar, J. S. Ingested Foreign Bodies in Children. In H. J. Kaufmann (ed.), *Progress in Pediatric Radiology* (2nd ed.). Chicago: Year Book, 1969. P. 256.

Campbell, J. B., and Davis, W. S. Catheter technique for extraction of blunt esophageal foreign bodies. *Radiology* 108:438, 1973.

Euler, A. R. How long should a foreign body stay in the stomach? *Pediatrics* 61:671, 1978.

Gans, S. L., and Austin, E. *Foreign Bodies.* In T. M. Holder and K. W. Ashcraft (eds.), *Pediatric Surgery*. Philadelphia: Saunders, 1980. P. 116.

Groff, D. B. III. Foreign Bodies and Bezoars. In K. J. Welch, et al. (eds.), *Pediatric Surgery*. Chicago: Year Book, 1986. P. 907.

Litovitz, T. L. Button battery ingestions. *J.A.M.A.* 249:2495, 1983.

Mandell, G. A., Rosenberg, H. J., and Schnaufer, L. Prolonged retention of foreign bodies in the stomach. *Pediatrics* 60:460, 1978.

Schreiber, H., and Filston, H. C. Obstructive jaundice due to gastric trichobezoar. *J. Pediatr. Surg.* 11:103, 1976.

Votteler, T. P., Nash, J. C., and Rutledge, J. C. The hazard of ingested alkaline disk batteries in children. *J.A.M.A.* 249:2504, 1983.

56 Chronic Abdominal Pain

I. **Definition.** *Chronic or recurrent abdominal pain* is defined as three or more episodes of abdominal pain occurring over a 3-month period not associated with symptoms of organ dysfunction.
   A. **One in ten children** comes to the doctor because of chronic abdominal pain.
   B. **Stress** is by far the most common cause of chronic abdominal pain (psychogenic abdominal pain).
   C. **Organic causes** of pain almost always produce additional symptoms, but there are rare exceptions; therefore, almost every abdominal disease must be considered. Appendiceal colic secondary to noninflammatory obstruction with a fecalith is an organic cause that is frequently missed.

II. **Pathophysiology.** Anxiety can cause abdominal pain by several physiologic mechanisms.
   A. **Increased secretion of gastric acid** can cause gastritis, duodenitis, or esophagitis, as well as ulcers of these organs.
   B. **Increased sympathetic tone** gives rise to intestinal hyperactivity.
   C. **Involuntary tensing of abdominal muscles** can cause spasm and pain.

III. **Clinical presentation.** Abdominal pain is considered chronic when the child is seen repeatedly for complaints of pain but physical examinations and screening laboratory tests show no abnormalities. X-rays are negative.
   A. **Organic causes** are more likely if:
      1. The pain is **consistently present** in the same place and can be well **localized** by the patient.
      2. Pain **awakens** the child at night.
      3. The occurrence of pain bears **no** relationship to **stress,** and there is no history of excess stress.
      4. Other **psychosomatic symptoms are absent.**
   B. **Psychogenic abdominal pain** is more likely if:
      1. The patient is a **girl** (80%) between the ages of 9 and 14.
      2. The pain is described vaguely or is **diffuse** and **ill-defined** in both nature and location.
      3. The pain **does not awaken** the child at night.
      4. The child is **not ill.**
      5. Other psychosomatic symptoms are present: pallor, dizziness, headache.
      6. **Growth and development are normal.**

Problems. Most parents assume the child's pain has an organic cause and expect the doctor to find it. However, 95% of the time the pain will be found to be psychosomatic, so extensive testing and x-rays are seldom indicated. The physician's dilemma is that he does not want to overlook the rare organic cause but that extensive testing reinforces the parental conviction that the pain has a physical cause. (Negative tests merely indicate to parents that you have not found it yet.) The solution is thorough clinical evaluation and early consideration of psychologic causes of the pain.

V. Diagnosis

   A. **A detailed history and thorough physical examination** provide evidence for or against both physical and psychosomatic causes while at the same time helping the physician gain the confidence of the patient and the family.

   B. **Psychogenic abdominal pain is not a diagnosis of exclusion.** It is just as important to have positive evidence in making a diagnosis of psychosomatic disease as it is in making a diagnosis of organic disease.

   C. **Psychologic causes must be considered and discussed from the beginning.** It is wise to begin by telling the parents the facts: In most children with chronic abdominal pain and no other symptoms, emotional stress is the cause. Therefore, the first thing to investigate is the possibility of emotional stress.

   D. **Seek causes of emotional stress.**
   1. Has there been a **recent change:** moving, starting a new school, and so on?
   2. Is there **marital discord?**
   3. Has there been a **recent loss?** A departure of a loved one from the household, death in the family, separation or divorce of parents?
   4. Are there problems in **school,** in **peer** relationships?

   E. A **family history** of psychosomatic illness is found in 60% of cases of psychogenic abdominal pain.

   F. **Hospitalization** is sometimes necessary to establish the diagnosis of stress-related abdominal pain. Separation of the child from the stressful environment often brings instant relief of symptoms. Nurses can evaluate whether the pain is "real" and the effect of parental visiting.

   G. If no evidence is found to support the diagnosis of psychogenic abdominal pain, further x-rays and testing for organic disease are indicated.

   H. **Point localization** of pain, particularly if associated with localized tenderness, indicates **organic** disease in most children.

VI. Medical treatment.
Sometimes discovery of the underlying stressful situation and realization of its importance by the parent is all that is necessary to bring about environmental changes that remove the stress and relieve the pain. In other children, psychiatric treatment is needed to uncover and deal with the causative factors.

VII. Indications for operation.
Few children with chronic abdominal pain need operative treatment. Clearly, if a surgical lesion is revealed by examination, x-rays, or other tests, the appropriate operation should be performed.

   A. **Laparoscopy** is sometimes of value in discovering an occult cause of abdominal pain, or at least in eliminating a number of possible causes. Its use has supplanted "exploratory laparotomy," which is no longer indicated.

   B. **Appendectomy** will relieve pain in a high percentage (80–85%) of children with chronic abdominal pain if the pain is **well localized** to the right lower quadrant. In most of these patients, the appendix shows signs of chronic inflammation or is obstructed with a fecalith.

VIII. Operative care (see Chap. 63).

Bibliography

Apley, J. *The Child with Abdominal Pains.* Oxford: Blackwell, *Scientific Publications,* 1959.

Apley, J., and Hale, B. Children with recurrent abdominal pain: How do they grow up? *Br. Med. J.* July 7, 1973. P. 7.

Barr, R. G., Levine, M. D., and Watkins, J. B. Recurrent abdominal pain of childhood due to lactose intolerance. *N. Engl. J. Med.* 300:1449, 1979.

Grossman, E. B. Chronic appendicitis. *Surg. Gynecol. Obstet.* 146:596, 1978.

Leape, L. L. Laparoscopy for Abdominal Pain: Laparoscopy for Gynecologic Disorders in Childhood. In S. Gans (ed.), *Pediatric Endoscopy.* New York: Grune & Stratton, 1982. PP. 169, 173.

Leape, L. L., and Ramenofsky, M. L. Laparoscopy in infants and children. *J. Pediatr. Surg.* 12:929, 1977.

Leape, L. L., and Ramenofsky, M. L. Laparoscopy in children. *Pediatrics* 66:215, 1980.

Schisgall, R. M. Appendiceal colic in childhood: The role of inspissated casts of stool within the appendix. *Ann. Surg.* 192:687, 1980.

57 Pyloric Stenosis

I. **Definition.** Hypertrophic *pyloric stenosis* is a thickening of the pyloric muscle that develops in the first month or so of life in 1 in 500 infants. It is familial in 5–20% of patients, and boys are affected 4 times as frequently as girls.

II. **Pathophysiology.** The etiology of pyloric stenosis is unknown. Immature functioning of the pylorus delays gastric emptying, causing increased peristalsis, which results in work hypertrophy and edema of the pylorus. Vomiting develops as a result of obstruction of the gastric outlet. As the muscle thickening increases, vomiting becomes progressively more severe and occurs after each feeding. Loss of food leads to **malnutrition and weight loss;** loss of gastric juice produces **dehydration** and **hypochloremic, hypokalemic alkalosis.** Jaundice is sometimes present, thought to be the result of starvation-induced decrease in glucuronyl-transferase activity.

III. **Clinical presentation**

   A. **Nonbilious vomiting** is the cardinal symptom of pyloric stenosis. It usually progresses within a few days to the point that every feeding is brought up. Vomiting is typically described as "projectile," but it may also be regurgitant. It is rarely intermittent.

   B. **Decreased urine output** and **reduced frequency of bowel movements** result from reduced intake, as does **weight loss.** The baby is hungry and fretful.

   C. **Physical examination** reveals evidence of **dehydration** (dry mucous membranes, poor tissue turgor), but the infant is usually obviously hungry. **Malnutrition** is evident. The enlarged pylorus can be felt in the upper abdomen.

IV. **Diagnosis**

   A. The **diagnosis** of pyloric stenosis is made by **palpation** of the olive-sized thickened and **enlarged pylorus,** which can be accomplished in almost every patient.

      1. The abdomen must be **relaxed** (as occurs when the infant sucks on a nipple), and the examiner must be gentle, persistent, and patient.

      2. The **"olive"** is felt in the **midepigastrium,** just cephalad to the umbilicus, near the spine. It is **mobile** which distinguishes it from the spine, liver, or tumor.

      3. Passage of a nasogastric catheter and decompression or inflation of the stomach may facilitate palpation.

      4. If the "olive" is felt, no further diagnostic studies are needed.

   B. **Ultrasound** examination may identify pyloric stenosis if the examiner is unable to palpate it. The length of the pyloric shadow must be at least 1.2 cm and the thickness of the wall, 0.4 cm, to meet the diagnostic criteria.

   C. **Upper GI series** findings of pyloric stenosis are the "track" sign, elongation of the pyloric channel, "shoulder" indentation of the thickened muscle, and failure of gastric emptying. UGIS will also demonstrate or rule out other causes of vomiting (such as gastroesophageal reflux, which is much more common than pyloric stenosis).

V. **Problems**

   A. **Malnutrition; dehydration; and hypochloremic, hypokalemic alkalosis** are always present to some degree and may be profound if the vomiting has been long-standing.

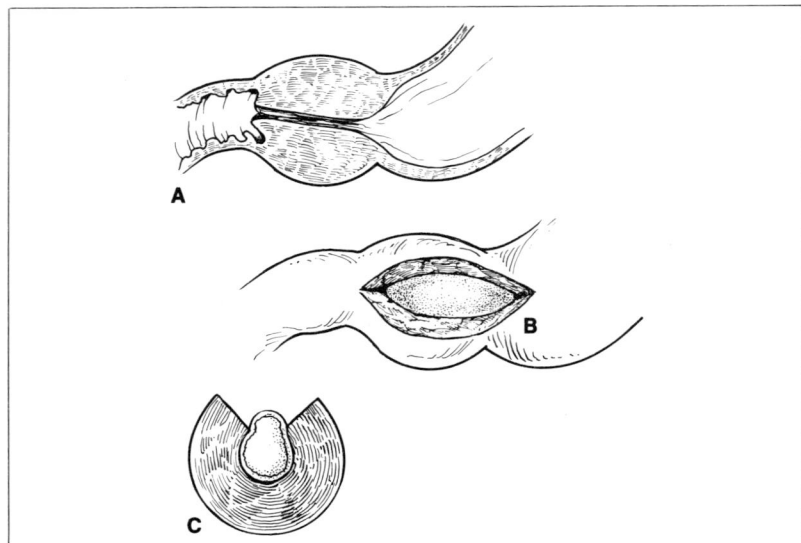

Fig. 57-1. Pyloric stenosis. A. Hypertrophied muscle constricting lumen at pylorus. B. Incision of muscle well up into stomach relieves obstruction. C. Cross section showing bulging of mucosa after myotomy.

- **B. Hematemesis** may result from gastritis caused by repeated vomiting and retching.
- **C. Jaundice** is seen in 5% of infants.

VI. **Indications for operation.** There is no effective medical treatent for pyloric stenosis. Demonstration of the enlarged pylorus by physical examination is the indication for operation. **A diagnosis based on positive ultrasound or barium study should always be confirmed by physical examination** since these studies have a measurable error rate.

VII. **Preoperative preparation**
- A. **Fluid and electrolyte balance must be corrected** before the operation; this can be accomplished in 12–24 hours in most infants.
- B. **Serum electrolytes** and bicarbonate are measured.
- C. Since pyloric obstruction is incomplete, **rehydration** and electrolyte replacement can be accomplished orally if the infant is not severely depleted and does not have gastritis. The infant is placed in a **chalasia chair** to facilitate gastric emptying. The **stomach is first emptied** of milk curds and barium by gavage with saline through a large (16F) catheter. Dextrose in half-normal saline is given, 60–90 ml every 2 hours.
- D. If vomiting persists or if there is severe dehydration, **electrolyte imbalance,** or **hematemesis,** the stomach is placed at rest by nasogastric tube, and fluid resuscitation is carried out by the **intravenous** route (5% D/1/2 NS, 200 ml/kg in 12–16 hours).

VIII. **Operative care** (Fig. 57-1)
- A. Pyloromyotomy is a simple operation with two specific technical **hazards: perforation** of the duodenum if the myotomy is extended too far distally, and **incomplete myotomy** if it is not extended sufficiently up onto the stomach wall.

B. After myotomy, air is introduced into the stomach by the anesthetist through the indwelling nasogastric tube and "milked" through the newly opened pylorus. If there is a perforation of the duodenal mucosa, air bubbles will leak out. A perforation must be closed but will heal readily.

X. Postoperative care. Feedings are **delayed for 8–12 hours** to allow return of gastric peristalsis. Electrolyte solution (Pedialyte) is given q2h, starting at 10 ml and doubling on alternate feedings if tolerated. Once full volumes are retained, half-strength and then full-strength formula or breast feedings may be commenced. The infant may then be discharged, usually on the second or third postoperative day. Vomiting once or twice a day for several days is seen in about half of infants following pyloromyotomy and is of no significance.

X. Complications

A. **Seizures, apnea, and cardiac arrest** have occurred from postoperative hypoglycemia in severely malnourished patients. Provision of adequate intravenous glucose until full feedings are resumed prevents this complication.

B. **Unrecognized perforation** of the duodenum can be disastrous, causing peritonitis. The diagnosis should be suspected if the infant shows any peritoneal signs, registers a fever, or rejects feedings. Contrast study will establish the diagnosis. Immediate reoperation for repair is necessary.

C. **Incomplete myotomy** results in unrelieved obstruction and persistent vomiting. At least a week should elapse before it is concluded that postoperative vomiting is pathologic. Barium study will reveal delayed or absent gastric emptying and the need for reoperation. The obstruction is usually at the gastric end.

D. **Recurrent pyloric stenosis** is exceedingly rare.

Prognosis. A normal life is expected.

Bibliography

Benson, C. O. Infantile Hypertrophic Pyloric Stenosis. In K. J. Welch, et al. (eds.), *Pediatric Surgery*. Chicago: Year Book, 1986. P. 811.

Blumhagen, J. D., and Noble, H. G. S. Muscle thickness in hypertrophic pyloric stenosis: Sonographic determination. *A.J.R.* 140:221, 1983.

Friesen, S. R., Boley, J. O., and Miller, D. R. The myenteric plexus of the pylorus: Its early normal development and its changes in hypertrophic pyloric stenosis. *Surgery* 39:21, 1956.

Henderson, B. M., et al. Hypoglycemia with hepatic glycogen depletion: A postoperative complication of pyloric stenosis. *J. Pediatr. Surg.* 3:309, 1968.

Hight, E. W., et al. Management of mucosal perforation during pyloromyotomy for infantile pyloric stenosis. *Surgery* 90:85, 1981.

Ravitch, M. M. The story of pyloric stenosis. *Surgery* 48:1117, 1960.

Scharli, A. F., and Leditschke, J. F. Gastric motility after pyloromyotomy in infants: A reappraisal of postoperative feeding. *Surgery* 64:113, 1968.

Scharli, A., Sieber, W. K., and Kiesewetter, W. B. Hypertrophic pyloric stenosis at the Children's Hospital of Pittsburgh from 1912 to 1967. *J. Pediatr. Surg.* 4:108, 1969.

Sieber, W. K. Gastric Outlet Obstructions. In T. M. Holder and K. W. Ashcraft (eds.), *Pediatric Surgery*. Philadelphia: Saunders, 1980. P. 313.

Woolley, M. M., et al. Jaundice, hypertrophic pyloric stenosis, and hepatic glucuronyl transferase. *J. Pediatr. Surg.* 9:359, 1974.

58 Gastrointestinal Bleeding

I. **Definition.** Gastrointestinal bleeding may range from massive to occult, result in circulatory collapse or be asymptomatic, and be continuous or intermittent. The cause may be difficult to determine.

II. **Clinical presentation.** The manner of presentation of bleeding is helpful in determining the source. **Massive** bleeding (more than one-half of the blood volume in 24 hours) is usually from the upper gastrointestinal tract (proximal to the jejunum) but can also occur in severe ulcerative colitis.

  A. **Hematemesis** indicates the bleeding source is in the upper gastrointestinal tract. Vomited blood may be fresh, clotted, or like **coffee-grounds** in appearance if altered by gastric acid.

  B. **Bright red rectal bleeding** results from anal and lower colon lesions. It is seldom massive.

  C. **Maroon, dark red, or "currant jelly"** stools indicate a colonic lesion or a source in the distal ileum such as a Meckel's diverticulum.

  D. **Tarry stools** results from bleeding from an upper gastrointestinal lesion such as peptic ulcer or esophageal varices.

  E. **Occult blood in stools** can result from a source of bleeding anywhere from the nasopharynx to the anus.

III. **Pathophysiology**

  A. **Massive gastrointestinal hemorrhage** causes profound hemodynamic effects.

   1. **Circulating blood volume** is rapidly depleted, causing hypotension, tachycardia, and poor tissue perfusion. If volume is not promptly replaced, these effects can be fatal.

   2. **Absorption of blood** from the intestine of a patient with liver failure can result in ammonia toxicity and coma from hepatic encephalopathy.

  B. **Chronic mild gastrointestinal bleeding** results in microcytic anemia. If the bleeding is occult, weakness, fatigue, and pallor may be the first effects recognized.

IV. **Differential diagnosis**

Type of Bleeding	Neonate	Toddler	Older child
Hematemesis or tarry stools (upper GI bleeding)	Gastritis Peptic ulcer Clotting disorder	Gastritis Peptic ulcer Clotting disorder Esophageal varices Nosebleeds	Gastritis Peptic ulcer Clotting disorder Esophageal varices Nosebleeds Mallory-Weiss tear
Bright red rectal bleeding in small amounts (lower GI bleeding)	Anal fissure Necrotizing enterocolitis (NEC)	Anal fissure Hemorrhoids Foreign body Rectal prolapse Colonic polyp	Anal fissure Hemorrhoids Foreign body Colonic polyp

Maroon, dark red, or "currant jelly" stools (lower GI bleeding)	NEC
	
	Hirschsprung's enterocolitis
	Duplication
		Intussusception
		Meckel's diverticulum
		Volvulus
		Hirschsprung's enterocolitis
		Duplication
		Colonic polyp
		Enterocolitis
		  Bacterial
		  Pseudomembranous
		  Radiation
			Meckel's diverticulum
			
			Duplication
			Colonic polyp
			Enterocolitis
			  Bacterial
			  Pseudomembranous
			  Radiation
			Ulcerative colitis
			Crohn's disease

Occult bleeding (upper or lower GI bleeding)	Swallowed maternal blood Gastritis Peptic ulcer Clotting disorder Hemangioma Duplication Formula intolerance NEC	Esophagitis Gastritis Peptic ulcer Clotting disorder Hemangioma Duplication Milk allergy Esophageal varices Colonic polyp Meckel's diverticulum Foreign body Nosebleeds Amebiasis	Esophagitis Gastritis Peptic ulcer Clotting disorder Hemangioma Duplication Milk allergy Esophageal varices Colonic polyp Meckel's diverticulum Foreign body Nosebleeds Amebiasis Ulcerative colitis Crohn's disease

V. **Diagnosis.** Determining the source of gastrointestinal bleeding, especially if it is occult, may tax the most experienced clinician. An orderly approach is helpful. The age of the patient limits the possibilities, as does the nature and rate of the bleeding. **Urgency** of evaluation depends on the rate of bleeding and its clinical effect (anemia, hypotension, weakness, pallor).

  A. **First,** the presence of **blood** in the vomitus or stool must be verified. Many ingested or passed substances resemble blood, "coffee grounds," or "tarry stools." A positive guaiac test is essential before embarking on an extensive workup.

  B. **Massive gastrointestinal bleeding** requires prompt diagnosis and treatment. (See sec. **VI**). If there has been no hematemesis, a nasogastric tube is passed and the aspirate is tested for blood to detect an upper gastrointestinal source. Further emergency diagnostic procedures depend on the presumed site of bleeding.

  C. A **history** of easy bruising or bleeding with minor operations suggests a clotting disorder. Painful defecation suggests the most common cause of red rectal bleeding: anal fissure. A family history of polyps or inflammatory bowel disease is relevant. Foreign travel raises the question of amebiasis.

  D. **Physical examination** is most helpful in lower gastrointestinal bleeding. Anal malformations and rectal polyps are easily detected. Portal hypertension is suggested by the presence of dilated abdominal wall veins, "spiders," ascites, or hepatosplenomegaly. Cutaneous hemangiomas or telangiectasia suggest, but do not establish, a similar internal lesion. Buccal pigmentation suggests Peutz-

Jeghers syndrome, and sebaceous cysts suggest Gardner's syndrome. Unsuspected bleeding from the nose may be noted on physical examination.
- **E. Laboratory studies** include as a minimum:
    1. CBC
    2. Platelet count
    3. Bleeding time
    4. Prothrombin time
    5. Partial thromboplastin time
    6. An **Apt test** on specimens from a neonate to exclude the possibility of swallowed maternal blood
- **F. Contrast x-rays** are indicated in most patients with significant or unexplained gastrointestinal bleeding. If there is no clear evidence pointing to an upper or lower site, obtain a barium enema first.
- **G. Endoscopy** is helpful in most patients with gastrointestinal bleeding. Biopsy will often establish a diagnosis.
    1. Esophagogastroduodenoscopy is the most reliable method for identifying an upper gastrointestinal source of bleeding. In patients with massive bleeding, it should precede contrast x-rays.
    2. Sigmoidoscopy or colonoscopy is indicated in unexplained lower gastrointestinal bleeding.

Management of massive gastrointestinal bleeding

- **A. Resuscitation takes precedence over diagnosis** if the patient is in shock.
    1. **First, establish a large-bore reliable intravenous** line. Place a catheter in the antecubital or saphenous vein; perform cutdown if necessary. Send a blood specimen for emergency **type and cross-match.**
    2. **Infuse lactated Ringer's** solution or normal saline rapidly to restore blood volume while blood is being cross-matched. O-negative blood should be used only if the hematocrit is very low and the patient responds slowly.
        a. **Bolus infusion** is the best way to assess the extent of the deficit and to correct it promptly. For shock to occur, blood volume must be contracted by at least 25%. This amount (20 ml/kg) can be safely given as rapidly as possible.
        b. A **repeat bolus** should be given if pulse and blood pressure do not respond. If only crystalloid is given, 2–3 times the deficit will be required.
    3. **Place a central venous catheter** to monitor the infusion rate and prevent overload.
    4. **Transfuse** packed cells and fresh frozen plasma as soon as available to restore the blood volume and the hematocrit to normal. Half of the calculated amount should be given as quickly as necessary to normalize pulse and blood pressure. The remainder is given over 4–6 hours.
- **B.** Insert a **nasogastric tube** and put to suction.
- **C. Monitor** pulse, blood pressure, central venous pressure, urine output, hematocrit, and blood loss.
- **D. Endoscopy** is the quickest and most reliable way to establish the diagnosis in acute bleeding. It should be performed as soon as the patient is stable. In obscure cases, **angiography** may be necessary to localize the bleeding source.
- **E. Treat** massive gastrointestinal bleeding according to the diagnosis.

1. **Acid-peptic disease: Gastric lavage** with iced saline will usually stop the bleeding. **Cimetidine** (10 mg/kg q4h IV) blocks acid production. Measure gastric pH hourly and give **aluminum hydroxide antacid** by nasogastric tube as necessary to keep pH above 5.
2. **Esophageal varices.** Give vasopressin **(Pitressin),** .005 µ/kg/minute IV. Use balloon tamponade if bleeding persists.
3. **Lower gastrointestinal bleeding.** Order bowel rest and high doses of steroids (**prednisone,** 1 mg/kg q6h) if the diagnosis is inflammatory bowel disease.
4. **Uncontrolled bleeding** from any source is an indication for operative treatment.

VII. **Management of rectal bleeding.** Passage of small amounts of red blood with the stool is commonly encountered in pediatric practice.
   A. **First, document** the presence of blood by guaiac test of the stool. Measure hemoglobin to assess severity of bleeding.
   B. **Anal fissure** (common), **hemorrhoids** (rare), and **rectal polyps** can be seen or felt on anorectal examination.
   C. **Barium enema** and **sigmoidoscopy** with biopsy are indicated if physical examination is negative.

VIII. **Management of occult gastrointestinal bleeding**
   A. **Etiology.** Any disease that causes gastrointestinal bleeding can produce occult bleeding. The most common are:
      1. Reflux esophagitis
      2. Inflammatory bowel disease
      3. Milk allergy
   B. **Symptoms** relate to the underlying cause, but in some patients anemia is the only finding.
   C. **Diagnosis.** Order upper and lower gastrointestinal contrast x-rays and endoscopy. If all studies are negative, a trial of a milk-free diet is indicated.

IX. **Management of the problem bleeder**
   A. **Definition.** *Problem bleeding* is persistent or recurrent bleeding, sufficient to require periodic transfusion, for which no cause is found by routine x-ray and endoscopic studies.
   B. **Additional diagnostic studies**
      1. Meckel scan (^{99}Tc pertechnetate)
      2. Angiography
   C. **Operative examination** of the intestine by endoscopy guided through the small bowel at laparotomy may be the only way to find the site of bleeding and correct it.

X. **Operative care.** Most patients with gastrointestinal bleeding do not require operative treatment. Details of operative and perioperative care are found in the sections on the specific diseases.

Bibliography

Arensman, R. M. Gastrointestinal Bleeding. In K. J. Welch, et al. (eds.), *Pediatric Surgery*. Chicago: Year Book, 1986. P. 904.

Chang, M., et al. Endoscopic examination of the upper gastrointestinal tract in infancy. *Gastrointest. Endosc.* 29:15, 1983.
Cox, K., and Ament, M. E. Upper gastrointestinal bleeding in children and adolescents. *Pediatrics* 63:408, 1979.
Holcomb, G. W. Gastrointestinal Bleeding. In T. M. Holder and K. W. Ashcraft (eds.), *Pediatric Surgery*. Philadelphia: Saunders, 1980. P. 433.
Holgersen, L. O., Mossberg, S. M., and Miller, R. E. Colonoscopy for rectal bleeding in childhood. *J. Pediatr. Surg.* 13:83, 1978.
Raffensperger, J. G., and Luck, S. R. Gastrointestinal bleeding in children. *Surg. Clin. North Am.* 56:413, 1976.
Sfakianakis, G. N., and Haase, G. M. Abdominal scintigraphy for ectopic gastric mucosa: A retrospective analysis of 143 studies. *A.J.R.* 138:7, 1982.
Sherman, N. J., and Clatworthy, H. W., Jr. Gastrointestinal bleeding in neonates: A study of 94 cases. *Surgery* 62:614, 1967.
Spencer, R. Gastrointestinal hemorrhage in infancy and childhood: 476 cases *Pediatr. Surg.* 55:718, 1964.

59   Peptic Ulcer

I. **Definition.** Ulceration of the duodenum, stomach, or esophagus can occur as a result of acid-peptic digestion by gastric juice. A lesser degree of injury results in esophagitis, gastritis, or duodenitis which can cause similar symptoms and complications (see Chap. 52 for discussion of esophagitis).

II. **Pathophysiology**
   A. Normally, the gastric mucosa is resistant to its own secretions, and the duodenum is protected by its highly alkaline secretions. Under a variety of conditions, but particularly physical or emotional stress, acid secretion increases, the mucosal barrier breaks down, and chemical inflammation results.
   B. **Stress ulcers** are most likely to occur when there is **increased intracranial pressure, a major burn, a massive injury, or life-threatening illness.**
   C. The mucosal barrier is also injured by **salicylates, corticosteroids,** and other drugs.

III. **Clinical presentation**
   A. **Pain** is the most common symptom. It is **epigastric** in location, with both duodenal and gastric lesions. The pain of inflammation is not distinguishable from that of ulceration. Pain comes on at times of maximal gastric acid production—before and after meals and at night—although it can occur anytime. **Acid-peptic disease is a major cause of chronic abdominal pain in children.**
   B. **Bleeding** from peptic ulcer or gastritis can vary from occult and minor to massive and life-threatening. It is usually painless. Massive bleeding results from ulceration into an artery but is also seen in severe diffuse gastritis. **Hematemesis** or **melena** results from massive bleeding. Minor bleeding is usually asymptomatic unless **anemia** results.
   C. **Perforation** of a gastric or duodenal ulcer can occur at any age, including the neonatal period. It is typically unheralded by pain or bleeding. Stress is the common proximal cause.
   D. **Obstruction** by a duodenal or pyloric ulcer is rare in childhood.

IV. **Diagnosis**
   A. **If perforation** is suspected, an upright film of the abdomen is obtained. If free air is demonstrated, no further studies are needed.
   B. **Upper gastrointestinal series** is performed in elective cases, in which symptoms are not life-threatening. Ulceration can be seen, but gastritis and duodenitis cannot be detected by x-ray. Duodenal irritability and pylorospasm suggest inflammation, however.
   C. **Endoscopy** permits more accurate evaluation of the disease and should be performed in any patient who has massive bleeding or persistent symptoms, or in whom the diagnosis is in doubt.

V. **Medical treatment.** Few children with acid-peptic disease require surgical therapy.
   A. **Cimetidine** is the drug of choice, given qid, 10mg/kg/dose, for a full 6 weeks to ensure complete healing. Patients with refractory ulcer may benefit from an aluminum hydroxide preparation (Mylanta, Gelusil, Maalox).
   B. **Dietary therapy** is of little value, difficult to endure, and not necessary. However, foods that cause symptoms are avoided.

VI. Indications for operation
   A. **Uncontrolled bleeding**
   B. **Perforation**
   C. **Refractory or recurrent pain**
   D. **Obstruction**

VII. **Preoperative preparation.** Routine. In patients with massive uncontrolled bleeding or perforation, the blood volume must be replaced before anesthesia is induced if possible.

VIII. **Operative care.** For acute perforation or bleeding, oversewing of the ulcer is all that is necessary. Patients with a long history of ulcer disease may require pyloroplasty and vagotomy. Gastric resection is seldom necessary.

IX. **Postoperative care.** Intensive care is needed for patients with perforation or life-threatening hemorrhage until they are stable. Feedings may be resumed once the postoperative ileus has subsided.

X. **Complications.** Bleeding, infection, and disruption of suture lines are more common in patients operated on in extremis. Pyloroplasty and vagotomy are generally well-tolerated by children. The dumping syndrome is rare.

XI. **Prognosis.** Fewer than 10% of patients have recurrent symptoms after operative treatment for acid-peptic disease.

Bibliography

Agunod, M., et al. Correlative study of hydrochloric acid, pepsin and intrinsic factor secretion in newborns and infants. *Am. J. Dig. Dis.* 14:400, 1969.

Bell, M. J., et al. Perforated stress ulcers in infants. *J. Pediatr. Surg.* 16:998, 1981.

Boley, S. J., et al. The effect of operations for peptic ulcer on growth and nutrition of puppies. *Surgery* 57:441, 1965.

Chattriwalla, Y., Colon, A. R., and Scanlon, J. W. The use of cimetidine in the newborn. *Pediatrics* 65:301, 1980.

Christie, D. L., and Ament, M. E. Diagnosis and treatment of duodenal ulcer in infancy and childhood. *Pediatr. Ann.* 5:673, 1976.

Grosfeld, J. L., et al. Acute peptic ulcer in infancy and childhood. *Am. Surg.* 44:13, 1978.

Habbick, B. F., Melrose, A. G., and Grant, J. C. Duodenal ulcer in childhood: A study of predisposing factors. *Arch. Dis. Child.* 43:23, 1968.

Johnson, D., L'Heureux, P., and Thompson, T. Peptic ulcer disease in early infancy: Clinical presentation and roentgenographic features. *Acta Paediatr. Scand.* 69:753, 1980.

Morden, R. S., et al. Operative management of stress ulcers in children. *Ann. Surg.* 196:18, 1982.

Nesser, J., et al. Association of adrenocorticosteroid therapy and peptic ulcer disease. *N. Engl. J. Med.* 309:21, 1983.

O'Neill, J. A., Jr., Pruitt, B. A., Jr., and Moncrief, J. A. Surgical treatment of Curling's ulcer. *Surg. Gynecol. Obstet.* 126:40, 1968.

Puri, P., et al. Duodenal ulcer in childhood: A continuing disease in adult life. *J. Pediatr. Surg.* 13:525, 1978.

Raffensperger, J. G., Condon, J. B., and Greengard, J. Complications of gastric and duodenal ulcers in infancy and childhood. *Surg. Gynecol. Obstet.* 122:1269, 1966.

Sieber, W. K. The Stomach. In T. M. Holder and K. W. Ashcraft (eds.), *Pediatric Surgery.* Philadelphia: Saunders, 1980. P. 313.

Ternberg, J. L. Peptic Ulcer: Acute and Chronic. In K. J. Welch, et al. (eds.), *Pediatric Surgery.* Chicago: Year Book, 1986. P. 815.

Wilson, S. D. The role of surgery in children with the Zollinger-Ellison syndrome. *Surgery* 92:682, 1982.

60. Meckel's Diverticulum

Definition. *Meckel's diverticulum* is a remnant of the vitelline duct, an outpouching on the antimesenteric border of the ileum in the distal third, which is sometimes attached to the umbilicus. It is found in 1–2% of the population. Males are affected 3 times as frequently as females.

Pathophysiology

A. **Ectopic gastric mucosa** is found in **50%** of Meckel's diverticula. Secretion of acid-peptic juice can result in **ulceration** of the adjacent ileal mucosa producing pain, bleeding, or perforation.

B. **Inflammation** (diverticulitis) may result from obstruction and bacterial overgrowth or from ulceration caused by ectopic gastric mucosa.

C. **Fibrous attachments** of the diverticulum to the umbilicus are sometimes present, permitting volvulus of a loop of intestine around the band with resulting intestinal obstruction.

D. Meckel's diverticulum can act as a **lead point** causing **intussusception.**

Clinical presentation.
In most patients, Meckel's diverticulum is silent, causing no complications and no symptoms. When complications occur, pain and bleeding are common symptoms (Fig. 60-1). Half of symptomatic patients are **under 2 years** of age.

A. **Abdominal pain** may be caused by obstruction or inflammation.
  1. **Intussusception** of a Meckel's diverticulum results in crampy abdominal pain, distention, vomiting, and passage of "currant jelly" stools.
  2. **Volvulus** of a loop of intestine around a band connecting the Meckel's diverticulum to the umbilicus produces typical symptoms of intestinal obstruction. The diagnosis is made at operation.
  3. **Diverticulitis** in a Meckel's diverticulum is clinically indistinguishable from appendicitis. Pain is initially umbilical, and later, in the lower abdomen.
  4. **Perforation** of an ulcer caused by Meckel's diverticulum is rare. As in diverticulitis, the symptoms are usually ascribed to appendicitis and the real cause is only discovered at operation.

B. **Lower gastrointestinal bleeding** from an ulcer caused by Meckel's diverticulum is typically **painless,** moderate-to-massive in amount, episodic, and burgundy-to-red in color. Signs of colitis (diarrhea, cramping, mucus) are absent.

Diagnosis

A. **Laboratory tests are usually negative** in patients with symptomatic Meckel's diverticulum. In most patients, the diagnosis must be made on clinical grounds. Fortunately, there are few other causes of episodic massive rectal bleeding in young children.

B. **Contrast x-rays** (small bowel series) seldom reveal a Meckel's diverticulum.

C. **Technetium 99 pertechnetate isotope scan** will demonstrate a Meckel's diverticulum if there is at least 2 cm^2 of gastric mucosa. It is negative in about half of symptomatic patients; a negative scan, therefore, does not rule out the disease.

Indications for operation

A. **A positive isotope scan** in a symptomatic patient

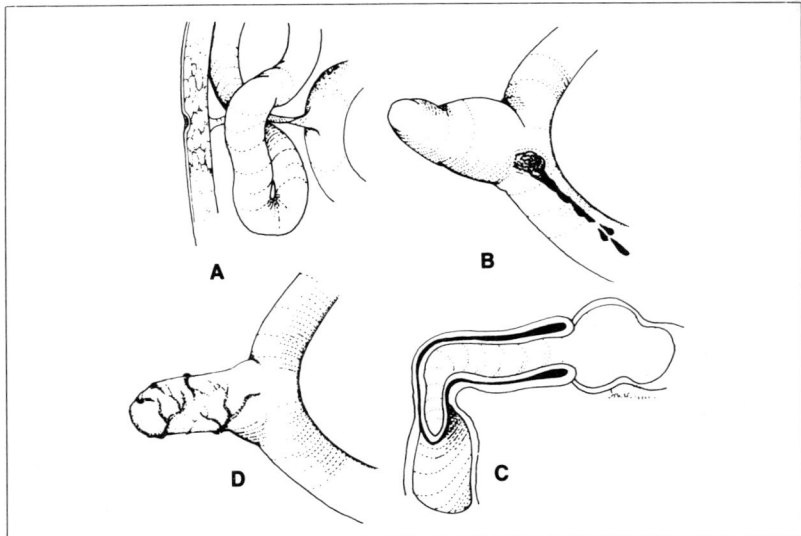

Fig. 60-1. Complications of Meckel's diverticulum. A. Intestinal obstruction due to volvulus of intestine at the attachment to the umbilicus. B. Bleeding from ulcer due to acid secretion from ectopic gastric mucosa. C. Intussusception caused by the diverticulum acting as a lead point. D. Diverticulitis.

- B. **A second episode of** moderate-to-massive **rectal bleeding** in an otherwise asymptomatic patient with normal sigmoidoscopy and barium enema examinations
- C. **Intestinal obstruction**
- D. **Signs of inflammation mimicking appendicitis**

VI. **Preoperative preparation**
- A. **Transfusion** as necessary to restore blood volume if bleeding has been massive
- B. **Correction of fluid and electrolyte deficits** in patients with intestinal obstruction

VII. **Operative care.** The diverticulum is resected with a small amount of adjacent normal ileum and the ulcer if one is present.

VIII. **Postoperative care.** Routine. Feedings can usually be resumed in 2 or 3 days.

IX. **Complications.** Rare. Those of laparotomy and intestinal resection.

X. **Prognosis.** Excellent. Resection is curative.

Bibliography

Amoury, R. A. Meckel's Diverticulum. In K. J. Welch, et al. (eds.), *Pediatric Surgery*. Chicago: Year Book, 1986. P. 859.

Berquist, T. H., et al. Specificity of 99m Te-pertechnetate in scintigraphic diagnosis of Meckel's diverticulum: Review of 100 cases. *J. Nucl. Med.* 17:465, 1976.

Canty, T., Meguid, M. M., and Eraklis, A. J. Perforation of Meckel's diverticulum in infancy. *J. Pediatr. Surg.* 10:189, 1975.

Cooney, D. R., et al. The abdominal technetium scan. *J. Pediatr. Surg.* 17:611, 1982.

DeBartolo, H. M., and van Heerden, J. A. Meckel's diverticulum. *Ann. Surg.* 183:30, 1976.

Jewett, T. C., Jr., Duszynski, D. O., and Allen, J. E. The visualization of Meckel's diverticulum with 99m Te-pertechnetate. *Surgery* 68:567, 1970.

Meguid, M., Canty, T., and Eraklis, A. J. Complications of Meckel's diverticulum in infants. *Surg. Gynecol. Obstet.* 139:541, 1974.

Seagram, C. G. F., et al. Meckel's diverticulum: A 10-year review of 218 cases. *Can. J. Surg.* 11:369, 1968.

Soltero, M. J., and Bill, A. H. The natural history of Meckel's diverticulum and its relation to incidental removal. *Am. J. Surg.* 132:168, 1976.

Tunell, W. P. Meckel's Diverticulum. In T. M. Holder and K. W. Ashcraft (eds.), *Pediatric Surgery*. Philadelphia: Saunders, 1980. P. 457.

61 Gastrointestinal Duplications

I. **Definition.** The term *duplication* applies to cystic or tubular structures that are lined with enteric mucosa, have a smooth muscle wall, and share a common blood supply. Duplications typically connect to the adjacent gut through the lumen or by a common muscle wall. They are found from the mouth to the anus. Multiple duplications may occur in one patient.

II. **Pathophysiology.** Expansion of the duplication and secretion of gastric juice account for most of the pathologic effects of duplications.

  A. **Expansion.** Most duplications have a lumen that is closed, or nearly closed. Continuous secretion by the lining mucosa leads inexorably to progressive enlargement. The expanding cystic mass compresses the neighboring gut, producing obstruction.

  B. **Ectopic gastric mucosa** is frequently found in duplications. Secretion of acid-peptic juice ulcerates the adjacent nongastric mucosa causing inflammation, pain, bleeding, or perforation.

III. **Clinical presentation**

  A. **Cervical.** A smooth, firm, somewhat cystic mass lateral in the neck, larger than an inflamed lymph node, deep to the muscles. Dysphagia may be present.

  B. **Mediastinal.** A discrete, round, asymptomatic posterior mediastinal mass discovered on chest x-ray. Large duplication cysts can cause dysphagia or respiratory distress. Spina bifida, hemivertebrae, or meningocele may be present.

  C. **Thoracoabdominal.** Some upper intestinal duplications communicate as long diverticula into the chest, passing behind the stomach and pancreas and through the esophageal hiatus. These often present as gastrointestinal bleeding or intraabdominal catastrophes.

  D. **Gastric.** Prepyloric duplications produce obstruction with vomiting. In other locations abdominal distention or a palpable mass may be the only evidence of a gastric duplication.

  E. **Duodenal.** Obstructive symptoms are the usual presenting complaint. Pyloric stenosis may be suspected. Ectopic gastric mucosa may cause perforation into the peritoneal cavity or pancreas, resulting in peritonitis or pancreatitis.

  F. **Jejunoileal.** An asymptomatic, movable mass in the abdomen is the most common presenting finding. **Cysts** may grow to a huge size without causing obstruction. Volvulus or intussusception may occur, however. **Tubular** duplications communicate with the intestinal lumen and can be as long as the entire intestine. Duplications with only a proximal communication may dilate massively; those with only a distal communication may be smaller than the normal intestine. Ectopic gastric mucosa may cause bleeding or perforation.

  G. **Colonic.** Findings and symptoms are similar to those of jejunoileal duplications.

  H. **Rectal.** Retrorectal duplications typically produce obstruction early in life if they are cystic, but they may be asymptomatic if there is an adequate distal communication. Hindgut duplication (distal ileum to anus) may drain normally through the anus or may be associated with imperforate anus. Duplication of the external genitalia or bladder may accompany this malformation.

Diagnosis. Duplication must be considered when a mass is found adjacent to the intestinal tract at any level and in the differential diagnosis of gastrointestinal bleeding. **CT** or **MRI** will demonstrate the cyst and its intimate association with the gut. Further studies are seldom helpful.

V. **Indications for operation.** The presence of a mass or obstruction is an indication for operative treatment.

VI. **Preoperative preparation.** Routine

VII. **Operative care**

   A. **Cystic duplications** are usually easily excised. If the cyst is in the mesentery of the intestine, a segmental excision of the adjacent normal bowel may be necessary.

   B. **Tubular duplications** pose a problem if they are long. Because they arise on the mesenteric side of the intestine, they cannot be removed without interfering with the blood supply to the normal bowel. An alternative is **mucosal stripping** of the mucosa of the duplication with retention of the common muscle wall. The stripping procedure is preferred to side-to-side anastomosis in duplication of the small intestine because ectopic gastric mucosa is usually present.

   C. **Thoracoabdominal** duplications require a thoracoabdominal incision and complete excision of the diverticular structure.

   D. **Gastric** and **duodenal** duplications may require marsupialization into neighboring duodenum to protect biliary and pancreatic drainage.

   E. **Rectal** duplications seldom contain gastric mucosa and therefore can be treated by creating a common lumen distally, similar to the Duhamel procedure for Hirschsprung's disease. Excision is dangerous and difficult.

VIII. **Postoperative care.** Routine

IX. **Complications.** Anastomotic leaks, bleeding, and infection may occur as after any intestinal resection. If marsupialization or side-to-side anastomosis is performed instead of resection and gastric mucosa is retained, bleeding or perforation may later result.

X. **Prognosis.** Excellent. Most patients have no sequelae.

Bibliography

Abrami, G., and Dennison, W. M. Duplication of the stomach. *Surgery* 49:794, 1961.

Ackerman, N. B. Duodenal duplication cysts: Diagnosis and operative management. *Surgery* 76:330, 1974.

Bower, R. J., Sieber, W. K., and Kiesewetter, W. B. Alimentary tract duplications in children. *Ann. Surg.* 188:669, 1978.

Moccia, W. A., Astacio, J. E., and Kaude, J. V. Ultrasonographic demonstration of gastric duplication in infancy. *Pediatr. Radiol.* 11:52, 1981.

Newmark, H., et al. Bleeding peptic ulcer caused by ectopic gastric mucosa in a duplicated segment of jejunum. *Am. J. Gastroenterol.* 75:158, 1981.

Ravitch. M. M. Duplications of the Gastrointestinal Tract. In K. J. Welch, et al. (eds.), *Pediatric Surgery*. Chicago: Year Book, 1986. P. 911.

Soper, R. T. Tubular duplication of the colon and distal ileum. *Surgery* 63:998, 1968.

Stockman, J. M., Young, V. T., and Jenkins, A. L. Duplication of the rectum containing gastric mucosa, *J.A.M.A.* 173:1223, 1960.

Teele, R. L., Henschke, C. I., and Tapper, D. The radiographic and ultrasonic evaluation of enteric duplication cysts. *Pediatr. Radiol.* 10:9, 1980.

Wrenn, E. L., Jr. Alimentary Tract Duplications. In T. M. Holder and K. W. Ashcraft (eds.), *Pediatric Surgery*. Philadelphia: Saunders, 1980. P. 445.

62 Intussusception

Definition. *Intussusception* is the telescoping of the intestine into itself. The common form is the terminal ileum into the colon, but colocolic and ileoileal intussusception may also occur.

Pathophysiology

A. **"Idiopathic" intussusception** is the typical form seen in infants. Hypertrophy of **lymphoid tissue** (Peyer's patches) is probably the cause of the intussusception in the majority of patients.
   1. Idiopathic intussusception typically follows an episode of gastroenteritis or an upper respiratory infection.
   2. Adenovirus can be cultured from the stool of half the patients with idiopathic intussusception.

B. **"Lead point" intussusception** is the common form in older children, but it is seen in only 5% of infants. Lesions that may cause intussusception include Meckel's diverticulum, intestinal polyp, hematoma from Henoch-Schönlein purpura or trauma, lymphoma, foreign bodies, and duplication. The abnormal stool in cystic fibrosis may result in intussusception.

C. **Postoperative intussusception** can occur after any abdominal or thoracic operation. Disordered motility is the presumed cause since no lead point is found.

D. Intussusception is almost invariably **progressive,** resulting in swelling of the intussusceptum, edema of the bowel, and obstruction of the venous outflow, causing the following:
   1. **Intestinal obstruction** with dilatation of the bowel and fluid loss into the gut wall, lumen, and peritoneal cavity
   2. **Bleeding** from congested mucosal veins
   3. **Infarction** if the strangulation is not promptly relieved

Clinical presentation. Idiopathic intussusception is a disease of infancy. Nearly 50% of instances occur in the **second 6 months of life,** and 85% by age 2 years. Lead point intussusception can occur at any age.

A. Typically the infant is **healthy** and **well-nourished** but may recently have had an episode of gastroenteritis or a respiratory infection.

B. **Intermittent pain** is the system that is most likely to bring the child to the doctor. He cries out and pulls his legs up in an episode lasting from 20 seconds to several minutes and then seems well. The spells are repeated at varying intervals up to an hour or two. Occasionally, intussusception is painless.

C. **Vomiting** occurs in about 90% of patients, sometimes with abdominal distention, followed by mucousy bloody **(currant jelly) stools** in 50%.

D. **Physical examination** reveals an infant who is fussy, in pain, sick and inconsolable during attacks but apparently well and quiet in between. He may be somewhat dehydrated.
   1. **A sausage-shaped mass** is palpable in the right upper quadrant in the majority of infants with intussusception.
   2. **Rectal** examination may reveal bloody mucus and may be the best way to palpate the mass.

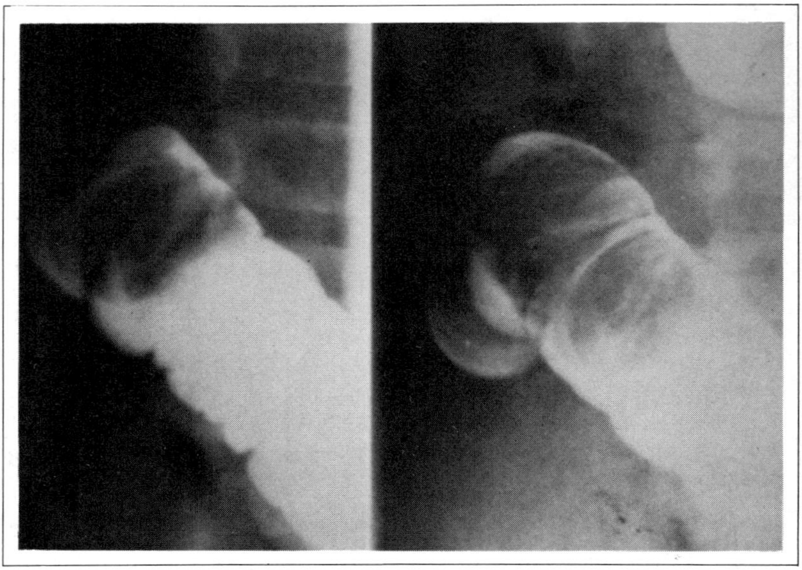

Fig. 62-1. Intussusception. Barium enema shows typical "coiled spring" appearance of reducing intussusceptum. (From L. L. Leape and T. M. Holder, Pediatric Surgery. In D. C. Sabiston (Ed.), *Textbook of Surgery*. Philadelphia: Saunders, 1981.

      3. Prolapse of the intussusceptum out the anus may occur; it is frequently mistaken for rectal prolapse (which is painless).

      4. Abdominal distention is present if there is significant intestinal obstruction.

      5. Dehydration, listlessness, and shock develop if the intussusception is not promptly diagnosed and treated.

   E. White blood count may be elevated to 20,000 or more, with a left shift.

   F. Intussusception in **older children** is frequently indistinguishable from other forms of intestinal obstruction.

   G. Postoperative intussusception occurs on the second to fifth day and is usually painless. It should be suspected when nasogastric drainage is unusually large and getting worse without apparent cause.

IV. Diagnosis

   A. Barium enema is the definitive diagnostic study for intussusception (Fig. 62-1). It is obtained unless the infant is in shock or there is evidence of perforation or intestinal gangrene.

      1. Barium enema should also be obtained in any infant with episodic pain of unknown etiology or mucousy bloody stools.

      2. Hydrostatic reduction of intussusception is accomplished with barium enema in over 50% of patients, so the diagnosis and treatment are carried out simultaneously.

   B. Ileoileal intussusception may not be diagnosed by barium enema. Signs of intestinal obstruction lead to the decision to operate.

V. Problems

- **A. The neglected child** who is toxic, dehydrated, and in shock because of intestinal obstruction and intestinal infarction.
- **B. The well child with intermittent pain** that is not localized. If there is any possibility of intussusception, barium enema should be obtained.
- **C. Prolapsed intussusception,** which can be mistaken for harmless rectal prolapse. In intussusception, but not in prolapse, the examining finger or a throat stick can be inserted into the rectum alongside the prolapsed bowel.

VI. Nonoperative treatment.
Barium enema (hydrostatic) reduction is successful in the majority of infants with idiopathic intussusception. It usually will not reduce a lead point intussusception.

- **A. The likelihood of success** of hydrostatic reduction is inversely related to the duration and severity of symptoms.
- **B. Contraindications.** Shock or sepsis, massive intestinal dilatation, peritonitis, perforation, intestinal gangrene.
- **C. Barium enema is ineffective** in the treatment of **ileoileal** intussusception.
- **D. Procedure.** Barium enema reduction of intussusception is a potentially hazardous procedure; **intestinal perforation** can result if it is not properly performed.
    1. The infant must be well-hydrated and stable. IV rehydration may be necessary before the study is done.
    2. The surgeon should be present.
    3. Hydrostatic pressure should be limited to 42 in. (106 cm).
    4. Manual pressure on the abdomen must not be used to reduce the intussusception.
    5. Continuous hydrostatic pressure is maintained as long as there is evidence of progression of reduction.
    6. Reduction is not considered successful unless barium is seen to reflux into the terminal ileum.
- **E.** A **repeat enema** is performed if the first attempt is unsuccessful.
- **F.** The infant shows **immediate clinical improvement** once the intussusception is reduced. The mass disappears.
- **G.** After successful reduction, the baby is **kept NPO,** given IV fluids, and observed **in the hospital overnight.**

VII. Indications for operation.
All patients with complications or intussusception that cannot be reduced by barium enema require emergency operation.

VIII. Preoperative preparation

- **A. Resuscitation** is necessary if the infant is in shock or dehydrated. Even apparently well patients benefit from preoperative fluid administration because of losses into the trapped gut.
- **B. A nasogastric tube** is inserted and placed on suction.
- **C. Antibiotics** are given if there is evidence of sepsis, perforation, peritonitis, or intestinal gangrene.

IX. Operative care

- **A. Manual reduction** of intussusception is performed by taxis (pressure and squeezing) of the proximal bowel, **not by traction.**

B. **Intestinal resection** and anastomosis is indicated if the intussusception is irreducible or if there is gangrene or perforation. Exteriorization or ileostomy is indicated if the infant is in extremis (rare).
   C. The reduced insussusception is carefully **examined for viability** and for a **lead point** (which must be resected).
X. **Postoperative care.** Routine
XI. **Complications.** If infarcted bowel is not resected, acidosis, toxicity, and intestinal perforation may occur.
XII. **Prognosis.** The risk of recurrent intussusception is 5% following hydrostatic reduction and 2% after surgical reduction. The risks of subsequent recurrences are about the same.

Bibliography

Beck, A. R., and Leichtling, J. J. Intussusception in Henoch-Schoenlein's purpura. *Mt. Sinai J. Med.* 39:397, 1972.
Bower, R. J., and Kiesewetter, W. B. Colo-colic intussusception due to a hemangioma. *J. Pediatr. Surg.* 12:777, 1977.
Brown, P. M., and Thronfeldt, R. Intussusception in the early postoperative period. *Am. J. Dis. Child.* 107:297, 1964.
Ein, S. H. Recurrent intussusception in children. *J. Pediatr. Surg.* 10:75, 1975.
Ein, S. H., and Stephens, C. A. Intussusception: 354 cases in 10 years. *J. Pediatr. Surg.* 6:16, 1971.
Ein, S. H., et al. Colon perforation during attempted barium enema reduction of intussusception. *J. Pediatr. Surg.* 16:313, 1981.
Hoy, G. R., Dunbar, D., and Boles, E. T., Jr. The use of glucagon in the diagnosis and management of ileocolic intussusception. *J. Pediatr. Surg.* 12:939, 1977.
Konno, T., et al. Human rotavirus infection in infants and young children with intussusception. *J. Med. Virol.* 2:265, 1978.
Lynn, H. B. Intussusception. In T. M. Holder and K. W. Ashcraft (eds.), *Pediatric Surgery*. Philadelphia: Saunders, 1980. P. 438.
Mollitt, D. L., Ballantine, T. V. N., and Grosfeld, J. L. Postoperative intussusception in infancy and childhood: Analysis of 119 cases. *Surgery* 86:402, 1979.
Mulcahy, D. L., et al. A two-part study of the aetiological role of rotavirus in intussusception. *J. Med. Virol.* 9:51, 1982.
Ravitch, M. M. *Intussusception in Infants and Children*. Springfield, Ill.: Thomas, 1959.
Ravitch, M. M. Intussusception. In K. J. Welch, et al. (eds.), *Pediatric Surgery*. Chicago: Year Book, 1986. P. 868.

63 Appendicitis

I. **Definition.** *Appendicitis,* inflammation of the vermiform appendix, is the most common surgical disease of the abdomen in childhood. It is uncommon in infancy, but the incidence increases steadily thereafter, peaking in the late teens.

II. **Pathophysiology.** Appendicitis is a progressive inflammatory disease, beginning with obstruction and, if not interrupted by surgical intervention, ending with gangrene and perforation.

   A. **Obstruction** of the lumen of the appendix is the initiating cause in most cases of appendicitis.
   1. A **fecalith** is the usual cause of obstruction, but lymphoid hyperplasia from a viral infection may also cause obstruction.
   2. Continuing **secretion** from the mucosa distends the lumen of the obstructed appendix and ultimately impairs the blood supply.
   3. **Nonobstructive inflammation** may occur. It is generally milder and may even subside spontaneously without treatment.

   B. **Bacterial invasion** by resident aerobes and anaerobes produces inflammation and pus formation. *Escherichia coli* and *Bacteroides* species are the usual culprits. The mucosa becomes ulcerated, and a fibrinopurulent exudate accumulates on the serosal surface.

   C. **Gangrene** eventually occurs as a result of progressive bacterial invasion and vascular impairment.

   D. **Perforation** follows, causing **peritonitis** or **abscess** formation.
   1. The **omentum** in the older child walls off the inflammation early, leading to localized abscess formation rather than free perforation in most cases.
   2. In the **toddler** the appendiceal wall is thinner and the omentum is a less effective guardian, so perforation occurs earlier and generalized peritonitis is more likely to result.

III. **Clinical presentation**

   A. The **history** of the details of onset of pain, anorexia, and vomiting is very helpful in making a diagnosis of appendicitis.
   1. **Pain** is the first and most important symptom of appendicitis. It is initially periumbilical in location and results from the luminal distention of the appendix early in the course of the disease. Progressive transmural inflammation and the formation of serosal exudates cause localized irritation of the parietal peritoneum and a shift of the pain to the right lower quadrant.
   2. **Nausea** and **vomiting** occur **after** the onset of pain, an important differential point in separating appendicitis from gastroenteritis.
   3. **Anorexia** almost invariably occurs with appendicitis; if the patient is hungry, the diagnosis is very much in doubt.

   B. **Physical examination** reveals a child who appears acutely ill, often with a slight flush of the cheeks. He walks slowly and bent over and may prefer to have his legs flexed when lying down. Mucous membranes may be dry.
   1. **Fever** is usually present, 38–39°C. Higher fever suggests the presence of perforation or another diagnosis.

2. **Point tenderness** in the right lower quadrant (RLQ) at McBurney's point, halfway between the anterior iliac spine and the umbilicus, is characteristic of acute appendicitis. Rebound tenderness is often seen.
3. **Muscle guarding** and **spasm** in the RLQ reflect significant peritoneal irritation. Rigidity may be present if perforation has occurred.
4. **Obturator** and **psoas signs** indicate inflammation from a posteriorly located appendix but are infrequently present.
5. **Rectal examination** will often reveal tenderness on the right side and not on the left. This tenderness may be a great deal more intense than the abdominal tenderness. An inflammatory mass or abscess may be felt.

C. **Only about half of patients** demonstrate the typical pattern of symptoms just described. Few acute, serious diseases show as much variation in symptoms and physical findings as acute appendicitis. In part this reflects the variable location of the appendix itself, as well as differences in response.

1. **Smoldering** or slowly progressive appendicitis may give rise to mild pain and nonprogressive symptoms for a week or more without perforation.
2. **Onset** of pain in the **RLQ** is sometimes seen, the periumbilical phase having been mild or not recognized.
3. **Fever** and **leukocytosis** are not infrequently **absent.**
4. **Retrocecal or pelvic appendicitis** may produce no abdominal signs and be detectable only by rectal examination.

D. **Perforated appendicitis** results in abscess formation or generalized peritonitis.

1. **Abscess** develops if the perforation is well contained by bowel or omentum or occurs in a rectrocecal appendix. The patient may not be severely ill, but leukocytosis and fever indicate the presence of sepsis. A **mass** is palpable by abdominal or rectal examination or can be demonstrated by imaging.
2. **Peritonitis** results from perforation into the free peritoneal space. The patient is acutely and seriously ill with high fever, leukocytosis, toxicity, and pain. There may be no localizing tenderness, but the abdomen is rigid.

IV. **Diagnosis.** The objective in appendicitis is to make the definitive diagnosis early enough that appendectomy can be performed before perforation occurs. Because of the variability of presentation, this is often more difficult than it may seem.

A. **Clinical findings** are of prime importance.

1. **Any patient with abdominal pain can have appendicitis.** To make the diagnosis one first has to think of it.
2. The diagnosis cannot be made in the **first few hours** after onset of symptoms. It takes time for peritoneal irritation to develop. The evaluation should be repeated in 4–8 hours.

B. **Physical findings are the key to diagnosis of appendicitis.**

1. Objective evidence of **localized peritoneal irritation** (involuntary guarding or muscle spasm) is essential.
2. Appendicitis is **a progressive disease.** The patient's findings typically worsen with time. The best way to detect progression of appendicitis is through repeated examinations at intervals of several hours performed by the same person.

C. **Laboratory tests** are of limited value in the diagnosis of appendicitis.

1. A **mild leukocytosis** (11,000–15,000) is typical but not universal. A left shift is common, even when the WBC is normal. A high WBC (20,000) in a patient with minimal findings suggests that another condition is responsible

for the symptoms. A **normal** WBC is found in a significant number of children with appendicitis.
    2. **Urinalysis** is usually normal, but both red and white cells may be found in the sediment if the inflamed appendix rests against the bladder.
  D. **Imaging** by x-rays or ultrasound may be helpful if the clinical picture is obscure, but it is unnecessary if the history and physical findings clearly indicate appendicitis.
    1. **Abdominal x-rays** may show a disordered gas pattern or a "mass effect" caused by absence of gas in the RLQ.
    2. A **fecalith** identified by x-ray examination (fewer than 10%) is very significant. If it is associated with symptoms of appendicitis rupture of the appendix will occur in a very high percentage of patients. Thus its presence is an indication for appendectomy.
    3. **Barium enema** may reveal a mass indenting the cecum and incomplete filling of the appendix (also seen with normal appendixes, however).
    4. **Ultrasound** or **CT scan** may be necessary to discover an abscess in patients who are obese, have equivocal symptoms, or are difficult to examine.
  E. **Laparoscopy** may be helpful in equivocal cases, in which the patient fails to improve but lacks peritoneal signs.
- **Differential diagnosis.** Virtually every disease that causes abdominal pain can masquerade as appendicitis, and vice versa.
  A. **Constipation. Fecal masses** palpable by abdominal examination and rectal impaction suggest the diagnosis even when the child or parent denies the possibility. There is no history of periumbilical pain shifting to the RLQ, and signs of peritoneal irritation are absent. Pain, fever, vomiting, and leukocytosis can be present, however. A large (1- to 2-liter) enema is given and is both diagnostic and therapeutic. Unlike cathartics, an enema is not harmful in appendicitis.
  B. **Gastroenteritis.** Vomiting or diarrhea must be present to make a diagnosis of intestinal "flu" or food intolerance. Vomiting precedes the onset of pain. There is no point tenderness in the RLQ. Others in the family may have similar symptoms.
  C. **Psychogenic abdominal pain,** although common, is seldom confused with appendicitis. Clinical and laboratory signs of inflammation are absent, and there is no objective tenderness.
  D. **Pelvic inflammatory disease** mimics appendicitis closely except there is no history of prior periumbilical pain. Tenderness and peritoneal irritation may be localized in the RLQ. Cervical and bilateral adnexal tenderness is usually present. The diagnosis can be confirmed if gonococci are found on smear of the cervical exudate. Laparoscopy may be necessary to make the diagnosis.
  E. **Mittelschmerz** (ovulatory pain) is common in teenaged girls. The findings are typically much milder than those of appendicitis, there is no prior periumbilical pain, and peritoneal signs are rarely present.
  F. **Miscellaneous causes** of abdominal pain that are easily confused with appendicitis include **urinary tract infection, Meckel's diverticulitis** (which can be differentiated only by operation or laparoscopy), right lower lobe **pneumonia** (no abdominal tenderness), **intussusception, measles, sickle cell crisis, regional enteritis, cholecystitis,** and **acid-peptic disease.**

Indications for operation. The diagnosis of appendicitis is the indication for appendectomy.
  A. Reproducible **objective** evidence of **localized peritoneal irritation in the RLQ** is the crucial clinical finding on which the diagnosis of appendicitis depends in most patients.

B. Appendectomy is **also indicated** for the following:
   1. Marked localized **rectal tenderness**
   2. A **RLQ or pelvic mass or fluid collection** demonstrated by physical examination, barium enema, ultrasound, or CT scan
   3. A **fecalith** in the RLQ
C. Patients with **persistent RLQ tenderness** who fail to develop peritoneal signs may or may not have appendicitis. Laparoscopy may be helpful in these children.
D. An **error rate of 5%** is customary in the diagnosis of appendicitis, but error should not exceed 10%.
E. **Chronic or recurrent localized RLQ pain,** occurring over several months or more, may be caused by mild recurrent inflammation of the appendix or a fecalith. Appendectomy is curative in most of these patients.

VII. **Preoperative preparation**
  A. **Uncomplicated appendicitis.** Intravenous rehydration should begin preoperatively, but the operation usually does not need to be delayed for this purpose.
  B. **Perforated appendicitis.** Resuscitation is essential in these patients, who may be toxic, dehydrated, and septic.
   1. **Rehydrate** with intravenous saline solutions and plasma if necessary.
   2. Give IV **antibiotics:** cefazolin sodium (Kefzol), 20 mg/kg, and clindamycin, 10 mg/kg.
   3. **Insert nasogastric tube** for decompression.
   4. **Control fever.** Intravenous fluids, pain medication, acetaminophen, and sometimes a cooling blanket are needed. The operation must not be carried out until the temperature is brought down to 39°C or lower.

VIII. **Operative care.** In uncomplicated appendicitis, appendectomy may be a simple, rapid operation. In other situations, it can be difficult and hazardous.
  A. **Incision.** A RLQ transverse incision is made just medial to the anterior iliac spine, and the muscles are split in gridiron fashion. If greater exposure is needed, the muscles can be cut and the incision extended medially as much as necessary. There is no need for a vertical incision.
  B. **Removal of the appendix** with inversion of the stump should be performed unless it is physically impossible, which is rare.
  C. A perforated appendix should also be removed. Pus is aspirated, and the peritoneum is irrigated with saline. If there is an **abscess** wall that cannot be removed, external **drainage** is needed. Drainage of the peritoneal cavity is useless.
  D. **The skin** is closed after the muscle layers unless there has been perforation or gross contamination, in which case delayed primary closure or drainage of the subcutaneous space is indicated.
  E. **Antibiotics** (cefazolin sodium and clindamycin) are given prophylactically for 24 hours to prevent wound infection in acute appendicitis and therapeutically (10 days) for perforated or gangrenous appendicitis.

IX. **Postoperative care**
  A. **Uncomplicated acute appendicitis.** The child usually recovers rapidly. Feedings can begin on the first postoperative day, and the patient is ready for discharge on the second or third day. Full activity may be resumed within the week (except for contact sports).

- **B. Complicated appendicitis.** These patients may be quite sick for several days or longer.
  1. **Intravenous fluids** are given for maintenance and to replace nasogastric losses. If there is severe peritonitis, plasma or albumin should also be given.
  2. **Nasogastric suction** decompression of the stomach is often needed for several days or more. Ileus may persist for a week after severe peritonitis.
  3. **Pulmonary physiotherapy** will help prevent atelectasis and consequent pneumonia.
  4. **Pain medication** may be needed for several days.
  5. **Ambulation** should begin on the first postoperative day if the child is hemodynamically stable.
  6. **Antibiotics** are continued for 10 days, with change as indicated by operative cultures.
  7. The superficial **wound** is closed with Steristrips on the third day if the wound pH is greater than 7.3. If not, saline dressings are applied until the wound closes secondarily.
  8. **Rectal examination** is performed every other day after the third day to detect abscess formation.

X. Complications

- **A. Abscess formation** is the most common complication after appendectomy, particularly if there was free perforation into the peritoneal cavity. It is much less common now that there are effective agents to treat anaerobes.
  1. **Fever** and **ileus** are the common signs of intraperitoneal abscess.
  2. **Leukocytosis** with a left shift suggests abscess.
  3. Most abscesses are **palpable**—in or under the wound or by rectal examination.
  4. **CT scan and ultrasound** are valuable in the diagnosis and treatment of an abscess. Imaging should be performed in any child with unexplained persistent postoperative fever.
  5. **Drainage** of an abscess can sometimes be done by percutaneous insertion of a catheter under radiologic guidance. If catheter drainage is ineffective, operative drainage is needed.
- **B. Intestinal obstruction** may occur early or late in the postoperative period; 90% occur within the first 3 months. It is caused by inflammation and adhesions, which may be very severe after perforated appendicitis.
  1. **Nasogastric suction** decompression, the primary treatment, is successful in all but a few patients, particularly in the imediate postoperative period.
  2. **Late obstruction** about an adhesive band usually requires operative treatment, although a day or two of tube decompression may be successful if there are no signs of vascular compromise of the bowel.
- **C. Sterility** has been reported in girls after perforated appendicitis, the result of inflammatory obliteration of the fallopian tubes.

XI. Prognosis.
The long-term outlook is excellent and late complications are rare in patients who have had appendectomy for uncomplicated appendicitis. Late abscess formation and adhesive intestinal obstruction occasionally occur after perforated appendicitis.

Bibliography

Bower, R. J., et al. Controversial aspects of appendicitis management in children. *Arch. Surg.* 116:885, 1981.

Cloud, D. T. Appendicitis. *J. Pediatr. Surg.* 925:498, 1980.

Cloud, D. T. Appendicitis. In T. M. Holder and K. W. Ashcraft (eds.), *Pediatric Surgery*. Philadelphia: Saunders, 1980. P. 498.

Giacomantonio, M., et al. Should prophylactic antibiotics be given perioperatively in acute appendicitis without perforation? *Can. J. Surg.* 25:555, 1982.

Grosfeld, J. L., et al. Acute appendicitis in the first two years of life. *J. Pediatr. Surg.* 8:285, 1973.

Holder, T. M., and Leape, L. L. The acute surgical abdomen in children. *N. Engl. J. Med.* 227:921, 1967.

Kottmeier, P. K. Appendicitis. In K. J. Welch, et al. (eds.), *Pediatric Surgery*. Chicago: Year Book, 1986. P. 989.

Leape, L. L., and Ramenofsky, M. L. Laparoscopy for questionable appendicitis: Can it reduce the negative appendectomy rate? *Ann. Surg.* 191:410, 1980.

Puri, P., and O'Donnell, B. Appendicitis in infancy. *J. Pediatr. Surg.* 13:173, 1978.

Schisgall, R. M. Appendiceal colic in childhood: The role of inspissated casts of stool within the appendix. *Ann. Surg.* 192:687, 1980.

Schwartz, M. Z., et al. Management of perforated appendicitis in children. *Ann. Surg.* 197:407, 1983.

Williams, G. R. A history of appendicitis. *Ann. Surg.* 197:495, 1983.

64. Primary Peritonitis

Definition. *Primary peritonitis* is infection of the peritoneal cavity that does not result from infection in an abdominal organ.

Pathophysiology. The cause of primary peritonitis is usually not found. Children with cirrhosis, nephrosis, or a ventriculoperitoneal shunt are more likely than others to develop primary peritonitis. Often there is a preceding upper respiratory infection. Since the majority of cases occur in girls, the genital tract has been suspected as a portal of entry. Organisms are typically *Escherichia coli, Pneumococcus, Streptococcus,* or *Meningococcus.* Blood cultures usually show the same organism as found in the peritoneal space.

Clinical presentation. Primary peritonitis is a rapidly progressive disease in which a previously well child suddenly develops fever, ileus, and peritoneal signs. There are no focal signs.

Diagnosis. Because of the much greater likelihood of peritoneal signs being secondary to perforated appendicitis, confident diagnosis of primary peritonitis may be difficult.

A. The presence of a known **predisposing cause** such as cirrhosis, nephrosis, or a ventriculoperitoneal (v-p) shunt should alert the clinician to the possibility of primary peritonitis.

B. **X-rays** are nondiagnostic. Generalized ileus is typical, often with fluid between the loops of bowel.

C. **Aspiration of peritoneal fluid** should be performed in questionable cases. If primary peritonitis is present, a **single organism,** often gram-positive, will be recovered. Mixed intestinal flora signifies intestinal perforation.

D. In doubtful cases, surgical **exploration** is indicated.

Treatment. Antibiotics are appropriate and sufficient therapy for primary peritonitis if the diagnosis is secure. The choice of agent is governed by smear and culture of the peritoneal fluid. Infection secondary to a v-p shunt may require removal of the shunt.

Indications for operation. Any child in whom the diagnosis of primary peritonitis is not reasonably certain should undergo exploration. In particular, this includes most children with no predisposing cause and those with mixed flora on peritoneal tap.

Preoperative preparation (see Chap. 63).

Operative care. If the appendix, terminal ileum, and adnexa are found to have a diffuse red serositis and there is an abundance of cloudy peritoneal fluid, primary peritonitis should be suspected. If smear of the peritoneal fluid shows a single organism, particularly *Pneumococcus* or *Streptococcus,* the appendix is removed and the patient is treated with antibiotics. If smear of the fluid shows mixed fecal flora, further exploration is necessary to make sure there is no perforation.

Postoperative care. Routine

Prognosis. Excellent. Death or recurrence is rare.

Bibliography

Clark, J. H., Fitzgerald, J. F., and Kleiman, M. B. Spontaneous bacterial peritonitis. *J. Pediatr.* 104:495, 1984.

Condon, R. E. Antibiotics in the management of peritonitis. In R. E. Condon and S. L. Gorbach (eds.), *Surgical Infections: Selective Antibiotic Therapy.* Baltimore: Williams & Wilkins, 1981. P. 83.

Ein, S. H. Primary Peritonitis. In K. J. Welch, et al. (eds.), *Pediatric Surgery.* Chicago: Year Book, 1986. P. 976.

Fine, R. N., et al. Peritonitis in children undergoing continuous ambulatory peritoneal dialysis. *Pediatrics* 71:806, 1983.

Fowler, R. Primary peritonitis: Changing aspects 1956–70. *Aust. Paediatr. J.* 7:73, 1971.

McDougal, W. S., Izant, R. J., Jr., and Zollinger, R. M., Jr. Primary peritonitis in infancy and childhood. *Ann. Surg.* 181:310, 1975.

Tchirkow, G., and Verhagen A. D. Bacterial peritonitis in patients with ventriculoperitoneal shunt. *J. Pediatr. Surg.* 14:182, 1979.

65   Crohn's Disease

I. **Definition.** *Crohn's disease* is a **granulomatous** inflammation of the small or large intestine of unknown etiology and with no known cure. As in ulcerative colitis, suggested etiologies include autoimmune mechanisms, infection, and stress. Like ulcerative colitis, Crohn's disease is much more common in whites, and specifically, in Jews, than in other racial and ethnic groups. Symptoms are most likely to begin in the second decade of life.

II. **Pathophysiology**

   A. In Crohn's disease the inflammation affects the **entire bowel wall,** with submucosal edema, fibrosis, and mucosal ulcers, which may penetrate the intestine causing **fistulas** and **abscesses. Stricture** formation may result in **intestinal obstruction.**

   B. **Both the ileum and the colon** are affected in over half the patients, but in 10% the disease is confined to the colon.

III. **Clinical presentation**

   A. **Weight loss,** abdominal **pain,** and bloody **diarrhea** are the most common presenting symptoms. **Fever** may be the only symptom.

   B. **Extraintestinal manifestations** are common **(25%)** and may cause the first symptoms. They are similar to those seen in ulcerative colitis: **arthritis, growth retardation, delayed sexual maturation, skin lesions, liver disease, uveitis, and oral ulcerations.**

   C. **Perianal ulcers, fistulas, or abscesses** may precede intestinal symptoms and are much more common than in ulcerative colitis.

   D. **Physical examination** may reveal a **mass** in the right lower quadrant: the thickened, inflamed terminal ileum.

   E. Crohn's disease is a **chronic continuing disease** in most patients. A small percentage of patients have an acute obstructive episode, requiring intestinal resection, after which they remain free of further symptoms for many years.

IV. **Diagnosis**

   A. **Barium contrast intestinal x-rays** frequently show ulcerations or strictures in the small intestine. A mass effect may be noted due to the thickened mesentery and lymph nodes. An intestinal **fistula** may be identified.

   B. **Sigmoidoscopy** is normal in many patients, for the rectum is frequently spared, unlike the situation in ulcerative colitis. If the rectum is involved, ulcerations with intervening normal mucosa may be seen. The presence of granulomas on biopsy confirms the diagnosis.

   C. **Laparoscopy or laparotomy** is diagnostic if thickening and inflammation of the terminal ileum are seen with **"creeping fat"** of the mesentery over the bowel wall.

V. **Problems**

   A. **Steroid dependence** with **growth arrest** and resultant short stature is distressingly common in adolescents with severe Crohn's disease. **Side effects** of corticosteroids are common: obesity, facial hair, acne, abdominal striae, and susceptibility to infection.

B. Intestinal obstruction.

C. Intestinal fistulas—to other parts of the intestine, the bladder, or the skin, particularly after laparotomy (e.g., for appendectomy).

D. Abscesses may result from intraabdominal perforation. Free perforation into the peritoneal cavity is rare.

E. Perianal fistulas, ulcers, and abscesses.

F. Obstruction of the right ureter from the inflammatory mass.

G. Adenocarcinoma may occur in either the small or large bowel. Malignant change is less common than in ulcerative colitis, but much more common than in the healthy population.

VI. Indications for operation. Unlike ulcerative colitis, there is no surgical (or medical) cure for Crohn's disease. The disease usually recurs after surgical resection, although long remission of symptoms may be achieved (average of 48 months). Repeated intestinal resections may result in insufficient small intestine to maintain nutritional status. Therefore, surgical treatment is reserved for acute complications and for patients whose symptoms cannot be controlled with medical therapy.

A. Emergency resection

1. **Perforation**—free, or causing abscess or fistula
2. **Intestinal obstruction**

B. Elective resection

1. **Growth failure.** The operation must be carried out before epiphyseal closure.
2. **Refractory disease.** Persistent symptoms despite medication. Most likely to be necessary in granulomatous colitis.
3. **Refractory extraintestinal manifestations.**

VII. Nonoperative therapy

A. Acute symptomatic Crohn's disease is treated with bowel rest, intravenous fluids, antidiarrheal drugs, and corticosteroids if necessary. Acute intestinal obstruction will also frequently respond to this therapy.

B. Chronic disease management requires dietary restriction (high-calorie, high-protein, low-roughage diet with nutritional supplements), antispasmodics, sulfasalazine (Azulfidine), and judicious use of corticosteroids.

C. Total parenteral nutrition can cause a dramatic, if temporary, remission in Crohn's disease. It is indicated for those with:

1. **Severe malnutrition**
2. **Refractory disease**
3. **Intestinal fistulas**
4. **Severe perianal disease**

VIII. Preoperative preparation

A. Emergency resection (intestinal obstruction, perforation, or abscess). Resuscitation with intravenous fluids, blood, and plasma as necessary. Antibiotics

B. Elective resection

1. **Nutritional status** should be optimized by use of TPN if necessary.
2. **Blood and plasma** transfusions are indicated if there is anemia or hypoproteinemia.

IX. Operative care

A. Objective. Permanent cure cannot be achieved in Crohn's disease as it can in ulcerative colitis. Because of the risk of loss of too much intestine from multiple resections, the objective of surgical treatment is to control the complications with as **few operations as possible,** removing no more intestine than necessary.

B. Resection includes the segment that is obviously diseased (together with a fistula, if present) plus some normal bowel. Because microscopic disease extends well beyond what the surgeon sees, an additional 20 cm of proximal and 10 cm of distal bowel must be removed to prevent early recurrence.

C. Colectomy for granulomatous colitis must include the rectum if it is involved. If the rectum is normal, subtotal colectomy with ileoproctostomy is rarely successful because of the frequency of recurrence. Endorectal pull-through with ileoanal anastomosis has not been successful for the same reason.

D. Diverting ileostomy is indicated for severe perianal disease that does not respond to TPN.

E. Exclusion or bypass procedures, once standard treatment, are now seldom appropriate in the treatment of Crohn's disease.

X. Postoperative care

A. If given preoperatively, **prednisone** is continued in therapeutic doses for 48 hours postoperatively and then reduced to maintenance dose (15 mg/day in a teenager), from which it can be tapered off over 6 weeks.

B. Nutritional supplements are usually indicated on a long-term basis.

XI. Complications

A. Intestinal obstruction

B. Wound infections

C. Ileostomy malfunction

D. Intestinal fistulas

XII. Prognosis.
Crohn's disease usually afflicts the patient for life, with relapses at variable intervals and a shortened life expectancy. Some patients with focal disease are apparently cured by surgical resection or have long periods of symptom-free existence. For most, operation controls a complication but has little or no effect on the course of the disease.

Bibliography

Becker, J. M., and Schneider, K. M. Inflammatory Bowel Disease. In T. M. Holder and K. W. Ashcraft (eds.), *Pediatric Surgery*. Philadelphia: Saunders, 1980. P. 465.

Benner, J., et al. Crohn's disease in children and adolescents: Is inadequate weight gain a valid indication for surgery? *J. Pediatr. Surg.* 14:325, 1979.

Castile, R. G., et al. Crohn's disease in children: Assessment of the progression of disease, growth, and prognosis. *J. Pediatr. Surg.* 15:462, 1980.

Crohn, B. B., Ginzburg, L., and Oppenheimer, G. D. Regional ileitis: A pathologic and clinical entity. *J.A.M.A.* 99:1323, 1932.

Farmer, R. G., and Michener, W. M. Prognosis of Crohn's desease with onset in childhood or adolescence. *Dig. Dis. Sci.* 24:752, 1979.

Fonkalsrud, E. W., et al. Surgical management of Crohn's disease in children. *Am. J. Surg.* 138:15, 1979.

Greenstein, A. J., et al. Reoperation and recurrence in Crohn's colitis and ileocolitis: Crude and cumulative rates. *N. Engl. J. Med.* 293:685, 1975.

Gryboski, J. D., and Spiro, H. M. Prognosis in children with Crohn's disease. *Gastroenterology* 74:807, 1978.

Karesen, R., et al. Crohn's disease: Long-term results of surgical treatment. *Scand. J. Gastroenterol.* 16:7, 1981.

Kelts, D. G., et al. Nutritional basis of growth failure in children and adolescents with Crohn's disease. *Gastroenterology* 76:720, 1979.

Raine, P. A. M. BAPS collective review: Chronic inflammatory bowel disease. *J. Pediatr. Surg.* 19:18, 1984.

Seashore, J. H., Hillemeier, A. C., and Gryboski, J. D. Total parenteral nutrition in the management of inflammatory bowel disease in children: A limited role. *Am. J. Surg.* 143:504, 1982.

Strobel, C. T., Bryne, W. J., and Ament, M. E. Home parenteral nutrition in children with Crohn's disease. *Gastroenterology* 77:272, 1979.

Telander, R. L. Crohn's disease. In K. J. Welch, et al. (eds.), *Pediatric Surgery*. Chicago: Year Book, 1986. P. 958.

66 Ulcerative Colitis

Definition. *Ulcerative colitis* (UC) is an *inflammatory disease* of the colon, mostly confined to the mucosa, causing ulceration, diarrhea, and bleeding. The **etiology is unknown.** Autoimmune mechanisms, infection, and stress have been implicated. **Genetic factors** are clearly important. There is a familial tendency, and UC is much more common in whites than in blacks and in **Jews** than gentiles. The peak incidence of onset is in the third decade, but over **20%** of patients develop symptoms **before** the age of **20** and 4% before the age of 10 years.

Pathophysiology

A. The inflammation of ulcerative colitis is **confined to the colon,** rarely affecting the terminal ileum ("backwash ileitis"). The **rectum** is involved in **95%** of patients.

B. Inflammation of the mucosa leads to **crypt abscesses,** which progress to **mucosal ulceration** and the formation of **pseudopolyps.** Rigidity and scarring of the bowel wall result from long-standing inflammation.

C. **Diarrhea** and **cramps** result from the inflammation and ulceration, with purulent discharge and **bleeding,** either overt or occult.

D. **Perforation** or **toxic megacolon** (acute dilatation of the colon with signs of systemic infection) may result from sudden progression of the disease.

Clinical presentation

A. **Diarrhea** and **abdominal pain** are the most common initial symptoms of ulcerative colitis, followed by **bleeding** and purulent discharge. In most cases, symptoms are easily controlled with medication.

B. An **acute toxic episode** may occur at any time and is the first indication of disease in 10% of children, with profuse bloody diarrhea, severe pain, high fever, and toxicity. An emergency operation may be required for toxic megacolon and perforation.

C. **Remissions** with prolonged symptom-free periods are common, followed by periodic exacerbations precipitated by stress or infection. Complete remission after a single attack occurs in only 5–10% of patients.

D. **Chronic UC,** with low-grade or "smoldering" symptoms, is associated with **anorexia, weight loss, growth failure, and lack of sexual maturation.** Continuous corticosteroid medication is necessary to control symptoms; the medication further inhibits growth.

E. **Extracolonic manifestations** may precede or follow the onset of colonic symptoms of ulcerative colitis and are seen in **25–40%** of patients: **arthritis, skin lesions (pyoderma gangrenosum and erythema nodosum), chronic hepatitis or cirrhosis, osteoporosis, uveitis, and oral ulcers.**

Diagnosis

A. Ulcerative colitis should be suspected in any child with **persistent noninfectious diarrhea,** particularly if there is **bleeding** or extracolonic symptoms.

B. **Barium enema** is normal early in the disease but later shows mucosal irregularity, pseudopolyps, or "thumbprinting." In chronic disease, there is loss of haustral markings, and the colon is shortened, narrowed, and rigid, especially on the left side. There may be evidence of backwash ileitis.

C. **Sigmoidoscopy** or colonoscopy is usually diagnostic since the rectum is almost always affected. Early on, only inflammation is seen. Later, mucosal ulceration develops with pseudopolyp formation. **Biopsy** should always be performed and is diagnostic if ulceration and crypt abscesses are seen.

V. **Problems.** Few diseases are more complicated than ulcerative colitis, even when symptoms can be controlled. Major concerns are as follows:

  A. **Complications of steroid therapy.**

   1. Permanent **short stature** occurs if medication is prolonged during the period of epiphyseal closure.

   2. Gastric or duodenal **ulcers** may develop.

   3. **Obesity, facial hair, acne, abdominal striae,** and susceptibility to **infection** are common side effects.

  B. **Toxic megacolon.**

  C. **Perforation** into the peritoneal cavity with acute peritonitis or into the retroperitoneal space with **abscess** formation.

  D. **Massive bleeding.**

  E. **Malignant change** occurs in 3% of patients in the first 10 years, increasing by 2%/year after that, even if the disease is quiescent.

VI. **Indications for operation.** Colectomy is curative in ulcerative colitis, eliminating both the disease and its extracolonic manifestations. Formerly, the need for a permanent ileostomy led to extreme measures to avoid surgical treatment. As new and more effective operations have been developed, the indications for colectomy have broadened.

  A. **Indications for emergency colectomy**

   1. **Toxic megacolon**

   2. **Perforation**—free air or abscess

   3. **Bleeding**—massive and life-threatening

  B. **Indications for elective colectomy**

   1. **Refractory disease**—persistent symptoms despite medication.

   2. Rectoperineal and rectovaginal **fistulae.**

   3. **Steroid-dependent** asymptomatic **disease,** especially if there is **growth failure** or delay in sexual maturation. It is mandatory that an operation be performed before epiphyseal closure if permanent stunting is to be avoided.

   4. **Prevention of carcinoma.** Colectomy is indicated in any child with disease of 10 years' duration.

   5. **Symptomatic extracolonic disease.**

VII. **Nonoperative therapy**

  A. **Acute** symptomatic UC is treated with **bowel rest** (intravenous fluids and nutrition); **antidiarrheal drugs** (diphenoxylate and atropine [Lomotil], 1–2 tablets qid, or loperamide [Imodium], 1 tablet qid); **antibiotics;** and **corticosteroids.** **Blood** or **plasma** transfusions may be necessary.

  B. **Chronic** disease management requires frequent attention by a concerned physician and includes **dietary restriction** (avoiding chocolate, citrus, raw fruits, vegetables, and nuts), **vitamin** supplements, **antispasmodics, antibiotics,** judicious use of **corticosteroids,** and in refractory cases, sulfasalazine **(Azulfidine)** or azathioprine **(Imuran).**

C. Total parenteral nutrition is the ideal means of obtaining complete bowel rest in refractory patients or in those with toxic megacolon.

III. Preoperative preparation

A. Emergency colectomy. Operation is performed as soon as the patient is **resuscitated**. Blood volume is restored with blood and plasma. Antibiotics are given intravenously (cephazolin sodium [Kefzol], 20 mg/kg q8h, and clindamycin, 10 mg/kg q8h).

B. Elective colectomy

1. **Nutritional status** should be optimal. A course of TPN is given for a week or two preoperatively if it is not.

2. **Blood** and **plasma** transfusions are given if there is anemia or hypoproteinemia.

3. **Prednisone** (30–60 mg/day) and Cortifoam enemas are administered as necessary to heal rectal disease as much as possible.

4. **Bowel preparation** preoperatively. Golitely, 1–4 liters intestinal lavage in the morning on the day before the operation, followed by intestinal antibiotics (kanamycin, 100 mg/kg or cefoxitin, 25 mg/kg) at 11 A.M., 12 noon, 1, 2, 6, and 10 P.M.

5. **Psychologic preparation** is essential if endorectal pull-through is planned. The patient must understand what is in store and be committed to the full program before the operation. Talking with another person of the same sex and similar age who has had a successful operative result is very helpful.

IV. Operative care

A. Objectives

1. **Removal of the entire colon.** If there is no colon, there is no disease and no risk of later malignancy. All of the colonic mucosa, including that in the rectum, must be removed.

2. **Avoidance** of a permanent **ileostomy** if possible.

B. Emergency colectomy. Subtotal colectomy with ileostomy is performed as a lifesaving measure. The rectum is left in place. At a later date it is removed or endorectal pull-through is performed (after mucosal healing).

C. Elective colectomy. Total colectomy with mucosal proctectomy and ileoanal endorectal pull-through is the operation of choice. There are two acceptable methods: **direct ileoanal anastomosis** and **formation of a pouch** of doubled-back ileum to increase the capacity of the neorectum (Fig. 66-1).

D. Total colectomy with a continent (Kock) **ileostomy** is an alternative operation for those for whom endorectal pull-through is unsuitable.

Postoperative care

A. Prednisolone is given in therapeutic doses (30 mg q6h) for 48 hours postoperatively and then reduced to maintenance level (15 mg/day in a teenager). The dose is slowly decreased over 3–6 weeks.

B. Rapid recovery is the rule. Nasogastric decompression can usually be stopped in 48 hours, and feedings can commence the following day. The drain is removed at 48 hours.

C. Training of the neorectum begins 6 weeks postoperatively and consists of balloon catheter dilatations, followed by water until the patient can hold **400 ml for 4 hours.** The ileostomy is then closed.

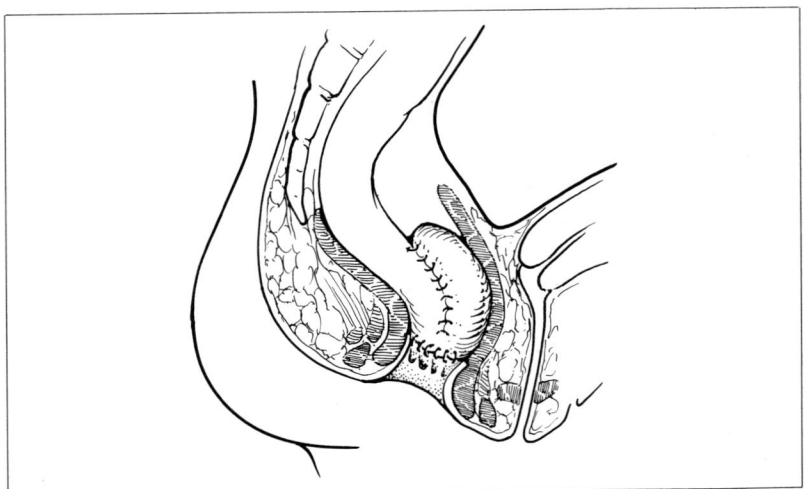

Fig. 66-1. Pull-through for ulcerative colitis. "J" loop of ileum is placed within the retained muscular rectal cuff with anastomosis just above the anal crypts.

    D. Antimotility drugs (diphenoxylate and atropine or loperamide) are used as necessary after the ileostomy is closed. The average patient will have **3–6 bowel movements a day** 1 year after the operation.

XI. Complications

    A. Bleeding from the rectal muscle cuff

    B. Cuff abscess

    C. Anastomotic leak if a diverting ileostomy has not been performed

    D. Pouch hematoma, infection ("pouchitis"), **leak, abscess**

    E. Stricture at the anoileal anastomosis or in the pouch

    F. Incontinence if the sphincters are damaged

XII. Prognosis.
Ulcerative colitis is cured by colectomy, rendering the patient free of the disease and of the risk of developing colon carcinoma. The child can lead a normal life, with **normal life expectancy.**

Bibliography

Aylett, S. D. Three hundred cases of diffuse ulcerative colitis treated by total colectomy and ileo-rectal anastomosis. *Br. Med. J.* 1:1001, 1966.

Becker, J. M., and Schneider, K. M. Inflammatory Bowel Disease. In T. M. Holder and K. W. Ashcraft (eds.), *Pediatric Surgery*. Philadelphia: Saunders, 1980. P. 465.

Coran, A. G., et al. The endorectal pull-through for the management of ulcerative colitis in children and adults. *Ann. Surg.* 197:99, 1983.

Fonkalsrud, E. W. Total colectomy and endorectal ileal pull-through with internal reservoir for ulcerative colitis. *Surg. Gynecol. Obstet.* 150:1, 1980.

Kock, N. G. Intra-abdominal "reservoir" in patients with permanent ileostomy: Preliminary observations on a procedure resulting in fecal "continence" in five ileostomy patients. *Arch. Surg.* 99:223, 1969.

Martin, L. W. Ulcerative Colitis. In K. J. Welch, et al. (eds.), *Pediatric Surgery*. Chicago: Year Book, 1986. P. 969.

Martin, L. W., and LeCoultre, C. Technical considerations in performing total colectomy and Soave endorectal anastomosis for ulcerative colitis. *J. Pediatr. Surg.* 13:762, 1978.

Martin, K. W., LeCoultre, C., and Schubert, W. K. Total colectomy and mucosal proctectomy with preservation of continence in ulcerative colitis. *Ann. Surg.* 186:477, 1977.

Michener, W. M., et al. The prognosis of chronic ulcerative colitis in children. *N. Engl. J. Med.* 265:1075, 1961.

Raine, P. A. M. BAPS collective review: Chronic inflammatory bowel disease. *J. Pediatr. Surg.* 19:18, 1984.

Ravitch, M. M. Anal ileostomy with sphincter preservation in patients requiring total colectomy for benign conditions. *Surgery* 24:170, 1948.

Seashore, J. H., Hillemeier, A. C., and Gryboski, J. D. Total parenteral nutrition in the management of inflammatory bowel disease in children: A limited role. *Am. J. Surg.* 143:504, 1982.

Telander, R. L., Hoffman, A., and Perrault, J. Early development of the neorectum by balloon dilatations after ileoanal anastomosis. *J. Pediatr. Surg.* 16:911, 1981.

Telander, R. L., and Perrault, J. Colectomy with rectal mucosectomy and ileoanal anastomosis in young patients. *Arch. Surg.* 116:623, 1981.

67 Colonic Polyps

Definition. *Colonic polyps* are the most common cause of rectal bleeding in the middle years of childhood. There are three major types.

- **A. Juvenile polyps** account for 97% of childhood polyps. The polyps are pedunculated mucoid hamartomas and have no tendency to malignant change. Eighty-five percent are **solitary.** The majority are in the rectum or lower sigmoid colon. In a rare variant, **juvenile polyposis,** the child has hundreds of polyps throughout the **entire intestinal tract.**
- **B. Familial polyposis** is an autosomal dominant disease in which multiple polyps are found throughout the colon. These are **premalignant** lesions, almost invariably changing to adenocarcinoma later in life.
- **C. Peutz-Jeghers syndrome** is also an autosomal dominant disorder, but with low (2–3%) malignant potential. Polyps are found **throughout the gastrointestinal tract,** most commonly in the small intestine. They are hamartomatous in nature and frequently asymptomatic.

Clinical presentation

- **A. Rectal bleeding** is the most common presenting symptom of colonic polyps. Bright red blood is noted on the stool or in the toilet. Bleeding is never massive and almost always occurs in association with a bowel movement. The polyp may **prolapse** through the anus during defecation.
- **B. Abdominal pain** from a polyp occurs if it is large and causes some degree of obstruction or serves as a lead point for intussusception. The pain is typically mild, crampy, and localized to the lower abdomen. Diarrhea sometimes occurs.
- **C. Juvenile polyposis** causes more severe symptoms. In addition to rectal bleeding, there may be **protein-losing enteropathy, malnutrition, recurrent intussusception** and **rectal prolapse.** Symptoms are particularly severe in infants.
- **D. Familial polyposis** is usually asymptomatic in the first decade of life, when only a small percentage of patients have developed the polyps. **Extracolonic manifestations** may predominate (Gardner's syndrome: benign soft and hard tissue tumors with familial polyposis). Because of the risk of carcinoma, **if either parent has the disease all children in the family should be checked annually starting at age 10 years.**
- **E. Peutz-Jeghers syndrome** is associated with pathognomonic **melanotic spots** on the lips and oral mucosa. Chronic bleeding and intussusception are the major complications.

Diagnosis

- **A. Rectal examination** will reveal about half of colonic polyps.
- **B. Barium enema with air contrast** will demonstrate almost all polyps above the reach of the examining finger. Even if a polyp is palpated, barium examination is performed to identify other polyps and rule out familial polyposis.
- **C. Colonoscopy** is indicated if physical examination and barium enema are negative. Colonoscopy is also indicated to obtain histologic diagnosis by **biopsy** in cases of polyposis.

Problems. Lymphoid hyperplasia is a common finding on barium study and must be distinguished from colonic polyps. The multiple filling defects are small (1–5 mm), are similar in size, and typically present an umbilicated profile on barium study. They are harmless and require no treatment.

V. Indications for operation

A. Isolated juvenile polyps. If the polyps are within the reach of the sigmoidoscope, they should be removed to prevent further symptoms and to rid the patient of the disease. Juvenile polyps tend to disappear or slough spontaneously, however, so removal is **not mandatory** if symptoms are mild and the polyps are inaccessible. Colonoscopy is used to remove higher polyps if they are persistently symptomatic. Laparotomy with colonotomy is seldom appropriate treatment.

B. Familial polyposis is cured by **total colectomy,** which should be performed by age 16 to prevent malignant degeneration.

C. Generalized juvenile polyposis may require operative treatment for recurrent bleeding or obstruction or to decrease the loss of protein and fluid from the mucinous polyps. Particularly in the infant, very aggressive therapy (colectomy and total parenteral nutrition) may be required as lifesaving measures.

D. Patients with **Peutz-Jeghers syndrome** also require operative treatment at times because of bleeding or intussusception.

VI. Operative care

A. Juvenile polyps. Isolated polyps are easily removed by sigmoidoscopy or colonoscopy under general anesthesia.

B. Familial polyposis. Total colectomy with ileoanal **endorectal pull-through** is the operation of choice (see Chap. 66). It eliminates the risk of malignant change by removing all of the mucosa, while avoiding ileostomy.

C. Juvenile polyposis. Partial or total colectomy as well as partial small-bowel resections may be necessary.

VII. Postoperative care.
Postoperative care is routine following colectomy for colonic polyps. See Chap. 66 for details of postoperative rectal training after ileoanal anastomosis.

VIII. Prognosis.
After colectomy for familial polyposis or removal of an isolated juvenile polyp, the risk of recurrence is exceedingly small.

Bibliography

Byrne, W. J., et al. Lymphoid polyps (focal lymphoid hyperplasia) of the colon in children. *Pediatrics* 69:598, 1982.

Dehner, L. P. *Pediatric Surgical Pathology.* St. Louis: Mosby, 1975.

Euler, A. R., and Seibert, J. J. The role of sigmoidoscoy, radiographs, and colonoscopy in the diagnostic evaluation of pediatric age patients with suspected juvenile polyps. *J. Pediatr. Surg.* 16:500, 1981.

Gardner, E. J., and Richards, R. C. Multiple cutaneous and subcutaneous lesions occurring simultaneously with hereditary polyposis and osteomatosis. *Am. J. Hum. Genet.* 5:139, 1953.

Kottmeier, P. K., and Clatworthy, H. W., Jr. Intestinal polyps and associated carcinoma in childhood. *Am. J. Surg.* 110:709, 1965.

Linos, D. A., et al. Does Peutz-Jeghers syndrome predispose to gastrointestinal malignancy? A later look. *Arch. Surg.* 116:1182, 1981.

Louw, J. H. Polypoid lesions of the large bowel in children with particular reference to benign lymphoid polyposis. *J. Pediatr. Surg.* 3:195, 1968.

Peutz, J. L. A. Very remarkable case of familial polyposis of mucous membrane of intestinal tract and nasopharynx accompanied by peculiar pigmentations of skin and mucous membrane. *Ned. Maandschr. Geneeskd.* 10:134, 1921.

Ravitch, M. M. Anal ileostomy with sphincter preservation in patients requiring total colectomy for benign conditions. *Surgery* 24:170, 1948.

Safaie-Shirazi, S., and Soper, R. T. Endorectal pull-through procedure in the surgical treatment of familial polyposis coli. *J. Pediatr. Surg.* 8:711, 1973.

Sandler, R. S., and Lipper, L. Multiple adenomas in juvenile polyposis. *Am. J. Gastroenterol.* 75:361, 1981.

Santulli, T. V., and Schullinger, J. N. Polypoid Diseases of the Gastrointestinal Tract. In K. J. Welch, et al. (eds.), *Pediatric Surgery*. Chicago: Year Book, 1986. P. 932.

Soper, R. T. Intestinal Polyps. In T. M. Holder and K. W. Ashcraft (eds.), *Pediatric Surgery*. Philadelphia: Saunders, 1980. P. 481.

Soper, R. T., and Kent, T. H. Fatal juvenile polyposis in infancy. *Surgery* 69:692, 1971.

Telander, R. L., and Perrault, J. Colectomy with rectal mucosectomy and ileoanal anastomosis in young patients. Its use for ulcerative colitis and familial polyposis. *Arch. Surg.* 116:623, 1981.

Velcek, F. T., et al. Familial juvenile adenomatous polyposis. *J. Pediatr. Surg.* 11:781, 1976.

68 Constipation

I. **Definition.** The term *constipation* has different meanings to different people. It may signify (1) **difficulty** moving the bowels, (2) **infrequent** bowel movements, and (3) **hard** stools. The three usually occur together, for when bowel movements occur infrequently they will become large, hard, and difficult to move.

II. **Etiology**
   A. **A wide variety** of conditions may result in constipation.
      1. Severely **brain-damaged** children are frequently constipated. Inability to respond consciously to sensations of rectal fullness, poor intestinal motility and sphincter function, and sedentary life patterns may be contributing factors.
      2. Rarely, **toxic, metabolic,** or **endocrine** diseases may be responsible for chronic constipation, e.g., hypokalemia, hypothyroidism, and lead poisoning.
      3. Unusual **diets,** supplemental **iron** in formula, and certain **drugs** will cause constipation.
   B. **In the vast majority of patients,** chronic constipation results from one of the three types of abnormalities: **anatomic, functional, and psychogenic.**
      1. **Anatomic anomalies** causing constipation are usually congenital and may be either neurologic or obstructive.
         a. **Neurologic malformations** include virtually any **spinal-cord** abnormality (e.g., myelomeningocele, occult spina bifida, traumatic spinal-cord injuries) and **Hirschsprung's disease** (aganglionosis).
         b. **Obstructive malformations** are more common than either of the neurologic types. **Anal stenosis** and **anterior ectopic anus** are the most common structural anomalies that cause difficulty in defecation. If undiagnosed at birth, **imperforate anus** with vestibular or perineal fistula may present as constipation.
      2. In **functional constipation** there is no evidence of an anatomic disorder. Sometimes called **"sluggish bowels,"** it is a disturbance of the physiology of defecation of unknown cause that is frequently manifested as infrequent stools in infancy. It is usually **familial.**
      3. **Psychogenic constipation** is the most common form of severe chronic fecal retention.
         a. Symptoms begin **after infancy,** often associated with some form of **psychic stress,** such as forceful toilet training or the birth of a sibling.
         b. **Excessive parental concern** over elimination may result in a parent-child struggle in which the child holds in bowel movements.
         c. **Progressive fecal retention** leads to decompensation, and the situation becomes **out of control** for both the child and the parent.

Pathophysiology

A. **Normal defecation** is the result of a complex interaction of voluntary and involuntary functions of the colon, rectum, and sphincters.
   1. Liquid products of digestion are transferred frequently from the ileum to the colon, where water is removed to produce solid stool.

2. **Propulsion of stool** in the colon results from mass action of the colonic musculature and contractions in response to the gastrocolic and ileocolic reflexes.
3. As the rectum fills, receptors in the rectal wall and in the puborectalis muscle are stimulated, resulting in the conscious urge to defecate.
4. Voluntary contraction of abdominal muscles and relaxation of the puborectalis and external sphincters results in defecation.
5. Suppression of the urge to defecate results in contraction of the external sphincter and the puborectalis, with retrograde emptying of the rectum and fecal retention.

B. **Chronic fecal retention** results if regular defecation (daily in a child, more frequently in an infant) does not take place. A predictable sequence of events occurs.
   1. **Stools become large and hard** as desiccation by the colon continues and more products of digestion are delivered into the colon from the small intestine.
   2. **Defecation** is **painful** when it occurs because the stools are large and hard. There may be tearing of the mucosa with **bleeding** and the development of an **anal fissure.**
   3. **Deliberate suppression** of defecation ("**holding**") results. Not surprisingly, as the child learns that defecation is painful, he seeks to avoid it, fighting the urge to defecate, making the stools larger and harder still. It is a true vicious cycle.
   4. **Decompensation** of the nerves and muscles of defecation develops.
      a. **Sensory inhibition** results in loss of the sensation of "having to go."
      b. **Stretching of the puborectalis and the external sphincters** results in incontinence (encopresis).
   5. The child is literally **unable to move his bowels** and unable to tell when he needs to.

C. **Encopresis** is almost always a sign of **chronic fecal retention,** the result of sensory and motor decompensation.

IV. **Clinical presentation.** A detailed history of the circumstances of the onset of constipation and the age at which it began is essential for accurate diagnosis and effective treatment. Patterns and causes of constipation differ considerably according to the age of onset of symptoms.

A. **Neonate.** The normal newborn infant has 2–6 "mushy" bowel movements a day. Constipation in the neonatal period suggests a congenital abnormality. Four patterns are seen.
   1. **Intestinal obstruction** suggests Hirschsprung's disease.
   2. "**Sluggish bowels**" is suspected if the infant has only one bowel movement a day and there is a family history of bowel dysfunction.
   3. **Hard stools** result from decreased frequency of bowel movements. Suspect familial functional constipation or the effect of diet or medications (particularly iron supplementation).
   4. **Straining and pain** with bowel movements, even when soft, is diagnostic of an **obstructive** lesion: **anal stenosis** or **anterior ectopic anus.**

B. **Toddler.** Most early childhood constipation is **functional** unless there is obsessive parental concern with toilet training, a common cause of psychogenic constipation. Rarely does an anatomic abnormality first become symptomatic this late.

C. **Older child.** Onset of symptoms after early childhood almost always indicates **psychogenic constipation.**

V. Diagnosis

A. **The age of onset** is the most critical factor in determining the cause of constipation. (See sec. **IV,** preceding.)

B. **Symptoms**
   1. **Straining at defecation** is a symptom of obstruction.
      a. **Large, hard stools are the most common cause of obstruction** in constipated patients.
      b. **Straining when stools are soft** indicates anatomic obstruction.
      c. **Hirschsprung's disease** does **not** cause straining because the rectum is typically empty.
   2. In an infant, **inability to defecate** despite effort suggests anal obstruction.
   3. **Pain and bleeding on defecation** result from large, hard stools. An anal fissure may be present.
   4. **Lack of the urge to defecate** may result from Hirschsprung's disease or decompensation from massive fecal retention.
   5. **Soiling (encopresis)** is almost always caused by chronic fecal retention and decompensation of the sphincters.
   6. **"Holding it"** (refusal to defecate) is caused by repeated painful experiences at defecation because of large, hard stools.
   7. **Bizarre behavior** results from attempts to conceal socially unacceptable behavior (holding, soiling), which result from decompensation.

C. **A family history** of constipation suggests a functional disorder.

D. **Social factors** are important. Birth of a sibling, divorce, death of a loved one, or forceful efforts at toilet training may be causes of **psychogenic constipation.**

E. **Physical examination** confirms the diagnosis suggested by the history in most patients. Findings of significance are as follows:
   1. **Malnutrition** caused by loss of appetite.
   2. **Abdominal distention.**
   3. **Palpable fecal masses** on abdominal examination.
   4. **Anterior displacement of the anus or anal stenosis.**
   5. **Anal fissure** is revealed by **digital eversion** of the anus.
   6. **Anal sensation and reflex sphincter contraction** are abnormal in neurologic causes of constipation.
   7. **Anal sphincter tone** is reduced in neurogenic constipation but also in some cases of chronic fecal retention with decompensation.
   8. **Rectal examination** reveals large, hard stools in chronic fecal retention, but the rectum is empty in Hirschsprung's disease.

F. **Laboratory studies** are not necessary if the history and physical examination are diagnostic.
   1. **Barium enema** contributes little to the evaluation or treatment of the patient with constipation. If Hirschsprung's disease is suspected, rectal biopsy will be required for confirmation anyway.

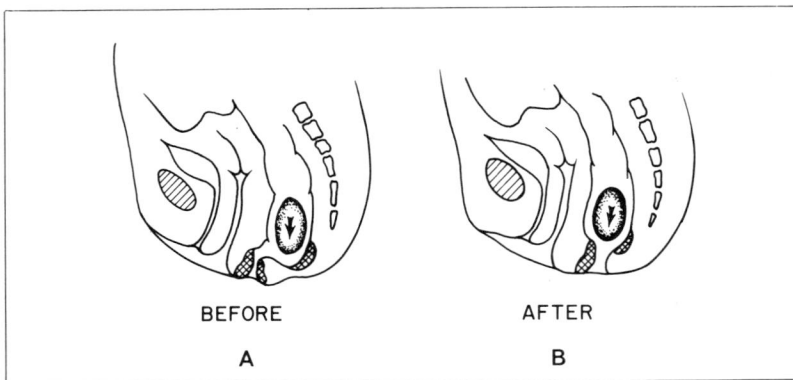

Fig. 68-1. Anterior ectopic anus. A. Anterior displacement results in diversion of defecatory force behind anus. B. After sphincterotomy force is directly into the anal canal.

   2. **Rectal punch biopsy** should be performed (as an office procedure) if there is any question of Hirschsprung's disease.
   3. **Manometric studies** may be indicated in patients with suspected neurologic disorders.

VI. Treatment
A. Anatomic malformations
   1. **Neurogenic constipation.** Stool softening is accomplished by changing the diet or giving milk of magnesia (15–60 ml bid). Daily enemas or suppositories may be necessary to control incontinence.
   2. **Hirschsprung's disease.** Resection of the aganglionic segment with endorectal pull-through procedure is curative.
   3. **Anal stenosis.** Daily dilatations for 1 to 3 months are usually all that is required. They can be performed by the parent.
   4. **Anterior ectopic anus.** Posterior sphincterotomy is curative (Fig. 68-1).
B. Functional (familial) constipation
responds to daily administration of stool softeners. Some children can be managed with prune juice or bran, but milk of magnesia is easier to give and well tolerated (see **VI.D.3.b**).
C. Psychogenic constipation.
If constipation has been present for some time, both the child and the parent are anxious to do something about it. The constipation itself has become the problem. Its correction will eliminate much of the focus of family concern. If the child is motivated, success is ensured. If he is not motivated, psychologic counseling should be obtained. No program of bowel control will work without the patient's cooperation and motivation.
D. Chronic fecal retention
   1. **Objectives.** Successful treatment must address the problems of **decompensation and discomfort.** The program must enable the bowel to recover its sensory and motor functions, enable the child to have a painless bowel movement, and ideally, result in a normal bowel pattern without the use of laxatives.
   2. **The physician's role** is to help the parent and child understand the problem, outline a program for its successful correction, and give emotional support.

3. **An effective program** must eliminate rectal distention, soften stool to make defecation painless, and establish a pattern of regular defecation. There are three steps in this process: evacuation of the colon, stool softening, and patterning.

   a. **Colon evacuation.** First, the colon must be emptied.

      (1) **Fecal impaction** may require **manual extraction.**

      (2) **Large-volume enemas** (1 quart in a 2-year-old) are required in most patients. Saline is used in a child under 3 years of age, soapsuds in an older child. Enemas such as Fleet Phospho-soda are usually inadequate. Two or three enemas may be required to completely empty the colon.

      (3) **In refractory cases, a milk and molasses enema** is usually effective (½ cup of molasses in 1 quart of milk).

   b. **Stool softening.** The bowel movements must be kept soft so they are painless.

      (1) **Milk of magnesia is the most effective agent** for softening stool. It is inexpensive, easy to take, and it works. It acts as a **hygroscopic agent,** not as a stimulant. **It must be given twice a day.** The dose is **titrated** to produce stool that is the consistency of cooked oatmeal. The starting dose in a 4-year-old child is 1 tablespoon twice daily.

      (2) **Stimulant laxatives** such as Senokot, cascara, castor oil, and Dulcolax **should be avoided** in long-term treatment of constipation for they induce dependency and prevent self-regulation.

      (3) **Dietary methods** (prune juice, bran) can be effective, but they are difficult to implement in a 2- or 3-year-old. One advantage of milk of magnesia is that its use does not entail limitation of diet.

   c. **Patterning.** Development of a normal habit of daily defecation may take months to achieve. Once the child discovers that bowel movements are no longer painful, however, progress may be amazingly fast.

      (1) Defecation should be planned for the **same time each day.** A convenient time for most families is after the evening meal; this plan takes advantage of the normal gastrocolic reflex.

      (2) If the child is unable to have a bowel movement within 5 or 10 minutes, an **enema** is given to empty the rectum.

      (3) **The rectum must be emptied each day**—either by a spontaneous bowel movement of adequate amount or by an enema. The enema is seen as an aid in defecation, **not** as a punishment.

4. **Support** is an essential part of the program. Although it is emphasized that **only the child can move his bowels,** it is equally important that he feel that the doctor and his parents are allies in helping him work with this problem and that it is not his fault.

5. **Follow-up** is essential. The child should return in **1 month** for assessment of progress and compliance. A daily **record** kept by the parent of medication dose, bowel movements, and when enemas were required is helpful in this assessment. **The program must be followed for at least 6 months** to establish a normal pattern of defecation. The milk of magnesia dose is then gradually tapered and eliminated.

Prognosis. It is not unreasonable for a child to expect to have easy, spontaneous, and painless bowel movements. This goal is almost always possible to achieve if sufficient attention is given to determining the cause of constipation and an appropriate program is devised for its correction.

Bibliography

Clayden, G. S., and Lawson, J. O. N. Investigation and management of long-standing chronic constipation in childhood. *Arch. Dis. Child.* 51:918, 1976.

Leape, L. L. Constipation and Encopresis. In S. S. Gellis and B. M. Kagan (eds.), *Current Pediatric Therapy*. Philadelphia: Saunders, 1982.

Leape, L. L. Other Disorders of the Rectum and Anus. In K. J. Welch, et al. (eds.), *Pediatric Surgery*. Chicago: Year Book, 1986. P. 1038.

Leape, L. L., and Ramenofsky, M. L. Anterior ectopic anus: A common cause of constipation in children. *J. Pediatr. Surg.* 13:627, 1978.

Martelli, H., et al. Mechanisms of idiopathic constipation: Outlet obstruction. *Gastroenterology* 75:623, 1978.

Meunier, P., Marechal, J. M., and DeBeaujeu, M. J. Rectoanal pressures and rectal sensitivity studies in chronic childhood constipation. *Gastroenterology* 77:330, 1979.

Schuster, M. M. Progress in gastroenterology: The riddle of the sphincters. *Gastroenterology* 69:249, 1975.

Shafik, A. A new concept of the anatomy of the anal sphincter mechanism and the physiology of defecation. *Invest. Urol.* 12:412, 1975.

Shandling, B., and Desjardins, J. G. Anal myomectomy for constipation. *J. Pediatr. Surg.* 4:115, 1969.

69 Rectal Prolapse

Definition. *Rectal prolapse* is herniation of the rectum through the anus; although alarming to the parents, the condition is less serious than it appears. Mucosal prolapse is common after operations for imperforate anus. Complete (full-thickness) prolapse may result from poor pelvic support, as in myelomeningocele or exstrophy of the bladder, from cystic fibrosis, or from any condition that results in straining at stool: constipation, diarrhea, overzealous toilet training, or rectal polyps. In many children, the etiology is unclear.

Pathophysiology. Herniation of the rectum, if not promptly reduced, leads to edema and venous stasis. The prolapse swells and turns blue. Rupture of superficial vessels causes bleeding. The swelling may make manual reduction difficult or impossible. If prolapse is unrelieved, swelling and stasis lead to infarction.

Clinical presentation

A. **Idiopathic** rectal prolapse tends to occur in **preschoolers,** with a peak incidence in the second year of life. Mucosal prolapse following repair of imperforate anus occurs in the first year.

B. Protrusion of the rectum usually takes place at the time of **defecation** when the child is straining. It is painless.

C. **Unreduced,** the prolapse becomes swollen, painful, and blue, and it bleeds.

D. **Recurrence** is common after reduction. The interval between recurrence varies tremendously. It may recur immediately, with the next bowel movement, or not for several months.

Diagnosis. The diagnosis of rectal prolapse is made by inspection and palpation. If reduction has occurred, one must rely on the parent's description. X-rays are of no value.

A. **Intussusception** can masquerade as prolapse in those rare instances in which the intussusceptum passes all the way through the anus. In these patients, the finger can be inserted into the rectum between the intussusceptum and the anus, whereas in prolapse it is not possible to insert the finger in the sulcus between the bowel and the anus.

B. **Rectal polyps** may protrude through the anus and be mistaken for prolapse. After reduction, the polypoid nature of the lesion is usually obvious on rectal examination.

C. **Hemorrhoids** are rare in children, do not involve the entire circumference of the anus, and are not reducible.

Treatment

A. **Reduction** of rectal prolapse is easy if done before edema forms. The herniated bowel is grasped with the fingertips of the gloved hand and squeezed. Steady pressure for a minute or two reduces the swelling and the bowel "pops" in. Digital rectal examination confirms complete reduction.

B. **Immediate recurrence** is treated by strapping the buttocks together with adhesive tape for several hours after reduction.

C. **The parents are taught** how to reduce the prolapse. Readily available plastic bags are good substitutes for gloves. A lubricant is not needed.

D. The **cause** of prolapse is treated. **Constipation and diarrhea** are the most common antecedents.

E. **Sweat test** for cystic fibrosis should be obtained in every child with prolapse.

VI. **Indications for operation. Recurrent prolapse** is the indication for more aggressive therapy. Since most children "grow out" of prolapse, rare recurrences that are easily reduced should be tolerated for some months before more extensive therapy is recommended. Constipation or diarrhea must be controlled before prolapse is considered refractory. Injection treatments should be tried before an operation is recommended.

VII. **Injection treatments**

A. **Injection of 5% phenol** in glycerine or peanut oil into the submucosa of the rectum is a simple and effective method of treatment.

B. **General anesthesia** is required, but the procedure can be performed on an outpatient basis and is painless postoperatively.

C. Ninety percent of children are **cured** by a single injection treatment and most of the remainder by a second treatment.

VIII. **Operative care**

A. More than **50 different operations** have been recommended for the cure of rectal prolapse, indicating that none are uniformly successful.

B. The **Ripstein procedure** is probably the best. The rectum is fixed to the hollow of the sacrum by a prosthetic or fascial graft sutured both to the bowel and to the presacral fascia.

IX. **Postoperative care.** Bowel movements are kept soft with milk of magnesia for several months following the operation.

X. **Complications.** If the fascia or prosthesis is too tight, obstruction results. Infection and fistula formation are other possible complications. If the operation is done in infancy, obstruction may develop as the child grows and the graft does not.

XI. **Prognosis.** Excellent. In the vast majority of children, rectal prolapse is a self-limited disease that disappears as mysteriously as it came. In refractory cases, injection treatments are usually successful; very few children ever need operative treatment.

Bibliography

Altemeier, W. A., and Culbertson, W. R. Technique for perineal repair of rectal prolapse. *Survey* 58:758, 1965.

Ashcraft, K. W., Amoury, R. A., and Holder, T. M. Levator repair and posterior suspension for rectal prolapse. *J. Pediatr. Surg.* 12:241, 1977.

Fowler, R. The anatomy and treatment of rectal prolapse in childhood. *Aust. Paediatr.* 3:90, 1967.

Holder, T. M., and Ashcraft, K. W. Acquired Anorectal Lesions. In T. M. Holder and K. W. Ashcraft (eds.), *Pediatric Surgery*. Philadelphia: Saunders, 1980. P. 429.

Leape, L. L. Other Disorders of the Rectum and Anus. In K. J. Welch, et al. (eds.), *Pediatric Surgery*. Chicago: Year Book, 1986. P. 1038.

Ripstein, C. B., and Lanter, B. Etiology and surgical therapy of massive prolapse of the rectum. *Ann. Surg.* 157:259, 1963.

Wyllie, G. G. The injection treatment of rectal prolapse. *J. Pediatr. Surg.* 14:62, 1979.

70 Anal Disorders

I. Anal fissure

A. Clinical presentation. Superficial tears at the anal mucocutaneous junction are the most common cause of rectal bleeding in childhood. Fissures are very common in infants.

1. **Constipation** is the usual cause of anal fissure. The large, hard stools cause a tear during defecation. Pain with subsequent bowel movements leads to holding of stools, which then get large and hard, causing further tears, perpetuating the disorder.
2. **Chronic anal fissure may be a symptom of Crohn's disease,** preceding the intestinal manifestations. Anal fissure is also common in children undergoing chemotherapy for **leukemia.**

B. Diagnosis. The diagnosis of anal fissure is made by inspection of the anus (**not** by anoscopy or sigmoidoscopy). The skin is everted by centrifugal traction with the patient bearing down. Chronic fissures are typically associated with a **skin tag** or hypertrophy of the anal papilla.

C. Treatment

1. **Stool softening** is the key feature of treatment of both acute and chronic fissures. In infants, addition of corn syrup, ½–1 teaspoon in each bottle, may be all that is necessary. Milk of magnesia, 1 teaspoon to 1 tablespoon, is the preferred medication in older children.
2. **Warm sitz baths** relax the anal muscle spasm and provide some relief.
3. **Topical analgesics** are seldom indicated but may be used.
4. **Chronic fissure requires excision** to eliminate the granulation tissue and indolent infection and to permit healing. Sphincterotomy is performed at the same time.
5. **Excision is not indicated for** fissures or ulcerations in **leukemic patients** since they do not heal.

II. Perianal abscess

A. Clinical presentation.

1. **Superficial perianal infection** is common in infants, presenting as a "boil" anywhere in the perianal region or the buttocks. The etiology is unknown. Common organisms are *Staphylococcus* or enteric bacteria.
2. **Perirectal infection** or infection in the anal canal usually results from a **crypt abscess.** Enteric organisms, particularly anaerobes, are the culprits. Abnormalities of defecation or hard stools are seldom responsible.
3. **Inflammatory bowel disease** may present as perianal sepsis in older children.
4. **Leukemia** and immunodeficiency states (e.g., resulting from chemotherapy) are other causes of perianal infection.

B. Diagnosis. Perianal or perirectal infection is usually obvious on examination. Redness, swelling, pain, and tenderness are present. Rectal examination may demonstrate a mass in the perirectal or ischiorectal space.

C. Treatment

1. **Superficial** perianal or buttock infections can sometimes be successfully treated with antibiotics. Incision and drainage is indicated if there is pus formation.
2. **Perirectal and ischiorectal abscesses** require incision and drainage as soon as diagnosed. Fluctuation may not be present yet. It invariably develops, but the abscess may expand a great deal first. Early drainage minimizes damage and hastens recovery.
3. Approximately **25%** of children with perirectal abscess will develop a **fistula-in-ano**.

III. Fistula-in-ano

A. Clinical presentation. Fistula-in-ano is the result of perianal infection that communicates between the skin and the mucosa of the rectum. It almost always follows a **crypt abscess.** The fistula may extend between the internal and external sphincters or may be lateral to the external sphincter. The typical symptom is **recurrent perianal infections** in the same location. Intermittent drainage of cloudy or purulent material is sometimes noted. Once established, the fistula seldom disappears spontaneously.

B. Diagnosis. The opening of the fistula on the perianal skin surface is usually evident. Recurrent infections in the same location near the anus are presumptive evidence of fistula. Contrast fistulogram is unnecessary and meddlesome.

C. Treatment. Fistulotomy, laying the fistula open so that it may epithelialize, is the appropriate treatment. Although this is a suitable outpatient procedure, general anesthesia is required. Excision of the fistula is not necessary unless there is excessive granulation tissue and inflammatory reaction. Postoperative sitz baths and stool softening aid healing and comfort.

IV. Condyloma acuminatum

A. Clinical presentation. Papillomas or "warts" in the perianal region are usually condyloma acuminatum, a viral infection that may be transmitted from an infected mother or result from **sexual abuse.**

B. Diagnosis. The appearance of the papilloma is characteristic.

C. Treatment. *Podophyllum* resin applications are effective, as is laser destruction. Surgical excision is not appropriate because of the high recurrence rate. Autoimmunization with autogenous vaccine made from the papilloma has been used in refractory cases. If sexual abuse is suspected, appropriate child protective measures must be taken.

Bibliography

Brook, I., and Martin, W. J. Aerobic and anaerobic bacteriology of perirectal abscess in children. *Pediatrics* 66:282, 1980.

De Jong, A. R., Weiss, J. C., and Brent, R. L. Condyloma acuminata in children. *Am. J. Dis. Child.* 136:704, 1982.

Enberg, R. N., Cox, R. H., and Burry, V. F. Perirectal abscess in children. *Am. J. Dis. Child.* 128:360, 1974.

Holder, T. M., and Ashcraft, K. W. Acquired anorectal lesions. In T. M. Holder and K. W. Ashcraft (eds.), *Pediatric Surgery.* Philadelphia: Saunders, 1980. P. 429.

Leape L. L. Other Disorders of the Rectum and Anus. In K. J. Welch, et al. (eds.), *Pediatric Surgery.* Chicago: Year Book, 1986. P. 1038.

McCoy, C. R., Applebaum, H., and Besser, A. S. Condyloma acuminata: An unusual presentation of child abuse. *J. Pediatr. Surg.* 17:505, 1982.

71 Mesenteric Cysts

I. **Definition.** Cysts arising in the mesentery or omentum are variants of cystic hygroma, resulting from malformations of the small lymphatics or the thoracic duct. They may be small or large, single or multiple, and filled with serous or chylous fluid.

II. **Pathophysiology.** The cysts are thin-walled and lined with mesothelium, unlike duplications, which have intestinal mucosa and muscular wall. Because they are soft and the abdominal contents are easily displaced, expansion of the cyst seldom interferes with the function of surrounding organs. Trauma may cause bleeding into a mesenteric cyst, but spontaneous rupture and torsion are very rare. Volvulus of the intestine can occur with intestinal infarction.

III. **Clinical presentation.** Mesenteric and omental cysts are usually asymptomatic until they are quite large. Abdominal distention is frequently the first sign. Chronic or acute abdominal pain may be a symptom of a mesenteric cyst. Vomiting, distention, and severe pain develop if the cyst and intestine have undergone volvulus.

IV. **Diagnosis.** Abdominal x-rays typically show a "blank" area in the midabdomen devoid of intestinal gas patterns. Ultrasound or CT scan will demonstrate the fluid-filled mass.

V. **Operative care.** Removal of the cyst may be very simple or very difficult. If the cyst cannot be removed without compromising the blood supply of the intestine, a partial intestinal resection may be required. Extensive cysts are best treated by open drainage into the peritoneal cavity and excision of as much of the cyst wall as possible. Some cysts recur and require repeat resection, but often no further treatment is needed. Internal drainage into the intestine is not necessary.

VI. **Postoperative care.** Routine

VII. **Complications.** Recurrent and chylous ascites are the most common complications, both fortunately rare.

VIII. **Prognosis.** Excellent

Bibliography

Arnheim, E. E., et al. Mesenteric cysts in infancy and childhood. *Pediatrics* 24:469, 1959.

Colodny, A. H. Mesenteric and Omental Cysts. In K. J. Welch, et al. (eds.), *Pediatric Surgery*. Chicago: Year Book, 1986. P. 921.

Fonkalsrud, E. W. Malformations of the Lymphatic System, and Hemangiomas. In T. M. Holder and K. W. Ashcraft (eds.), *Pediatric Surgery*. Philadelphia: Saunders, 1980. P. 1042.

Handelsman, J. C., and Ravitch, M. N. Chylous cysts of the mesentery in children. *Ann. Surg.* 140:185, 1954.

Mollitt, D. L., Ballantine, T. V. N., and Grosfeld, J. L. Mesenteric cysts in infancy and childhood. *Surg. Gynecol. Obstet.* 147:182, 1978.

72 Biliary Atresia and Choledochal Cyst

I. **Definition.** *Biliary atresia* is a progressive sclerosing obliteration of the bile ducts producing cholestatic jaundice and cirrhosis. Biliary atresia accounts for approximately 20% of jaundice in neonates after 2 weeks of age.

   A. The **etiology** of biliary atresia is unknown, but there is considerable evidence that it is an inflammatory process caused by a viral infection. Congenital absence of bile ducts—true atresia—is very rare.

   B. The inflammation may extend into the liver, obliterating intrahepatic bile ducts as well.

II. **Pathophysiology.** The interference with excretion of bile produces severe liver damage and a host of pathologic consequences.

   A. **Liver cell damage** from bile stasis (and perhaps also from the primary insult) results in decreased synthetic and conjugating functions of the liver. Numerous functions are affected, including detoxification of metabolites and drugs and the production of proteins and clotting factors. Growth failure results.

   B. **Hepatomegaly** develops from cellular swelling due to the intense inflammatory response.

   C. **Jaundice** results from backup of conjugated bilirubin into the bloodstream.

   D. **Cirrhosis,** scarring of the liver, develops from the inflammatory fibrosis, causing **portal hypertension, splenomegaly,** and **ascites**.

   E. **Fat-soluble vitamins** cannot be absorbed because of the absence of bile in the intestine, augmenting the **coagulopathy** from decreased synthesis of clotting factors.

III. **Clinical presentation**

   A. **Persistent jaundice** is the presenting symptom in infants with biliary atresia. "Physiologic" jaundice, common in newborns, almost always disappears by 5–7 days.

   B. **Hyperbilirubinemia** in a neonate that develops or persists **beyond 2 weeks of age is pathologic** and requires evaluation.

   C. **Clay-colored stools** and a large, **hard liver** are typical associated findings. A normal liver is almost never found in infants with biliary atresia.

   D. **Cholestatic jaundice** (conjugated bilirubin levels of 5–15 mg/dl, with a normal or slightly elevated unconjugated fraction) suggests biliary atresia.

IV. **Differential diagnosis of cholestatic jaundice.** Neonatal hepatitis or biliary atresia is the cause of cholestatic jaundice in three-fourths of infants. Many other causes make up the remainder (Table 72-1).

V. **Diagnosis.** The problem is to separate biliary atresia from hepatitis, which is common, and from other causes of jaundice, which are rare.

   A. **Laboratory tests** are used to evaluate liver function and to identify the cause of jaundice if possible (Table 72-2).

   B. **Radiologic studies** are carried out if infectious and genetic disorders have been excluded, in the hope of separating extrahepatic biliary obstruction from hepatitis.

Table 72-1. Causes of cholestatic jaundice

Congenital infections	Genetic syndromes	Miscellaneous
TORCH syndromes Hepatitis A and B Coxsackie virus B Echovirus 11, 14, 19 Syphilis *Listeria* Group B *Streptococcus* Gram-negative infection Urinary tract infection	Galactosemia Tyrosinemia Congenital fructose intolerance $Alpha_1$-antitrypsin deficiency Cystic fibrosis Niemann-Pick disease Trisomy 17, 18, 21 Hypopituitarism Alagille's syndrome Zellweger's syndrome Byler's syndrome Menkes' syndrome Polysplenia syndrome	Hemolytic disease TPN Congestive heart failure Necrotizing enterocolitis Respiratory distress syndrome Neonatal hepatitis Biliary atresia

1. **Ultrasound** of the liver and porta hepatis is useful to reveal a **choledochal cyst** or dilated intra- or extrahepatic ducts.
2. **Hepatic scintiscan** using ^{99m}Tc-labeled iminodiacetic acid derivatives (e.g., **HIDA, PIPIDA, DISIDA**) is the most accurate method of demonstrating excretion from the liver. Infants with biliary atresia show no excretion, while those with hepatitis should excrete isotope. A choledochal cyst may be demonstrated. Unfortunately, nonexcretion does not prove extrahepatic obstruction, since severe hepatitis or intrahepatic obliteration of the bile ducts will also result in lack of excretion.
C. **Liver biopsy** has been used to differentiate biliary atresia from neonatal hepatitis, but its use is not recommended since there is an unacceptably high error rate.

VI. **Indications for operation**
A. **Biliary atresia can be corrected in a high percentage of infants** by means of the Kasai portoenterostomy, provided the operation is done before irreversible liver damage has occurred. Thus it is essential that this diagnosis be made or

Table 72-2. Laboratory tests for evaluating jaundice

General screening tests	Hematologic tests	Liver function tests	Etiologic tests
CBC, urinalysis Blood types—parent and child BUN, creatinine	Platelet count Reticulocyte count Prothrombin time Partial thromboplastin time	Bilirubin, D/T SGOT SGPT LDH Alkaline phosphatase Albumin, globulin Cholesterol, triglycerides Vitamin E level	Sweat test $Alpha_1$-antitrypsin TORCH titers Urine reducing substances Hepatitis B Ag and Ab Alpha fetoprotein Urine amino acids

excluded in timely fashion, by **6 weeks** of age if possible. **There is essentially no chance of cure if operation is delayed beyond 10 weeks of age.**

1. **Bile flow** is more likely to occur after portoenterostomy if the operation is done earlier.
2. **Jaundice** is more likely to disappear when the operation is done in the younger patient.
3. **Cirrhosis** is less severe if the operation is done early.

B. **A positive DISIDA scan** (no excretion of isotope) in a jaundiced infant who has no evidence of infectious or genetic disorders to explain the jaundice **is an indication for operative exploration** to determine presence of biliary atresia.

VII. Preoperative preparation

A. **Coagulation abnormalities,** anemia, and hypoproteinemia should be corrected, if possible, before exploration.

B. **Parents** must understand the severity of the disorder and realize that our current methods of treatment are far from satisfactory. They need to know that portoenterostomy may not be successful but that there is little else to offer these unfortunate infants.

VIII. Operative care

A. **Exploration of the porta hepatis** for the presence of bile ducts is the initial operative procedure.

B. **Cholangiogram** is obtained if a gallbladder is present. The gallbladder is cannulated and dye is injected. Rarely, a true atresia may be found with dilatation of the proximal common hepatic duct, and cholangiography may be performed by direct injection of dye.

C. If an **intact biliary system** is demonstrated with flow up into the liver as well as into the duodenum, the diagnosis of biliary atresia is excluded. **Liver biopsy** is obtained, and the operation is terminated.

D. **Portoenterostomy** (Fig. 72-1) is performed if the bile ducts are not patent. (They may be absent or represented by fibrous cords.) A loop of jejunum is isolated and anastomosed to the porta after fibrotic tissue has been cut away in the region of the confluence of the left and right hepatic ducts.

IX. Postoperative care

A. **Bile flow** may occur immediately after the operation but is often slow to appear, presumably due to resolution of inflammation.

B. **Jaundice** also disappears slowly after successful portoenterostomy; it may take 6–12 weeks to disappear.

C. **Phenobarbital,** 1 mg/kg/day, and **cholestyramine,** 0.25 gm tid, may be of value in stimulating bile flow.

D. **Cephalosporins** or trimethoprim-sulfamethoxazole **(Bactrim)** is given prophylactically for 6–12 months to prevent cholangitis.

X. Complications.
Results of portoenterostomy are variable. If the operation is highly successful (return of bilirubin and liver function tests to near normal), there are fewer complications. Incomplete success usually results from preexisting severe liver damage that is not completely reversible by the operation.

A. **Cholangitis** occurs in many patients following portoenterostomy. Persistent **obstruction,** either extra- or intrahepatic, and ascending infection are the most significant etiologic factors. Resident intestinal flora—coliforms and *Klebsiella* species—are the usual culprits. External venting of the enterostomy and use of prophylactic antibiotics may decrease the frequency of cholangitis.

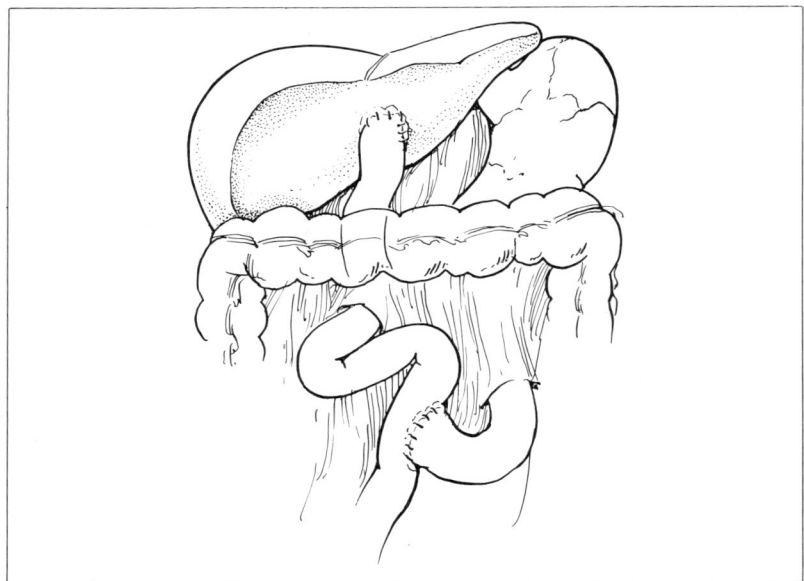

Fig. 72-1. Kasai portoenterostomy. Roux-en-Y jejunostomy with anastomosis of the intestine to the hilum of the liver.

- **B. Persistent jaundice** is evidence of failure or partial success of portoenterostomy. It may reflect either an inadequate operation or, more typically, an irreversible situation.
- **C. Return of jaundice** after successful portoenterostomy usually indicates mechanical obstruction. Reoperation is indicated.
- **D. Portal hypertension** develops from progressive cirrhosis in a significant fraction of patients who have had an apparently good result from portoenterostomy.
- **E. Hepatic failure, ascites, and hepatic encephalopathy** may occur as a result of progressive cirrhosis, despite initially favorable results.
- **F. Growth retardation** is often seen after portoenterostomy, even when it is otherwise apparently successful. It is worst in the first year.
- **G. Osteomalacia** may result from impaired absorption of vitamin D.

XI. **Prognosis**

- **A. Effective bile flow with disappearance of jaundice can be expected in nearly 75%** of infants with biliary atresia who undergo portoenterostomy within the first 6 weeks of life. Results decline rapidly with advancing age at the time of operation beyond that point.
- **B. Long-term survival rates are 30–50%** in large series.
- **C. Progressive cirrhosis** develops in at least half of the children who survive following portoenterostomy. Life expectancy is highly variable. Some children live relatively well with significant hepatic failure. Others have a fairly rapid downhill course.
- **D. Liver transplantation** has been employed successfully in children in whom liver failure has developed after portoenterostomy.

Biliary hypoplasia

A. Biliary exploration sometimes reveals an intact biliary tract that is small but patent. Hypoplasia may extend into the intrahepatic biliary radicals.

B. Biliary hypoplasia results from **low bile flow states** ($alpha_1$-antitrypsin deficiency, hepatitis, and intrahepatic biliary atresia) and from **inflammation** of the extrahepatic ducts themselves, an early or aborted stage of biliary atresia.

C. Low flow states are not improved by operation, but corticosteroids may be of some benefit. If the patient does not improve within a few weeks, reexploration and portoenterostomy may be indicated.

Choledochal cyst

A. **Dilatation of the common hepatic duct,** causing extrahepatic biliary obstruction and the formation of a cyst, may be caused by an inflammatory process related to biliary atresia. It is much less common but more easily corrected.

B. Only **half** of choledochal cysts are **diagnosed in infancy.** The symptoms are similar to biliary atresia. The cyst is found by ultrasound or HIDA scan.

C. **Clinical findings** in older children are the triad of **abdominal pain, jaundice,** and an epigastric **mass** by physical examination or radiologic studies.

D. **Ultrasound, CT, or MRI** demonstrates the cyst most accurately, but the cyst often will also be evident on contrast study of the duodenum and stomach (upper GI series).

E. **Excision** of the cyst with Roux-Y anastomosis of a loop of jejunum to the dilated proximal hepatic duct is the operation of choice. If the cyst is not removed, there is a significant risk of later development of bile duct carcinoma.

Bibliography

Adelman, S. Prognosis of uncorrected biliary atresia. *J. Pediatr. Surg.* 13:389, 1978.

Alonzo-Lej, F., Revor, W. B., and Pessagno, D. J. Congenital choledochal cyst, with a report of 2, and an analysis of 94 cases. *Surg. Gynecol. Obstet. Int. Abst. Surg.* 108:1, 1959.

Altman, R. P. Results of re-operation for correction of extrahepatic biliary atresia. *J. Pediatr. Surg.* 14:305, 1979.

Altman, R. P., Chandra, R., and Lilly, J. R. Ongoing cirrhosis after successful porticoenterostomy in infants with biliary atresia. *J. Pediatr. Surg.* 10:685, 1975.

Barkin, R. M., and Lilly, J. R. Biliary atresia and the Kasai operation: Continuing care. *J. Pediatr.* 96:1015, 1980.

Filler, R. M., and Stringel, G. Treatment of choledochal cyst by excision. *J. Pediatr. Surg.* 15:437, 1980.

Hays, D. M. Biliary Tract and Liver. In T. M. Holder and K. W. Ashcraft (eds.), *Pediatric Surgery.* Philadelphia: Saunders, 1980. P. 509.

Hitch, D. C., and Lilly, J. R. Identification, quantification, and significance of bacterial growth within the biliary tract after Kasai's operation. *J. Pediatr. Surg.* 13:563, 1978.

Ishida, M., et al. Primary excision of choledochal cysts. *Surgery* 68:884, 1970.

Iwatsuki, S., Shaw, B. W., Jr., and Starzl, T. E. Liver transplantation for biliary atresia. *World J. Surg.* 8:51, 1984.

Kant, R. J., Jr., et al. Biliary atresia survey, surgical section. In Proceedings of the American Academy of Pediatrics, 1965.

Kasai, M. Advances in treatment of biliary atresia. *Jpn. J. Surg.* 13:265, 1983.

Kasai, M., Watanabe, I., and Ohi, R. Follow-up studies of long-term survivors after hepatic portoenterostomy for "noncorrectable" biliary atresia. *J. Pediatr. Surg.* 10:173, 1975.

Kasai, M., et al. Surgical treatment of biliary atresia. *J. Pediatr. Surg.* 3:665, 1968.

Kim, S. H. Choledochal cyst: Survey by the Surgical Section of the American Academy of Pediatrics. *J. Pediatr. Surg.* 16:402, 1981.

Klotz D., Cohn, B. D., and Kottmeier, P. K. Choledochal cysts: Diagnostic and therapeutic problems. *J. Pediatr. Surg.* 8:271, 1973.

Lilly, J. R. The surgical treatment of choledochal cyst. *Surg. Gynecol. Obstet.* 149:36, 1979.

Lilly, J. R. Biliary Atresia: The Jaundiced Infant. In K. J. Welch, et al. (eds.), *Pediatric Surgery*. Chicago: Year Book, 1986. P. 1047.

Ohi, R., et al. Reoperation in patients with biliary atresia. *J. Pediatr. Surg.* 20:256, 1985.

O'Neill, J. A., Jr. Choledochal Cyst. In K. J. Welch, et al. (eds.), *Pediatric Surgery*. Chicago: Year Book, 1986. P. 1056.

73 Portal Hypertension

I. Definition. Increased pressure in the portal venous system results from obstruction, which may be either intrahepatic or extrahepatic.

   A. Intrahepatic portal hypertension usually results from cirrhosis, most commonly caused by hepatitis or biliary atresia. Other causes are cystic fibrosis, Wilson's disease, alpha$_1$-antitrypsin deficiency, and congenital hepatic fibrosis.

   B. Extrahepatic portal hypertension results from thrombosis of the portal vein. In most cases the cause is unknown, but neonatal omphalitis or cannulation of the umbilical vein may be responsible.

   C. Hepatic vein obstruction, constrictive pericarditis, congestive heart failure, and cor pulmonale may also cause portal hypertension.

Pathophysiology

   A. Obstruction to portal venous flow within the liver or in the portal vein results in flow through **collateral** channels, principally the coronary vein and short gastrics, which empty into the veins of the lower esophagus, which connect with the azygos vein. The **esophageal** veins dilate, forming submucosal **varices.**

   B. Consequences of portal hypertension are **hemorrhage** from ruptured esophageal varices, **hypersplenism, ascites,** and **encephalopathy.**

   C. Esophageal varices tend to rupture and bleed. The precipitating factors are not well understood, but most episodes are preceded by an upper respiratory infection or aspirin ingestion.

   D. Hypersplenism is induced by the reversal of flow through the splenic vein causing splenic congestion and splenomegaly. Leukopenia and thrombocytopenia develop.

   E. Ascites results from several factors: intrahepatic obstruction to lymph flow, increased portal filtration pressure, decreased serum albumin, and hormonal factors such as increased production of aldosterone and antidiuretic hormone (ADH).

   F. Encephalopathy only occurs in patients with cirrhosis. It is caused by the impaired ability of the liver to metabolize ammonia to urea and clear intestinal amines, as well as other less understood mechanisms. Coma is most commonly precipitated by a protein load, such as blood from bleeding esophageal varices.

Clinical presentation. Intrahepatic portal hypertension is but one of many manifestations of progressive cirrhosis in a sick child. Extrahepatic portal hypertension may be unsuspected until the child has a sudden episode of massive hemorrhage from esophageal varices or splenomegaly develops.

   A. Upper gastrointestinal hemorrhage from ruptured esophageal varices is the most dramatic manifestation of portal hypertension. Bleeding may be massive and rapid, with vomiting of large quantities of clotted and changed blood, or it may be slow and occult, with melena or anemia the only evidence.

   B. Hemorrhoids occasionally may be the presenting complaint.

   C. Splenomegaly is usually present, with hypersplenism manifested as low leukocyte and platelet counts.

   D. Abnormal liver function tests, jaundice, and growth failure are frequently found if the child has cirrhosis.

- E. **Ascites** may precede or follow bleeding from esophageal varices.
- F. **Malabsorption** and protein-losing enteropathy are seen in long-standing portal hypertension.
- G. **Physical findings**
  1. **Splenomegaly.** If the liver is not palpable and liver function tests are normal, portal hypertension is extrahepatic.
  2. **Enlarged, hard, nodular liver.**
  3. **Dilated abdominal veins** (caput medusae).
  4. **Hemorrhoids.**
  5. **Ascites.**

IV. Diagnosis

- A. **Esophageal varices** are demonstrated by **barium swallow.** Esophagoscopy is seldom necessary.
- B. **Liver function tests** distinguish intra- from extrahepatic portal hypertension.
- C. **Leukopenia** and **thrombocytopenia** indicate hypersplenism.
- D. **Elevated blood ammonia** (>1000 μg/liter) confirms the diagnosis of hepatic encephalopathy.
- E. **CT scan** will usually demonstrate the portal and splenic veins and inferior vena cava. Angiography is seldom necessary.

V. Medical management

- A. **Bleeding esophageal varices.** Because hemorrhage from varices almost always stops spontaneously, treatment is resuscitation and support.
  1. **Blood volume is restored** by rapid and adequate transfusion, with monitoring of pulse, blood pressure, hematocrit, and urine output.
  2. **Nasogastric intubation** and cold saline gastric lavage may be necessary.
  3. **Cimetidine,** 10 mg/kg, is given to block gastric acid production.
  4. **Vasopressin** is used if bleeding continues. (Starting dose: 0.005 μ/kg/minute, increased as necessary to .02 μ/kg/minute.)
  5. **Balloon tamponade** of the esophagus may be necessary to stop bleeding in extreme cases, but this is seldom necessary in children.
  6. **Cathartics and enemas** are given to empty the intestine of blood to prevent absorption and possible encephalopathy.
  7. If clotting factors are abnormal, transfusions of fresh frozen **plasma** and **platelets** are given.
  8. **Sclerotherapy**—endoscopic injection of varices with sclerosing solution—is an effective means of control in most children.
  9. **Aspirin** should never be given to a child with esophageal varices.
- B. **Hypersplenism** from portal hypertension is seldom severe enough to require treatment. Splenectomy is not indicated.
- C. **Ascites** can usually be managed by use of chlorothiazide (Diuril), 10–15 mg/kg, q12h; spironolactone (Aldactone), 0.5–1.0 mg/kg, qid; and a low-salt diet. Occasionally paracentesis is indicated to relieve respiratory distress. Fortunately, the ascites disappears spontaneously in most patients.

VI. Indications for operation.
Some children only bleed once or have only a few easily controlled episodes; operation is not indicated. When recurrent bleeding from esoph-

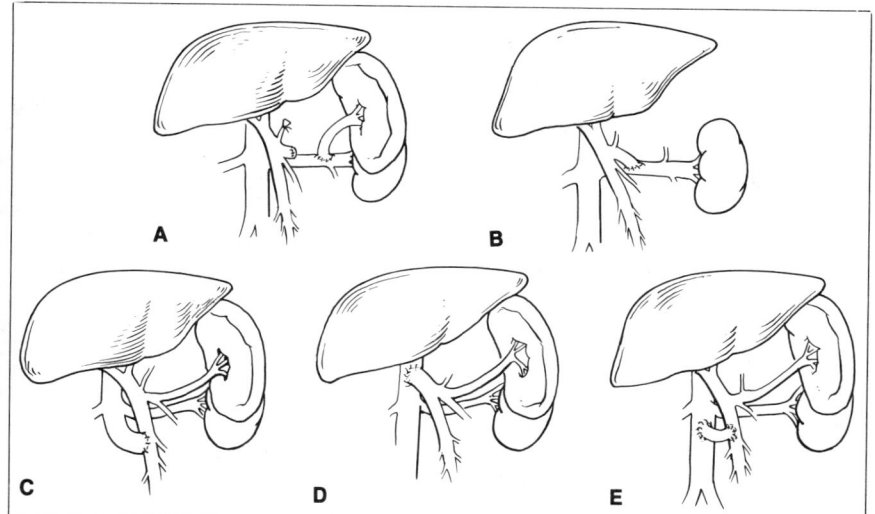

Fig. 73-1. Shunts for portal hypertension. A. Distal splenorenal shunt. B. Central splenorenal shunt. C. Side-to-end mesocaval shunt. D. End-to-side portacaval shunt. E. Interposition mesocaval shunt.

ageal varices is life-threatening, however, a **shunting procedure** should be considered.

- **A. Sclerotherapy** has eliminated the need for shunting in many patients and allowed shunting to be delayed in others.
- **B. Liver transplantation** is preferred to a shunting procedure if the patient has irreversible, progressive liver failure.
- **C. Current indications for a shunt**
    1. **Absence of liver disease** (extrahepatic portal hypertension) **or stable,** nonprogressive **cirrhosis** with good synthetic function.
    2. **Recurrent** episodes of **variceal hemorrhage** that are **life-threatening** and uncontrolled by other means.
    3. **Age of 10 years or more,** if possible. Shunts have a low long-term patency rate when performed in young children.

VII. Preoperative preparation. A shunt is an elective operation performed after the patient is resuscitated and stable.
- **A. Clotting factors** should be restored to as close to normal as possible.
- **B. Albumin** level should be low normal or better.
- **C. Encephalopathy** must be reversed.
- **D. Venogram** must demonstrate a vein with a diameter of at least **1 cm** in the portal system.

VIII. Operative care
- **A. Portal-systemic venous shunts** (Fig. 73-1) can be constructed in several ways, each of which has its advocates and detractors. The condition of the veins often dictates which procedure may be followed.

1. **Splenorenal** shunts may be constructed by anastomosis of the splenic vein to the renal vein, either centrally or distally. The spleen does not have to be removed.
2. **Portacaval** shunts entail end-to-side or side-to-side anastomosis of the portail vein to the vena cava. This type of shunt is not possible if there is portal vein thrombosis.
3. **Mesocaval** shunts connect the dilated superior mesenteric vein (SMV) to the inferior vena cava, either by division of the cava and end-to-side anastomosis to the SMV or by interposition of a graft of vein or prosthetic material.

B. **Sugiura procedure.** Radical devascularization of the stomach and the esophagus with esophageal transection (and reanastomosis) and splenectomy has a high success rate and surprisingly low mortality. Postoperative encephalopathy has not been seen as a result of this procedure. It is indicated if the patient is unsuitable for a shunt because of thrombosis of the splenic and mesenteric veins, or if the shunt fails.

C. **Esophagectomy** can also be used to control bleeding varices in patients who are unsuitable for shunt. Colonic interposition is required to reestablish continuity. This operation is well-tolerated by children.

D. **Transthoracic ligation** of varices is not a satisfactory long-term solution to bleeding from portal hypertension but is sometimes employed as an emergency procedure before shunting. Sclerotherapy has made it nearly obsolete.

IX. **Postoperative care.** Because of preexisting liver disease in many of these patients, postoperative care is demanding and critical.

A. **Maintain blood volume** with transfusions of blood, plasma, and albumin solution. Hypotension may cause shunt thrombosis.

B. **Monitor** and correct **clotting factor deficiencies.** Fresh frozen plasma and platelet transfusions are usually necessary.

C. **Monitor blood ammonia** levels.

D. Give **cimetidine,** 10 mg/kg q4h, to help prevent gastritis and ulcer.

X. **Complications**

A. **Encephalopathy** may occur in the immediate postoperative period or at any time later. The risk of its occurrence is related to the severity of the liver disease.

B. **Shunt thrombosis** is most likely to occur if the veins are too small. Deferring operation to the age of 10 or later minimizes this risk.

XI. **Prognosis.** The prognosis after shunting procedures in general is good. Most patients have no further bleeding episodes. The shunt has no effect on the underlying liver disease, however. Radical procedures (esophagectomy and Sugiura procedure) also have good long-term results but a higher incidence of mechanical complications (e.g., stricture).

Bibliography

Altman, R. P. Portal Hypertension. In K. J. Welch, et al. (eds.), *Pediatric Surgery.* Chicago: Year Book, 1986. P. 1075.

Altman, R. P., and Krug, J. Portal hypertension: American Academy of Pediatrics, Surgical Section Survey. *J. Pediatr. Surg.* 17:567, 1982.

Alvarez, F., et al. Portal obstruction in children. I. Clinical investigation and hemorrhage risk. *J. Pediatr.* 103:696, 1983.

Alvarez, F., et al. Portal obstruction in children. II. Results of surgical portosystemic shunts. *J. Pediatr.* 103:703, 1983.

Baum, S. I., and Nusbaum, M. The control of gastrointestinal hemorrhage by selective mesenteric arterial infusion of vasopressin. *Radiology* 98:497, 1971.

Bismuth, H., Franco, D., and Alagille, D. Portal diversion for portal hypertension in children: The first ninety patients. *Ann. Surg.* 192:18, 1980.

Boles, E. T. Portal Hypertension. In T. M. Holder and K. W. Ashcraft (eds.), *Pediatric Surgery*. Philadelphia: Saunders, 1980. P. 530.

Boles, E. T., Jr., and Birken, G. Extrahepatic portal hypertension in children: Long-term evaluation. *Chir. Pediatr.* 24:23, 1983.

Clatworthy, H. W., Jr. Extrahepatic Portal Hypertension. In C. G. Child (ed.), *Major Problems in Clinical Surgery*, Vol. 14. Philadelphia: Saunders, 1974.

Fonkalsrud, E. W. Surgical management of portal hypertension in childhood. *Arch. Surg.* 115:1042, 1980.

Howard, E. R., Stamatakis, J. D., and Mowat, A. P. Management of esophageal varices in children by injection sclerotherapy. *J. Pediatr. Surg.* 19:2, 1984.

Koop, C. E., and Roddy, R. Colonic replacement of distal esophagus and proximal stomach in the management of bleeding varices in children. *Ann. Surg.* 147:17, 1958.

Lilly, J. R., Van Steigmann, G., and Stellin, G. Esophageal endosclerosis in children with portal vein thrombosis. *J. Pediatr. Surg.* 17:571, 1982.

Sugiura, M., and Futagawa, S. Further evaluation of the Sugiura procedure in the treatment of esophageal varices. *Arch. Surg.* 112:1317, 1977.

Terblanche, J., et al. Acute bleeding varices: A 5-year prospective evaluation of tamponade and sclerotherapy. *Ann. Surg.* 194:521, 1981.

74 Gallbladder Disease

Cholelithiasis

I. **Definition.** *Cholelithiasis,* stones in the gallbladder, is not rare in childhood; it almost always requires surgical treatment.
   A. **Hemolytic anemias** are well-known causes of cholelithiasis. Stones occur in 30% of children with hereditary spherocytosis, 20% of those with sickle cell disease, and up to 25% of children with thalassemia major.
   B. **Nonhemolytic cholelithiasis** is associated with obesity, teenage pregnancy, terminal ileal resection, cystic fibrosis, chronic hepatitis, leukemia, TPN, and malformations of the biliary tree such as choledochal cyst or duplication of the gallbladder.

Pathophysiology
   A. **Gallstones** in patients with **hemolytic anemia** result from **excessive pigment** load, which causes precipitation as the bile is concentrated in the gallbladder.
   B. **Nonpigment gallstones** develop as a result of chemical or physical alterations in gallbladder bile, which may be caused by hormonal effects (gallstones are 10–20 times more common in girls than boys), abnormalities of cholesterol metabolism (obesity), interference with enterohepatic circulation of bile salts (distal ileal resection), or biliary stasis (pregnancy, TPN).
   C. **Obstruction** of the cystic duct by a stone can precipitate an attack of acute cholecystitis. Obstruction of the common bile duct causes jaundice and sometimes cholangitis; a stone at the ampulla can cause pancreatitis.
   D. **Gallstones are foreign bodies** that cause irritation and inflammation of the gallbladder and predispose to infection. They are the most common cause of acute cholecystitis.

Clinical presentation
   A. **Gallstones may be asymptomatic** and discovered accidentally, particularly if they are large and do not obstruct. Pigment stones may be asymptomatic for a long time.
   B. **Abdominal pain** is the most common symptom of cholelithiasis or cholecystitis, usually localized to the right upper quadrant and often, but not necessarily, precipitated by ingestion of fatty foods.
   C. **Right upper quadrant tenderness,** fever, and leukocytosis are frequently present if there is acute cholecystitis. The gallbladder may be palpable.
   D. **Jaundice** signifies obstruction in the common bile duct.
   E. **Pancreatitis** may be the presenting evidence of cholelithiasis. The child should be evaluated for possible biliary stones after the acute episode subsides.

Diagnosis
   A. **Ultrasonography** is the simplest method of identifying gallstones and is accurate in more than 90% of cases. Sometimes very small stones or "sludge" will be detected.
   B. **Radionuclide** imaging with technetium-99m-labeled iminodiacetic acid derivatives (e.g., HIDA, DISIDA) is the most accurate method of evaluating gallblad-

der function and thus of making the diagnosis of acute cholecystitis in the absence of stones.

   C. Oral cholecystography is a good diagnostic method for evaluating gallbladder function in the older child but has been largely supplanted by simpler radionuclide studies.

V. Indications for operation

   A. Cholecystectomy is advised for any child with **symptomatic cholelithiasis**. Experiments with chemical dissolution have been discouraging.

   B. The gallbladder should be removed at the time of **splenectomy** for spherocytosis if stones are present to prevent later symptomatic cholecystitis.

   C. Asymptomatic stones in children with sickle cell disease or thalassemia major and in infants undergoing TPN probably do not require cholecystectomy, although this is controversial.

VI. Preoperative preparation. Routine

VII. Operative care. Cholecystectomy is a standardized operation that is well-tolerated and has a low risk of complications. Operative cholangiography is indicated if jaundice has occurred.

VIII. Complications. Rare

Acalculous Cholecystitis

Definition. *Acalculous cholecystitis,* inflammation of the gallbladder in the absence of stones, is not rare. It may occur spontaneously but is more commonly associated with an acute illness, such as a major burn, severe trauma, or septicemia, or with patients undergoing total parenteral nutrition. *Hydrops of the gallbladder* refers to acute severe distention of the gallbladder in the absence of stones or inflammation. It is seen in acute febrile illnesses.

Pathophysiology. Acalculous cholecystitis usually results from gallbladder stasis, which in turn is caused by dehydration, sepsis, or gastrointestinal ileus or disuse.

Clinical presentation

A. Acalculous cholecystitis affects boys and girls equally.

B. **Abdominal pain,** nausea, and vomiting are the usual symptoms. Fever and leukocytosis are common.

C. **Tenderness** and muscle guarding in the right upper quadrant are found on physical examination.

Diagnosis

A. **Ultrasonography** may reveal a dilated gallbladder.

B. **Radionuclide** study (^{99m}Tc-IDA) demonstrates nonfunction of the gallbladder.

Indications for operation. Unless the symptoms are mild or the child has other serious disease, operative removal of the gallbladder is the quickest and safest method of treatment of acalculous cholecystitis. Hydrops of the gallbladder does not require treatment unless it is symptomatic.

Operative care. Cholecystectomy. Common duct exploration is not indicated. Cholecystostomy may be employed in the treatment of hydrops if the clinical condition is perilous, but cholecystectomy is usually needed later.

Bibliography

Chamberlain, J. W., and Hight, D. W. Acute hydrops of the gallbladder in childhood. *Surgery* 68:899, 1970.

Hays, D. M. Biliary Tract and Liver. In T. M. Holder and K. W. Ashcraft (eds.), *Pediatric Surgery.* Philadelphia: Saunders, 1980. P. 509.

Holcomb, G. W., Jr. Gallbladder Disease. In K. J. Welch, et al. (eds.), *Pediatric Surgery.* Chicago: Year Book, 1986. P. 1060.

Holcomb, G. W., Jr., O'Neill, J. A., Jr., and Holcomb, G. W. III. Cholecystitis, cholelithiasis and common duct stenosis in children and adolescents. *Ann. Surg.* 191:626, 1980.

Lau, G. E., Andrassy, R. J., and Mahour, G. H. A thirty year review of the management of gallbladder disease at a children's hospital. *Am. Surg.* 49:411, 1983.

Marks, C., Espinosa, J., and Hyman, L. J. Acute acalculous cholecystitis in childhood. *J. Pediatr. Surg.* 3:608, 1968.

Takiff, H., and Fonkalsrud, E. W. Gallbladder disease in childhood. *Am. J. Dis. Child.* 138:565, 1984.

Ternberg, J. L., and Keating, J. P. Acute acalculous cholecystitis. *Arch. Surg.* 110:543, 1975.

Todd, D. W., Rosen, W. C., and Miller, R. H. Hydrops of the gallbladder in children: Diagnosis and management. *Minn. Med.* 66:81, 1983.

Touloukian, R. J., and Downing, S. E. Cholestasis associated with long-term parenteral hyperalimentation. *Arch. Surg.* 106:58, 1973.

Whitington, P. F., and Black, D. D. Cholecystitis in premature infants treated with parenteral nutrition and furosemide. *J. Pediatr.* 97:647, 1980.

75 Pancreatitis

Definition. *Pancreatitis,* or inflammation of the pancreas, is uncommon in childhood. Infection, biliary tract disease, congenital anomalies, steroid therapy, and trauma may be responsible, but in most patients the cause is unknown.

Pathophysiology.

A. **Release of pancreatic enzymes**—amylase, elastase, phospholipase, and vasoactive peptides—results in autodigestion within the gland, which produces an intense inflammatory response, edema formation, fat necrosis, and sometimes, hemorrhagic necrosis of all or part of the pancreas.

B. **Absorption of enzymes** and cell breakdown products produces toxicity, fever, leukocytosis, and elevation of pancreatic enzymes in the serum.

C. **Severe inflammation** results in release of enzymes into the peritoneal cavity, causing a chemical **peritoneal burn,** with resultant hypovolemia, acidosis, and hypoproteinemia.

Clinical presentation

A. **Acute upper abdominal pain** is the usual presenting symptom in pancreatitis. Low-grade fever, nausea, and vomiting may also be present.

B. **Physical examination** reveals upper abdominal tenderness, which is not well-localized.

C. In **severe hemorrhagic pancreatitis,** the patient is seriously ill with hypovolemic **shock, hypoxia, and lethargy.**

Diagnosis

A. **Elevation of the serum amylase** confirms the diagnosis of pancreatitis. The rise in amylase often precedes symptoms, and sometimes serum values are normal.

B. **Urinary amylase and lipase** will be found to be elevated and are more accurate indicators of the degree of inflammation. The ratio of amylase clearance to creatinine clearance is elevated.

C. **Hypoglycemia, hypocalcemia,** and elevation of LDH and SGOT indicate very severe pancreatitis. Metabolic acidosis and hypoxemia follow.

Treatment

A. **Supportive care** consists of decreasing pancreatic stimulation by nasogastric suction, intravenous feedings, and use of analgesics. Antibiotics are traditionally given, although the evidence of their efficacy is poor.

B. **Deterioration** clinically and by laboratory tests is an indication for more aggressive therapy because of the substantial risk of fatality.

  1. **Peritoneal lavage** will reduce the peritoneal contamination, diluting the irritating enzymes.
  2. **Pancreatectomy,** partial or complete, is indicated in progressive severe hemorrhagic pancreatitis, although the mortality rate is high in these desperately ill children.
  3. **Parenteral nutrition** is necessary for several weeks.

Complications

Pancreatic pseudocyst may develop after severe pancreatitis (see Chap. 99).

B. Abscess in the pancreas, subphrenic space, or lesser sac may be seen after severe necrotic pancreatitis. CT or MRI is the preferred method of diagnosis, followed by catheter or operative drainage.

VII. **Prognosis.** Recurrent pancreatitis may indicate a structural abnormality of the pancreatic duct but is most commonly seen in patients with cystic fibrosis and hyperlipidemia. If the latter are absent, endoscopic pancreatogram is indicated.

Bibliography

Bluestein, P. K., et al. Endoscopic retrograde cholangiopancreatography in pancreatitis in children and adolescents. *Pediatrics* 68:387, 1981.

Folkman, J., and Tapper, D. The Pancreas. In T. M. Holder and K. W. Ashcraft (eds.), *Pediatric Surgery*. Philadelphia: Saunders, 1980. P. 551.

Ghishan, F. K., et al. Chronic relapsing pancreatitis in childhood. *J. Pediatr. Surg.* 102:514, 1983.

Hendren, W. H., Jr., Greep, J. M., and Patton, A. S. Pancreatitis in childhood: Experience with 15 cases. *Arch. Dis. Child.* 40:132, 1965.

Krauste, A., et al. Peritoneal lavage as a primary treatment in acute form of pancreatitis. *Surg. Gynecol. Obstet.* 156:458, 1983.

O'Neill, J. A., Green, H., and Ghishan, F. K. Surgical implications of chronic pancreatitis. *J. Pediatr. Surg.* 17:920, 1982.

Scott, H. W., et al. Longitudinal pancreaticojejunostomy in chronic relapsing pancreatitis with onset in childhood. *Ann. Surg.* 199:610, 1984.

Welch, K. J. The Pancreas. In K. J. Welch, et al. (eds.), *Pediatric Surgery*. Chicago: Year Book, 1986. P. 1086.

76 Splenectomy

Definition. *Splenectomy,* removal of the spleen, is performed for a number of diseases that cannot be managed medically. Primarily these are hematologic disorders: idiopathic thrombocytopenia, hereditary spherocytosis, thalassemia major, immune hemolytic anemia, and aplastic anemia. Other indications are certain metabolic diseases, parasitic disease, cyst or torsion of the spleen, some operations for portal hypertension, and staging of Hodgkin's disease. Splenic trauma (including operative) rarely requires splenectomy unless the organ is avulsed or pulverized.

Risk of splenectomy. Although there is a slight operative risk with splenectomy, the significant risk of removal of the spleen is that of **overwhelming sepsis.** Splenectomy deprives the child of the spleen's protective mechanisms.

A. Protective and immunologic functions of the spleen

1. Production of lymphoid cells
2. Production of antibodies, particularly IgM
3. Filter for bacteria and other foreign material
4. Production of opsonin
5. Production of tuftsin

B. Postsplenectomy sepsis

1. The **incidence** of severe infection is increased after splenectomy regardless of the reason for removal.
2. The **course** of postsplenectomy sepsis is **rapid** and the **mortality** from severe infection is high **(30–70%).** Most deaths follow overwhelming meningitis and occur within hours of the onset of symptoms.
3. The risk of sepsis after splenectomy is significantly **higher in very young children.**
4. *Streptococcus pneumoniae* is the cause of fatal postsplenectomy sepsis in more than half the patients. *Neisseria meningitidis* and *Haemophilus influenzae* are the other major organisms responsible.
5. **Prophylactic immunization** with polyvalent pneumococcal vaccine may prevent postsplenectomy sepsis, but the vaccine is of much less value if it is given after splenectomy.
6. **Prophylactic penicillin** decreases the rate of infection after splenectomy and may diminish the mortality.

Indications for operation. Splenectomy is indicated when the benefits of removal of the spleen outweigh the risk of postsplenectomy sepsis. In considering elective splenectomy, an individual decision must be made in each case based on response to medical therapy, risk of alternative therapy (e.g., chronic steroid administration), and age of the patient. If possible, splenectomy should be **deferred until after the age of 4.**

A. Idiopathic thrombocytopenia (ITP).
Inability to maintain a satisfactory platelet count without continuous steroid therapy.

B. Hereditary spherocytosis.
Elective splenectomy is performed after the age of 6 to prevent complications of hemolysis (gallstones and hemochromatosis).

Splenectomy is indicated at an earlier age if there is severe anemia requiring repeated transfusions.
- C. **Thalassemia major.** Splenectomy is sometimes advised to decrease the need for repeated transfusions, reduce the risk of gallstones and hemochromatosis, and decrease the risk of rupture of the large spleen.
- D. **Parasitic disease.** To decrease the risk of traumatic rupture of a huge spleen.
- E. **Other anemias** that are unresponsive to medical therapy.
- F. **Hodgkin's disease.** Splenectomy is part of staging laparotomy in stage I or II Hodgkin's disease of the neck or mediastinum. If subdiaphragmatic nodes or the spleen is involved, it is stage III disease and chemotherapy will be added to the radiotherapy regime.

IV. **Preoperative preparation**
- A. **Pneumovax** pneumococcal vaccine is given 3 weeks in advance of elective splenectomy. Adequate antibody formation requires the presence of the spleen.
- B. **Platelets** and packed **red cells** must be available for use in the operating room if thrombocytopenia is not arrested by splenectomy in patients with ITP. Platelets are not given until the spleen is removed and not then if clotting is adequate.

V. **Operative care.** Splenectomy is a simple operation. However, a careful search is necessary to remove any **accessory spleens,** found in 16% of patients. A retained accessory spleen will function and nullify the results of splenectomy. Cholecystectomy is performed if gallstones are present.

VI. **Postoperative care.** Immediate care is routine. Prophylactic penicillin is given at discharge to prevent postsplenectomy sepsis.

VII. **Complications**
- A. **Subphrenic abscess** may occur after splenectomy, particularly following bleeding in the splenic bed.
- B. **High platelet counts** are to be expected (up to one million/mm^3 by the tenth day) after splenectomy; since thromboembolism does not result, heparinization is not indicated.

VIII. **Prognosis**
- A. **Results** following splenectomy vary with the disease. Seventy-five to eighty percent of patients with ITP have sustained return of the platelet count to normal values. Children with spherocytosis can expect a 100% successful result.
- B. **The late mortality risk** from splenectomy is 20–60 times greater than for the normal population: about 0.5%. The risk is high because of the high mortality of postsplenectomy sepsis. It is higher in patients undergoing splenectomy for metabolic errors, tumor, thalassemia, and posthepatic splenomegaly. Prophylactic penicillin probably diminishes these risks significantly.

Bibliography

Appelbaum, P. C., et al. Fatal pneumococcal bacteremia in a vaccinated, splenectomized child. *N. Engl. J. Med.* 300:203, 1979.

Balfanz, J. R., et al. Overwhelming sepsis following splenectomy for trauma. *J. Pediatr.* 88:458, 1976.

Boles, E. T., Jr. The Spleen, In K. J. Welch, et al. (eds.), *Pediatric Surgery.* Chicago: Year Book, 1986. P. 1107.

Chilcote, R. R., et al. Septicemia and meningitis in children splenectomized for Hodgkin's disease. *N. Engl. J. Med.* 295:798, 1976.

Eraklis, A. J. The Spleen. In T. M. Holder and K. W. Ashcraft (eds.), *Pediatric Surgery.* Philadelphia: Saunders, 1980. P. 563.

Eraklis, A. J., and Filler, R. M. Splenectomy in childhood: A review of 1413 cases. *J. Pediatr. Surg.* 7:382, 1972.

Eraklis, A. J., et al. Hazard of overwhelming infection after splenectomy in childhood. *N. Engl. J. Med.* 276:1225, 1967.

Huntley, C. C. Infection following splenectomy in infants and children. *Am. J. Dis. Child.* 95:477, 1958.

King, H., and Shumacker, H. B., Jr. Splenic studies. I. Susceptibility to infection after splenectomy performed in infancy. *Ann. Surg.* 136:239, 1952.

McClure, P. D. Idiopathic thrombocytopenia purpura in children: Diagnosis and management. *Pediatrics* 55:69, 1975.

Najjar, V. A., and Nishioka, K. "Tuftsin": A natural phagocytosis stimulating peptide. *Nature* 228:672, 1970.

77 Inguinal Hernia

I. **Definition.** *Inguinal hernia* is the protrusion of an abdominal viscus into a peritoneal sac (the **processus vaginalis**) in the inguinal canal (Fig. 77-1). The contents of the sac are usually intestine but may be omentum or ovary and fallopian tube. Repair of inguinal hernia is the most common operation performed in children. Boys outnumber girls 6:1. The incidence of inguinal hernia is increased in premature infants and in patients with Ehlers-Danlos syndrome, exstrophy of the bladder, or a ventriculoperitoneal (V-P) shunt.

II. **Pathophysiology.** As the testis (or round ligament in the female) descends in the last month of prenatal life, a peritoneal pouch, the **processus vaginalis,** is brought down with it through the internal inguinal ring, along the inguinal canal, and through the external inguinal ring into the scrotum (labium). The distal-most sac wraps around the testis, forming the **tunica vaginalis,** and the proximal sac is normally obliterated. Failure of this obliteration results in a patent processus vaginalis into which intestine, ovary, or other viscera can protrude, forming an **indirect** inguinal hernia.

   A. A **hernia** only exists when something protrudes into the sac.
   B. A **patent processus vaginalis (not** a hernia) is present in 80% of boys at birth, in 40% at 2 years, and in 20% of adult men.
   C. **Other types of groin hernias**
      1. **Direct inguinal hernia.** Protrusion through the posterior wall of the inguinal canal, medial to the deep inferior epigastric vessels
      2. **Femoral hernia.** Protrusion through a defect that is deep to the inguinal ligament, medial to the femoral vessels

III. **Clinical presentation**

   A. Nearly half of all inguinal hernias are noted in the first year of life, most in the first 6 months.
   B. A **bulge in the groin** (sometimes extending into the scrotum) that comes and goes is almost always an inguinal hernia.
      1. Typically, the hernia appears when the child cries or strains but disappears when he relaxes. After a hernia has been present for a long time, it may remain "out" constantly.
      2. Hernias are **seldom symptomatic** except when they are incarcerated.
   C. **Physical examination** reveals a soft bulge in the groin that can be made to disappear by digital pressure. The "silk glove" sign and "thickening" of the cord noted by palpation are unreliable signs of hernia.
   D. A **femoral hernia** presents as a bulge in the groin that is actually on the anterior thigh deep to the inguinal ligament, medial to the femoral vessels.
   E. A **direct hernia** is usually indistinguishable from an indirect one by physical examination, although it will not progress into the scrotum.

IV. **Diagnosis.** The diagnosis of an inguinal hernia is made by the history and the finding of a reducible bulge in the groin. Nothing else feels like a hernia. **Needle aspiration is contraindicated!** If the mass is a hernia, intestinal perforation by the needle may produce peritonitis. Other conditions that must be considered and their distinguishing characteristics include the following:

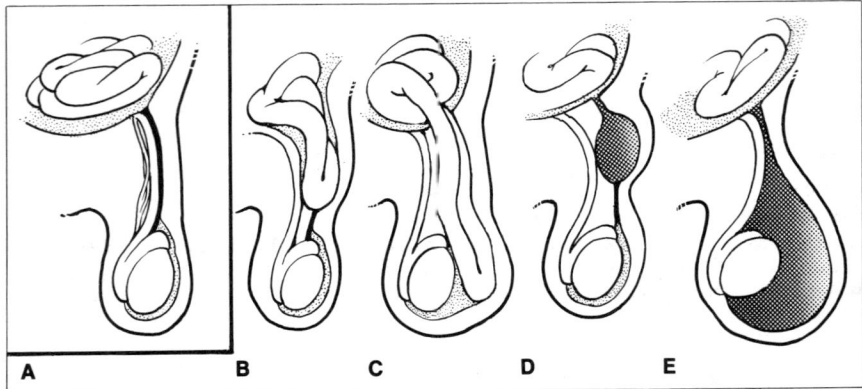

Fig. 77-1. Hernias and hydroceles. A. Normal anatomy. The processus vaginalis is obliterated between the abdominal peritoneum and the scrotum. B. Inguinal hernia into patent processus vaginalis. C. Inguino-scrotal hernia. The processus is patent into the scrotum. D. Hydrocele of the cord. A tiny proximal communication permits fluid to accumulate in a patent segment of the processus. E. Scrotal hydrocele (most common lesion). Incomplete obliteration of the processus permits accumulation of fluid distally (communicating hydrocele).

- **A. Enlarged lymph node.** Firm, immobile, nonreducible.
- **B. Abscess.** Tender, firm, immobile, nonreducible.
- **C. Undescended testis.** Firm, grapelike mass that sometimes can be "reduced" or manipulated into the scrotum.
- **D. Hydrocele.** Fluid in the scotum with no mass in the groin above, soft or firm, nonreducible.
- **E. Hydrocele of the cord** (or canal of Nuck). Firm, mobile, grapelike nontender mass that cannot be reduced or manipulated into the scrotum. (Note: Transillumination is unreliable in differentiating a hernia from a hydrocele.)

V. **Incarcerated inguinal hernia**

  A. **Mechanism.** Incarceration results if the intestine gets stuck in the internal inguinal ring.

   1. If the hernia is not promptly reduced, the **intestine swells** and becomes edematous causing compression of the blood supply of the testis or obstruction of the bowel.
   2. Once the blood supply to the testis is cut off, **infarction** will occur within a few hours.
   3. An **ovary** may become incarcerated but seldom infarcts because of the small size of the vascular pedicle.

  B. **Characteristics** of an incarcerated hernia

   1. **Sudden onset.**
   2. **Severe pain.**
   3. A hard, tender, **fixed mass** in the groin.
   4. Symptoms of **intestinal obstruction:** vomiting and distention.
   5. Often, there is **no prior history** of a hernia.
   6. Incarceration is **most likely in infants.**

C. **Diagnosis.** In young children with incarcerated inguinal hernia, it is possible to confirm the diagnosis by digital **rectal examination.** The intestine may be palpated as it exits the internal ring.

D. **Differential diagnosis**
   1. **Hydrocele of the cord** is the condition most commonly mistaken for an incarcerated hernia. Hydroceles are **painless** and the mass is **nontender and mobile.**
   2. **Abscess** has a slow onset, and there are no intestinal symptoms.
   3. An enlarged **lymph node** is usually painless and mobile.

E. **Reduction** of an incarcerated hernia should always be attempted, for operation on an incarcerated hernia carries a significantly **increased risk of complications** (primarily wound infection) and recurrence.
   1. **Almost all** incarcerated hernias **can be reduced.**
   2. Hydroxyzine **(Vistaril),** 1 mg/kg and meperidine hydrochloride (Demerol), 1 mg/kg, are given for pain relief and sedation in older children but are unnecessary in infants.
   3. **Firm, steady pressure** is applied to the mass with the fingertips of both hands for several minutes.
   4. **As the edema is squeezed out** of the bowel wall, it becomes smaller; suddenly (**not** gradually), it reduces.
   5. **If the hernia cannot be reduced, immediate operation is required.**

F. **After reduction** of the hernia, the child should be **admitted** to the hospital and checked hourly to be certain there is no damage to the **intestine or testis** and to reduce a **recurrent incarceration** promptly if it occurs.

G. **Herniorrhaphy is performed after 48 hours** to allow tissue edema to subside.

I. Indications for operation

A. **All inguinal hernias** should be promptly repaired unless there is another medical condition that makes the anesthetic risk prohibitive. There are several reasons for avoiding delay, especially in infants:
   1. **Spontaneous disappearance** of inguinal hernias **does not occur.**
   2. The **risk of incarceration** is greater in smaller patients.
   3. The operation is **technically more difficult** and the risk of injury to the vas or testicular vessels greater in long-standing hernias.
   4. Increasing age does not decrease the **risk of anesthesia,** provided an experienced pediatric anesthetist is available.

B. In normal **newborn** infants, repair should be performed before the infant goes home from the hospital, but after several days have elapsed to allow for discovery of other congenital anomalies that may exist. **Premature infants** should also undergo repair before discharge, but after resolution of other medical problems.

C. **Indeterminate hernias.** To make the diagnosis of a hernia it is essential that a knowledgeable person see it. If the surgeon has not seen the hernia personally and the diagnosis is in doubt, there is no harm in waiting until the hernia is unequivocally present. The parent should be informed of what to look for and be made aware of the need for emergency treatment in case of incarceration.

D. **Bilateral exploration** and repair is indicated in patients with bilateral hernias and in **infants** under the age of 1 year who have a unilateral hernia.
   1. The incidence of **"second side" hernia** appearing at some time after unilateral repair is **50% in infants** under the age of 1 year.

2. Bilateral repair is **not indicated for older children** with unilateral hernia because the incidence of "second side" hernias after the age of one year is only 10%.

VII. Preoperative preparation

1. Inguinal herniorrhaphy is ideally suited for **day-surgery** (outpatient) repair in most patients, although general anesthesia is indicated in children.
2. Since it is an elective operation, the patient should be in a state of **optimal health.** Specifically, the child should be free of fever, upper respiratory infection, and otitis, and an infant should not have a severe diaper rash.

VIII. Operative care

A. Ligation of the sac (processus vaginalis) at the internal ring is all that is needed to repair an indirect inguinal hernia in a child. Since there is no fascial defect, fascial repair is not required as it is in adults.

B. Direct and femoral hernias require a Cooper's ligament repair.

IX. Postoperative care

A. The preschool child has little pain, recovers quickly, and does not need to have any restrictions whatever on activity, bathing, or feeding.

B. The older child may need pain medicine for a day or two, but after that can return to school. He should avoid contact sports for 2 weeks.

C. The premature infant should be kept in the intensive care unit for 24 hours with continuous cardiac and respiratory monitoring because of the risk of postanesthetic apnea.

X. Complications.

A. Wound infection

B. Bleeding in the incision or into the scrotum

C. Acute hydrocele

XI. Prognosis. The risk of recurrence is less than 1 in 200.

Bibliography

Bock, J. E., and Sobye, J. V. Frequency of contralateral inguinal hernia in children. *Acta Chir. Scand.* 136:707, 1970.

Holder, T. M., and Ashcraft, K. W. Groin hernias and Hydroceles. In T. M. Holder and K. W. Ashcraft (eds.), *Pediatric Surgery*. Philadelphia: Saunders, 1980. P. 594.

Janik, J. S., and Shandling, B. The vulnerability of the vas deferens. II. The case against routine bilateral inguinal exploration. *J. Pediatr. Surg.* 17:585, 1982.

Kaplan, G. W. Iatrogenic cryptorchidism resulting from hernia repair. *Surg. Gynecol. Obstet.* 142:671, 1976.

Kiesewetter, W. B. Unilateral inguinal hernias in children. *Arch. Surg.* 115:1443, 1980.

Liu, L. M. P., et al. Life-threatening apnea in infants recovering from anesthesia. *Anesthesiology* 59:506, 1983.

McGregor, D. B., Halverson, K., and McVay, C. B. The unilateral pediatric inguinal hernia: Should the contralateral side be explored? *J. Pediatr. Surg.* 15:313, 1980.

Murdoch, R. W. G. Testicular strangulation from incarcerated inguinal hernia in infants. *J. R. Coll. Surg. Edinb.* 24:95, 1979.

Puri, P., Guiney, E. J., and O'Donnell, B. Inguinal hernia in infants: The fate of the testis following incarceration. *J. Pediatr. Surg.* 19:44 1984.

Rescoria, F. J., and Grosfeld, J. L. Inguinal hernia repair in the perinatal period and early infancy: Clinical considerations. *J. Pediatr. Surg.* 19:832, 1984.

Rowe, M. E., and Lloyd, D. A. Inguinal Hernia. In K. J. Welch, et al. (eds.), *Pediatric Surgery.* Chicago: Year Book, 1986. P. 779.

Steward, D. J. Preterm infants are more prone to complications following minor surgery than are term infants. *Anesthesiology* 56:304, 1982.

78   Hydrocele

I. **Definition.** *Hydrocele* means "water cyst." The term is used to refer to accumulation of fluid in the scrotum next to the testis. Fluid accumulation in the groin is called a **hydrocele of the cord.** Hydroceles may be **communicating** or **noncommunicating,** depending on whether there is a patent connection with the peritoneal cavity (see Fig. 77-1).

II. **Pathophysiology.** In children, hydroceles are almost always communicating since they are formed by the same mechanism as an indirect inguinal hernia: failure of obliteration of the processus vaginalis. A narrowed processus is too small for intestine to enter, but fluid from the peritoneal cavity easily passes through. The narrow channel acts like a one-way valve: fluid passes into the scrotum with increases in intraabdominal pressure. When the processus closes completely, the fluid is absorbed and the hydrocele disappears.

III. **Clinical presentation**
   A. The **sudden appearance** of swelling in the scrotum is the typical presenting finding. There is **no pain or tenderness.**
   B. Babies are frequently noted to have hydroceles **at birth** or develop them in the first few months.
   C. Hydrocele may occur at almost any time in **early childhood,** and rarely after the fifth year.
   D. **Acute hydrocele** is sometimes seen after herniorrhaphy and is thought to be caused by an inflammatory reaction. It usually subsides within 4 weeks.

IV. **Diagnosis**
   A. The diagnosis is made by **examination.** Fluid in the scrotum may be soft or tense but is never tender.
      1. Hydroceles vary widely in size; some are huge.
      2. **Diurnal variation in size** may be noted in the older child. The hydrocele may be larger in the evening after he has been upright all day.
      3. **Compressing** a hydrocele does not make it smaller. The communication is too narrow to permit rapid fluid shifts.
      4. **Transillumination** is the time-honored method of confirming the diagnosis but is unreliable in separating hydrocele from hernia.
   B. **Differential diagnosis**
      1. **Inguinal hernia** is most commonly confused with hydrocele. Scrotal hernias must pass through the inguinal canal to get into the scrotum; thus there is a **mass in the groin** as well as in the scrotum. A hydrocele, on the other hand, is confined to the scrotum alone.
      2. **Testicular tumor** is usually firm but not tense. Failure of transillumination is suggestive. Tumors are very rare in infants when hydroceles are most common.
      3. **Spermatocele** and **varicocele** are found almost exclusively in older children and adults. They do not transilluminate.
      4. Hydrocele of the cord is often mistaken for an **incarcerated hernia.** It is distinguished by the fact that it is **nontender** and **mobile,** and the patient is

asymptomatic. Transillumination is unreliable, but rectal examination reveals no intestine exiting the internal ring.

V. Indications for operation
  A. **Surgical treatment is rarely indicated for hydroceles.** More than **90% will spontaneously disappear.**
  B. Operation is indicated for hydroceles that have not disappeared by the age of 5 and those that are huge or symptomatic (rare).

VI. Preoperative preparation. As in hernia (day surgery)

VII. Operative care
  A. In preadolescent children, one may assume the hydrocele is a **communicating** one. The operation is identical to that for indirect inguinal hernia: isolation, division, and high ligation of the processus.
  B. In teenagers, or in patients in whom a hydrocele recurs after division of the processus, the hydrocele is usually **noncommunicating.** Scrotal exploration and excision of the tunica vaginalis is required.

VIII. Postoperative care. As in inguinal hernia
IX. Complications. As in inguinal hernia
X. Prognosis. As in inguinal hernia

Bibliography

Holder, T. M., and Ashcraft, K. W. Groin Hernias and Hydroceles. In T. M. Holder and K. W. Ashcraft (eds.), *Pediatric Surgery.* Philadelphia: Saunders, 1980. P. 594.

79 Undescended Testis

I. **Definition.** An *undescended testis*, or *cryptorchid*, is one that is not in the scrotum. It is to be distinguished from the more common **retractile** testis, seen in young boys, in which the testis tends to stay in the inguinal canal but can be brought into the scrotum by gentle manipulation. An **ectopic** testis is one that has strayed from the inguinal canal, usually to the thigh or perineum.

The **incidence** of cryptorchism is 3% at birth in full-term infants, decreasing to 1% after 1 year of age. It is more common in premature infants, approaching 100% at gestational age of 32 weeks or less.

II. **Pathophysiology**

   A. **Normal descent** of the testis occurs at about the seventh month of fetal life when the gubernaculum swells and shortens, drawing the testis through the inguinal canal into the scrotum. Gonadotropin (maternal) and testosterone (testis) are required.

   B. **Failure of descent** may occur if there is:

   1. **Hormonal** failure. Inadequate gonadotropin or inadequate secretion of testosterone by the stimulated testis
   2. **Dysgenesis** of the testis
   3. An **anatomic abnormality** such as abnormal development of the gubernaculum, obstruction of the inguinal canal or scrotum, or short vas or vessels

   C. **Abdominal testes** are frequently **dysgenetic,** are less likely to function after orchidopexy, and have a higher incidence of later malignant degeneration.

   D. **Spermatogenesis** will not occur if the testis is not in the scrotum prior to the onset of puberty. **Testosterone** production is unaffected by position. Thus a male with bilateral undescended testes will develop secondary sexual characteristics but will be sterile.

   E. **Cancer of the testis is 10–20 times more common** in adult men with undescended testes than in the normal male population. However, an individual's risk of a malignancy developing is only 1 in 1000–5000. Malignant degeneration correlates with the degree of dysplasia. The risk of malignant degeneration is not altered by orchidopexy.

III. **Clinical presentation**

   A. **Diagnosis** of cryptorchism is usually made by the pediatrician on routine examination. There are no symptoms. Parents are frequently unaware of the condition in their child.

   B. **Spontaneous descent** of undescended testes occurs in the first year of life in two-thirds of full-term cryptorchid infants, less often in prematures. Spontaneous descent probably does not occur after the first year of life.

   C. **Bilateral cryptorchism** at birth may represent a diagnostic emergency. If neither testis is palpable, the patient may either have bilateral undescended testes or be a virilized female. Immediate differentiation is indicated (see Chap. 34).

IV. Diagnosis

A. Physical examination is the primary method of diagnosis. The patient must be relaxed, and the examiner must have warm hands! Gentle bimanual palpation in the groin will usually reveal the testis, which is then "milked" toward the scrotum. If it cannot be manipulated well into the scrotum, cryptorchism is present. Use of the cross-leg sitting position, warm baths, and other maneuvers is unnecessary if the examiner is gentle and patient.

B. Retractile testes must be distinguished from true cryptorchism. The testis is retractile if it can be manipulated deep into the scrotum but retracts into the groin when released. No therapy is necessary. Spontaneous descent ultimately occurs in most of these boys.

C. Bilateral absent testes may represent bilateral intraabdominal undescended testes or anorchism. Serum levels of luteinizing hormone (LH) and follicle-stimulating hormone (FSH) are elevated in anorchism. If a testis is present, serum testosterone levels will increase rapidly to 5–25 times normal following the injection of human chorionic gonadotropin (HCG) (2000 IU daily for 3 days).

D. Angiography, isotope scans, and CT x-rays have been used with mixed results to identify an intraabdominal testis.

V. Problems

A. Torsion of the testis is more likely to occur in an undescended testis because it lacks fixation. Groin or abdominal pain in a patient with an empty scrotum on the same side suggests the diagnosis. Unfortunately, few such testes are salvageable.

B. Inguinal hernia commonly accompanies cryptorchism and may require repair before the optimal age for orchidopexy. Orchidopexy should be performed at the time of herniorrhaphy, however, for it is more difficult and hazardous as a later procedure.

VI. Indications for operation

A. Bilateral undescended testes require orchidopexy if the patient is to have any hope of fertility. Results are poor in this group, with reported fertility rates of only 40%.

B. In **unilateral undescended testis**, the purposes of operation are to establish a **normal body image** and to provide "insurance" against unilateral testicular injury.

1. **Fertility** is not significantly enhanced by orchidopexy if the opposite testis is descended.
2. **Testosterone production** is not affected by testicular position.
3. The risk of **malignancy** is **not** an indication for orchidopexy, since the incidence is low and is not altered by operation.

C. Operation is **not indicated in confirmed anorchism** (no response to HCG) since there is no testicular tissue.

D. Timing of orchidopexy is somewhat controversial.

1. **Functionally,** orchidopexy must be performed before puberty for spermatogenesis to occur. Fertility rates after unilateral prepubertal orchidopexy are 75–80%. Earlier orchidopexy will probably give better results, since **biopsy studies** show progressive lag of growth and development of the undescended testis after 1 year of age.
2. **Psychologically,** the emotional effects of orchidopexy are related to the pain of the operation, separation from parents, and castration anxieties surrounding an operation on the genitals.

a. **Pain** is less in the younger patient. The 2-year-old can walk out after the operation, while the 10-year-old needs a day or two in bed.

b. **Separation** of the child from the parent is the major cause of psychic distress in the child less than 5 years of age. It can be eliminated by having the parents with the child at the time of anesthesia induction.

c. **Castration anxieties** are rarely seen before 3 years of age but become important by 5 or 6.

3. **Technically,** the younger the boy is, the easier it is to mobilize the testis and place it in the scrotum.

4. From every standpoint, the **ideal age for orchidopexy appears to be between 1 and 3 years.** At this age the operation is well-tolerated and can be done on a day-surgery basis. Initial results are excellent.

VII. **Hormonal therapy.** Descent of undescended testes sometimes occurs following injections of HCG. Results are best in low-lying inguinal testes. Since the therapy is frequently unsuccessful, it is not widely used.

A. **HCG** is given intramuscularly, 1000 IU, 3 times weekly for 10 doses. Descent occurs within the next week if treatment is successful.

B. **Side effects.** Penile growth and frequent erections are usually seen, but premature closure of epiphyses is not.

C. **Contraindications.** Abdominal, retractile, and ectopic testes; undescended testes with hernias; and prior hernia repair.

D. **Descent** occurs in **20–50%** of reported cases, but measured fertility after hormonal therapy is only 46%. In 10%, the testis retracts into the groin and requires later orchidopexy.

VIII. **Preoperative preparation.** For young children, simple explanations are all that are needed. In older children, attention should be given to the unspoken castration fears.

IX. **Operative care**

A. **Orchidopexy** by the dartos pouch technique is preferred. After mobilization of the testis, a pouch is created in the scrotal wall between the dartos fascia and the skin. The testis is secured in the pouch by suturing the fascia around the cord.

B. **Orchiectomy** instead of orchidopexy is indicated if the testis is dysplastic or high in the abdomen and in the postpubertal male in whom the risk of malignancy outweighs the benefits of orchidopexy.

C. **Prosthetic replacement** can be performed if the testis is absent or must be removed.

X. **Postoperative care.** Normal activity can be resumed the day following the operation, with avoidance of activities that might injure the scrotum (e.g., riding a bicycle or hobby horse). Contact sports are prohibited for 3 weeks.

XI. **Complications**

A. **Scrotal hematoma** or **wound infection** occurs in 1–2%.

B. **Ischemic loss** of the testis results from accidental division of the blood supply or tension on the spermatic cord due to inadequate mobilization of the testis.

C. **Traumatic infarction** can occur if there is trauma to the scrotum in the immediate postoperative period.

XII. **Prognosis**

A. **Anatomic:** 2% recurrence, 2–5% atrophy, 80% normal growth of testis

B. **Functional:** 75–80% fertility after unilateral orchidopexy, 40% fertility after bilateral orchidopexy

Bibliography

Altman, B. K., and Malament, M. Carcinoma of the testis following orchiopexy. *J. Urol.* 97:498, 1967.

Atkinson, P. M. A followup study of surgically treated cryptorchid patients. *J. Pediatr. Surg.* 10:115, 1975.

Campbell, J. R. Undescended Testes. In T. M. Holder and K. W. Ashcraft (eds.), *Pediatric Surgery.* Philadelphia: Saunders, 1980. P. 816.

Cywes, S., Retief, P. J. M., and Louw, J. H. Results following Orchiopexy. In E. W. Fonkalsrud and W. Mengel (eds.), *The Undescended Testis.* Chicago: Year Book, 1981.

Fonkalsrud, E. W. The undescended testis. *Curr. Probl. Surg.* 15:5, 1978.

Fonkalsrud, E. W. Undescended Testes. In K. J. Welch, et al. (eds.), *Pediatric Surgery.* Chicago: Year Book, 1986. P. 793.

Fonkalsrud, E. W., and Mengel, W. (eds.). *The Undescended Testis.* Chicago: Year Book, 1981.

Fowler, R., and Stephens, F. D. The role of testicular vascular anatomy in the salvage of high undescended testis. *Aust. N.Z. J. Surg.* 29:92, 1959.

Hadziselimovic, F., Herzog, B., and Seguchi, H. Surgical correction of cryptorchidism at 2 years: Electron microscopic and morphologic investigation. *J. Pediatr. Surg.* 10:19, 1975.

Lattimer, J. K., et al. The optimum time to operate for cryptorchidism. *Pediatrics* 53:96, 1974.

Lipshultz, L. I. et al. Testicular function after orchiopexy for unilaterally undescended testis. *N. Engl. J. Med.* 295:15, 1976.

Mengel, W., et al. Studies on cryptorchidism: A comparison of histological findings in the germinative epithelium before and after the second year of life. *J. Pediatr. Surg.* 9:445, 1974.

Scorer, C. G. Descent of the testes in the first year of life. *Br. J. Surg.* 27:374, 1955.

Scorer, C. G. The incidence of incomplete descent of the testicle at birth. *Arch. Dis. Child.* 31:198, 1956.

80 Torsion of the Testis

I. **Definition. Torsion of the testis is a surgical emergency.** Occlusion of the blood supply can result in testicular infarction in just a few hours. Early recognition and immediate emergency operation are necessary if the testis is to survive.

There are two major forms of torsion of the testis: intravaginal and extravaginal.

   A. **Intravaginal torsion** takes place within the tunica vaginalis and results from an abnormally high investment of the tunica on the spermatic cord within the scrotum. Sometimes referred to as a "bell-clapper" deformity, it is the most common abnormality associated with torsion.

   B. **Extravaginal torsion** results when the testis and the cord twist because of nonfixation of the testis, cord, and processus vaginalis, as in newborns and patients with undescended testes.

   C. **Torsion of an appendix testis** may also occur. There are four appendices, but the one most likely to undergo torsion is the hydatid of Morgagni.

II. **Pathophysiology.** Twisting of the testis first causes occlusion of the spermatic veins, then of the artery.

   A. **Venous obstruction** results in passive congestion of the testis with swelling and pain. Prolonged occlusion leads to thrombosis.

   B. **Arterial occlusion** ultimately occurs, followed by **testicular infarction.**

   C. **The duration of symptoms** before infarction occurs varies and depends on the degree of torsion (360 versus 720 degrees). Testicular loss has been reported as early as 2 hours after the onset of symptoms. Few testes can survive torsion of more than 12 hours.

III. **Clinical picture**

   A. **Pubertal boys** are more susceptible to torsion of the testis, although it can occur at any age. About 1 in 160 males are affected.

   B. **Neonatal torsion** usually results from a prenatal event. The scrotum is red and swollen at birth, and the testis is almost always necrotic. Testicular salvage has been possible only in neonates in whom the torsion occurred after delivery.

   C. **A history of trauma** is present in 20% of patients, but in most there is no precipitating event. About a third have had **prior episodes of testicular pain,** usually of short duration.

   D. **Symptoms**

      1. **Pain** is almost always the first symptom of torsion of the testis. It may begin suddenly or gradually but increases with time. Although there is considerable individual variation, the pain is usually severe.

      2. **Erythema and swelling of the scrotum** develop rapidly, sometimes involving the opposite side.

      3. **Nausea, vomiting, and fever** may develop.

   E. **Physical examination**

      1. **The scrotum is swollen and red,** sometimes with a bluish hue.

      2. **The testis is exquisitely tender,** often so much so that accurate palpation is impossible.

3. A **"transverse lie"** of the testis may be noted.

F. **Torsion of the appendix testis** causes milder but similar symptoms. Since the pain is mild, the patient may not be seen until the second day of symptoms; by that time edema and erythema may make differentiation from torsion of the testis impossible.

G. **Torsion of an undescended testis** occurs more readily than torsion of a descended testis because of lack of fixation. Pain in the groin is the usual symptom. The finding of a **tender mass** in the groin in association with an **empty scrotum** should alert the examiner to the possibility of this diagnosis.

IV. **Diagnosis.** Since testicular salvage can be achieved in patients with torsion of the testis only if the diagnosis is promptly made, no time should be wasted in unnecessary tests or examinations. The problem is differentiating torsion of the testis from nonsurgical scrotal afflictions.

   A. **Epididymoorchitis** is most commonly confused with torsion of the testis. There are several clues to their distinction.
      1. **Age of the patient.** Epididymitis and orchitis are rarely seen before puberty.
      2. **The rate of onset of the pain** is of little value despite teachings to the contrary. Patients in each group can have pain of either sudden or gradual onset.
      3. **Fever and urinary symptoms** are more common in orchitis.
      4. **Previous episodes of pain are rare** in orchitis but fairly common in torsion of the testis.
      5. **Physical examination is unreliable.** Erythema, edema, and testicular pain may be similar.
   B. **Torsion of the appendix testis** can be diagnosed by palpation of a **tender pea-sized mass** separate from the testis. If the testis itself is not tender, the diagnosis is secure. The infarcted appendix may be seen through the skin: the **blue dot sign.**
   C. **Other diagnostic possibilities:** strangulated hernia, traumatic hematocele, fat necrosis, acute hydrocele, torsion of a hernial sac within the scrotum, testicular tumor, idiopathic scrotal edema, acute varicocele, Henoch-Schönlein purpura, leukemic infiltration, and scrotal abscess.
   D. **Laboratory tests**
      1. **Doppler ultrasound** may demonstrate an absent testicular pulse in torsion. The test is unreliable when there is scrotal hyperemia, however.
      2. **Radionuclide scan** of the scrotum, using ^{99m}Tc pertechnetate, may demonstrate absent testicular blood flow if there is torsion of the testis. Its limitations are the same as those of the Doppler.
      3. **CT scan and B-scan ultrasound** have not been of consistent value in differentiating torsion of the testis from inflammatory conditions.

V. **Indications for operation.** The decision to operate is made on clinical grounds. Laboratory tests and imaging have not proved sufficiently reliable to replace clinical judgment in deciding which patients need operation.

   A. **Any patient with a tender testis must be presumed to have torsion of the testis** unless another diagnosis can be positively established. Surgical exploration is harmless in epididymoorchitis but critically essential in torsion.
   B. **Neonatal torsion,** if present at delivery, will not benefit from operation. The testis is long gone. Torsion occurring after birth requires prompt operation.
   C. **Torsion of the appendix testis** does not require surgical treatment if the diagnosis is certain. However, if the pain is severe, surgical removal of the necrotic

tissue brings instant relief and spares the patient a week or two of discomfort and medication.

D. **Recurrent testicular pain** is an indication for surgical orchidopexy. Many of these patients will otherwise develop torsion and risk testicular loss.

E. **Patients with torsion of the testis should undergo scrotal exploration,** even when symptoms have been present for more than 12 hours. Because of individual variation in the degree of torsion, salvage may still be possible.

Preoperative preparation

A. **Manual detorsion** should be carried out if at all possible. It shortens the testicular ischemic time, relieves pain, and if successful, makes orchidopexy an elective operation. Lidocaine **(Xylocaine) block analgesia** may be achieved by the injection of 5–10 ml of 1% lidocaine around the external inguinal ring. Following this, manipulation of the testis can usually be carried out painlessly. If the torsion can be reduced, operation can be scheduled electively within 48 hours.

B. **Laboratory tests or imaging must not delay corrective surgery.** Testicular survival depends on prompt operation, and the best results are obtained when operation is performed within 6 hours of the onset of symptoms.

Operative care

A. **A scrotal incision** permits direct examination of the testis, detorsion, and fixation orchidopexy.

B. **The tunica vaginalis is opened,** and the testis is untwisted and observed for return of circulation. Up to 20 minutes' observation may be necessary to be sure about the viability of the testis. Incision of the tunica albuginea and examination of the parenchyma may assist in determining if the tissue can recover.

C. **Bilateral fixation orchidopexy** is carried out to prevent contralateral torsion at a later date.

D. **Use of nonabsorbable sutures** and excision of a window of tunica vaginalis are necessary to provide secure fixation. Alternatively, a Lord procedure (eversion of the tunica vaginalis) can be performed.

E. **Orchiectomy should be performed if the testis is not viable.** The ischemic testis has the capacity to stimulate production of antibodies that inhibit spermatogenesis by the **contralateral testis** and render the patient sterile. Only a testis that is clearly viable should be retained.

Postoperative care. Scrotal support and analgesics are necessary for a few days following operation, but there is no need for bed rest. The patient may be discharged from the hospital within a day or two.

Early complications

A. **Suppuration and slough** may occur if a necrotic testis is retained.

B. **Bleeding** into the scrotum can form a large hematoma.

Late complications

A. **Testicular atrophy** may result from ischemic damage. Testicular biopsy shows little or no spermatogenesis.

B. **Sterility** may occur after orchidopexy for torsion of the testis when an ischemic testis is retained, even when the opposite testis is normal. Current evidence indicates that this is an autoimmune phenomenon that is not seen when orchidectomy is performed for torsion.

C. **Endocrine failure** is not seen unless there is bilateral torsion and complete infarction of both testes.

Bibliography

Bartsch, G., et al. Testicular torsion: Late results with special regard to fertility and endocrine function. *J. Urol.* 124:375, 1980.

Cass, A. S. Elective orchiopexy for recurrent testicular torsion. *J. Urol.* 127:253, 1982.

Guiney, E. J., and McGlinchey J. Torsion of the testes and the spermatic cord in the newborn. *Surg. Gynecol. Obstet.* 152:273, 1981.

Harris, B. H., et al. Protection of the solitary testis. *J. Pediatr. Surg.* 17:950, 1982.

Leape, L. L. Torsion of the testis. *J.A.M.A.* 200:93, 1967.

Leape, L. L. Torsion of the Testis. In K. J. Welch, et al. (eds.), *Pediatric Surgery.* Chicago: Year Book, 1986. P. 1330.

Riley, T. W., et al. Use of radioisotope scan in evaluation of intrascrotal lesions. *J. Urol.* 116:472, 1976.

Rodriguez, D. D., et al. Doppler ultrasound versus testicular scanning in the evaluation of the acute scrotum. *J. Urol.* 125:343, 1981.

Skoglund, R. W., et al. Torsion of testicular appendages: Presentation of 43 new cases and a collective review. *J. Urol.* 104:598, 1970.

Sonda, L. P., and Lapides, J. Experimental torsion of the spermatic cord. *Surg. Forum* 12:502, 1961.

Tank, E. S. Testicular Torsion. In T. M. Holder and K. W. Ashcraft (eds.), *Pediatric Surgery.* Philadelphia: Saunders, 1980. P. 824.

Thomas, W. E. G., and Williamson, R. C. N. Diagnosis and outcome of testicular torsion. *Br. J. Surg.* 70:213, 1983.

81 Circumcision

Definition. *Circumcision* is removal of the foreskin. It may be performed at any age for disease, and it is a ritual requirement of Judaism and Islam, as well as many primitive tribes.

Neonatal circumcision. Circumcision shortly after birth was formerly a routine practice in the United States. The reasons are unclear. It has been defended as a measure to promote cleanliness and to prevent cancer of the cervix and penis. Available evidence does not support either of these as valid reasons. Circumcision is not medically indicated in the absence of disease of the foreskin.

Clinical presentation. The medical indications for circumcision are phimosis, recurrent posthitis, and paraphimosis.

A. *Phimosis* is excessive tightness of the foreskin preventing retraction behind the glans. It occurs in 1–2% of males. The foreskin normally **cannot** be **retracted** in infants; nonretractability of the foreskin is not pathologic until age 2. Forced retractions may cause phimosis by producing tears in the foreskin, which heal with scarring and contraction.

B. *Posthitis* is inflammation of the foreskin, caused by poor hygiene or by phimosis. The foreskin is edematous, red, and sore. In infants, similar findings occur with a diaper rash and respond to its treatment. The term **balanitis,** which means inflammation of the penis, is often incorrectly used for posthitis.

C. *Paraphimosis* refers to a foreskin that has been retracted and is caught behind the glans. It usually results from phimosis and forcible retraction. The foreskin may be massively swollen and painful.

Operative care. The skin and underlying mucosa are amputated, and the raw edge is sutured. General anesthesia is required.

Complications. Although it is a simple operation, circumcision has more than its share of complications.

A. **Bleeding** is usually caused by inadequate surgical technique: failure to secure the submucosal blood supply. Resuture is sometimes needed.

B. **Infection** of the suture line.

C. **Bisection or amputation of the glans** can occur if the foreskin is not mobilized adequately before being cut by the scissors. Prompt suture is necessary but not always successful.

D. **Dehiscence** occurs if too much foreskin is removed, resulting in separation and retraction, leaving the penile shaft denuded.

E. *Concealed penis* refers to retraction of the penis into the prepubic fat because of excessive removal of foreskin or scarring of the suture line.

F. **Meatal stricture** is a common late complication of circumcision. It results from diaper trauma to the thin scale of the glans and is almost never seen in uncircumcised males. Meatotomy may be necessary.

Bibliography

Aitken-Swan, J., and Baird, D. Circumcision and cancer of the cervix. *Br. J. Cancer* 19:217, 1965.

Hospital Care of Newborn Infants (5th ed.). Evanston, Ill.: American Academy of Pediatrics, 1971. P. 110.

Leape, L. L. Circumcision. In T. M. Holder and K. W. Ashcraft (eds.), *Pediatric Surgery*. Philadelphia: Saunders, 1980. P. 793.

Patel, H. The problem of routine circumcision. *Can. Med. Assoc. J.* 95:576, 1966.

Preston, E. N. Whither the foreskin? A consideration of routine neonatal circumcision. *J.A.M.A.*, 213:1853, 1970.

Trier, W. C., and Drach, G. W. Concealed penis: Another complication of circumcision. *Am. J. Dis. Child.* 125:276, 1973.

VII Tumors

82 Tumors: General Principles

Introduction

A. **The outcome** following treatment of childhood malignancies has improved dramatically in the past 2 decades. This change has resulted less from specific advances in surgery, chemotherapy, or radiation therapy than from the increasingly sophisticated application of these modalities as a result of cooperative studies.

B. Because all solid tumors in childhood are relatively **rare** in comparison with the major adult cancers, pooling of results of **standardized treatment programs** has been the key to progress. The various children's tumor study groups, and the intergroup studies in particular, have produced exceptional results.

C. In many cases tumor treatment protocols have been developed that simultaneously improve outcomes and make treatment safer.

   1. **Pulse therapy** of short-course high-dose chemotherapy is often more effective than prolonged low-dose treatment.
   2. **Mutilative surgery** is rarely necessary for cure.
   3. **Death on the operating table** should rarely if ever happen anymore. Heroic measures to "get it out at any cost" are not needed.
   4. Dangerous or **unresectable tumors** often become resectable after treatment with chemotherapy or radiation.
   5. **Growth deformities** from radiation have been minimized by selective and carefully calibrated use, the development of more effective and specific energy modes, and the elimination of radiation treatment in cases in which it proved of no value.

Diagnosis

A. **The profusion of imaging techniques** within the past decade has immensely improved the accuracy of preoperative diagnosis as well as its safety. Invasive studies and the complications they entail are becoming extinct, their passing mourned by few.

B. **Selection** from this generous "menu" of the one or two studies that will furnish the information needed to provide safe and optimal treatment expeditiously can be a formidable challenge.

   1. **Angiograms** are seldom needed for the diagnosis or treatment of soft-tissue malignancies in children.
   2. **CT and MRI**, noninvasive imaging modalities of great clarity and definition, have revolutionized the radiologic approach to tumors. They provide details of origin; involvement of surrounding organs, blood vessels, and lymph nodes; and often the histologic nature of the tumor. For most pediatric tumors, no further preoperative studies are needed.
   3. **The metastatic survey**, involving "total body x-rays" and isotope scan, often can be postponed until after the operation, when the known histologic findings will accurately predict the likely sites for spread.

Treatment

A. **Malignant tumors have individual characteristics** of growth, method of spread, and response to therapy. Effective therapy requires an understanding of these factors for each tumor and the tailoring of treatment to host and disease.

B. **Host immune mechanisms** are key both to the development of malignancy and to its control. The finest surgery or chemotherapy almost always leaves behind some tumor cells that the patient must destroy if recurrence is to be prevented. Lymphocytes, particularly T cells, appear to be a major factor in this destruction.

C. Every child with a malignancy should be treated by **pediatric cancer specialists.** A cooperative effort is necessary to plan the timing and interrelationship of the various forms of treatment.

D. Most maglignant tumors require **multimodal therapy,** typically given as part of a study protocol. Surgery is usually the **primary** treatment. Chemotherapy and radiation therapy are referred to as **adjuvant** therapy, often essential for cure but seldom curative alone.

IV. Surgery

A. **Removal of the tumor,** if it can be accomplished, is almost always the first form of treatment. It is the only hope of cure for many tumors for which there is no chemotherapy or in which chemotherapy will be effective only if the tumor burden is small.

B. Major tumor surgery, however traumatic and painful, is **less disturbing** to the patient and associated with fewer intermediate and long-term ill effects than the other two, seemingly simpler, modalities. Usually, once an operation is over, it is over, while aftereffects of chemotherapy and radiation treatment can be long-lasting and troublesome.

C. **Surgical removal** of the tumor alone is often **not sufficient** therapy, however, since many malignant tumors have already metastasized by the time of operation. Microscopic residual disease is usually present even when the surgeon "got it all out." Adjuvant therapy is needed to provide the best possible chance of cure.

D. **Operative principles**

1. **Careful exploration** of the entire abdominal or chest cavity is first performed to assess the extent of tumor spread, thus determining the **stage,** which in turn determines the extent of adjuvant treatment required.

2. **Total resection** of the tumor by careful anatomic dissection is the goal of a cancer operation. Care is taken to encompass the tumor totally and not enter it or cause rupture or spillage of tumor cells if at all possible. Adjacent lymph nodes should be taken en bloc with the specimen. Regional nodes are removed if tumor involvement is suspected.

3. *Primum non nocere*—first of all, do no harm. This hallowed aphorism is the first principle of modern cancer surgery. Total removal of the tumor is the desired objective, but heroic efforts to "get the tumor out at any cost," including damage to neighboring organs, are no longer appropriate.

4. **Unresectable tumors** involving critical structures are subjected to biopsy and treated with chemotherapy and/or radiation to shrink the tumor. Resection of the entire tumor is often possible at a **"second-look" operation.** If not, reduction in tumor bulk by partial resection will enhance the effectiveness of adjuvant therapy.

5. Similarly, if tumor resection requires removal of an organ such as the bladder or uterus, biopsy or partial resection is usually the appropriate first procedure. After tumor shrinkage has been accomplished by chemotherapy total resection of the tumor without removal of the organ may be possible

6. **Metastatic spread** does not necessarily mean the tumor is incurable. Infants with **neuroblastoma** with metastases to the liver, marrow, or skin (stage IV-S) often survive after removal of the primary tumor. **Pulmonary metastases** of Wilms' tumor, osteosarcoma, and selected other tumors,

isolated, can sometimes be surgically removed or eradicated by chemotherapy or radiation treatment.

I. Chemotherapy

A. **Drugs that kill cancer** cells are referred to as chemotherapeutic agents. They are sometimes dramatically successful, making the tumor appear to "melt away."

B. Chemotherapeutic agents are most effective at the time of **cell division.** Since not all of the tumor cells in a patient replicate at one time, repeat drug courses are necessary, fractionally reducing the cancer cell population with each dose. Since the tumor cells are never 100% eliminated, the host immune mechanisms must destroy the remaining malignant cells.

C. Anticancer drugs are also more effective when the **tumor burden is small.** The best results occur when the drugs are given after an operation in which the tumor has been grossly removed.

D. **Types of chemotherapeutic agents**

1. **Antimetabolite.** An agent that is structurally similar to a normal cell component, which it replaces, and thereby interferes with normal cellular function. Example: methotrexate.

2. **Alkylating agent.** A compound that contributes an alkyl group (R-CH-), which replaces a hydrogen atom in the molecules of DNA and RNA, interfering with their functions. Examples: cyclophosphamide, chlorambucil.

3. **Antibiotic.** An agent that alters DNA function by intercalating in the DNA molecule or binding to it. Examples: actinomycin D, daunorubicin, bleomycin, mithramycin.

4. **Vinca alkaloid.** A plant derivative that interferes with cell division but whose anticancer mechanism is incompletely understood. Examples: vincristine, vinblastine.

5. **Miscellaneous** agents. A number of diverse chemicals have been discovered that have anticancer effects of unknown mechanism. These include cisplatin, decarbazine (DTIC), and procarbazine.

E. **Side effects.** No anticancer agent has been developed that affects only the malignant cells in the body. Normal cells, particularly those that have high mitotic activity, are also damaged, sometimes profoundly. Interference with normal cellular function is the cause of most of the side effects seen with the use of anticancer drugs.

1. **Myelosuppression,** stomatitis, skin rashes, alopecia, diarrhea, nausea, vomiting, hepatic dysfunction, and renal dysfunction are the most common side effects, but an almost limitless variety of side effects can occur.

2. Different classes of drugs have **specific complications** related to their individual actions. Examples: neurotoxicity from *Vinca* alkaloids, hypocalcemia from mithramycin, cardiotoxicity from doxorubicin (Adriamycin).

3. Chemotherapeutic agents may induce **malignant change,** particularly when given in combination with radiation therapy. Fortunately, this is a rare complication, although clearly a most serious and distressing one.

F. **Protocols** are used for the treatment of most tumors, usually the result of multiinstitutional studies. These prescribe the drug dose and schedule, the use of multiple agents, the tests for monitoring tumor effects and toxicity, and the procedures for altering treatment when toxic complications develop.

Radiation therapy

A. **Ionizing radiation will destroy tumor cells.** Like chemotherapy, the effect is proportional to the mitotic activity and immaturity of the cells. Normal dividing cells are also susceptible to the effects of radiation, however, limiting its usefulness.

B. Modern radiotherapy is both **safer** and **more effective** than its counterpart of a decade or two ago. Use of high-voltage energy, refinement of dosage, and increasingly sophisticated and accurate methods of delivery have greatly enhanced its efficacy while diminishing side effects.

C. **Major side effects** of radiation therapy result from damage to normal tissue within the radiation field. They include retardation of skeletal growth; impairment of renal, hepatic, or pulmonary function; damage to the gonads (although genetic effects have not been seen in offspring of radiated patients); and oncogenesis. The risk of a **second malignancy** developing is greater when the patient receives both radiation therapy and chemotherapy: of the order of magnitude of 1 in 100.

VII. **Prognosis.** The long-term disease-free survival rate after treatment is gratifyingly high in Wilms' tumor, rhabdomyosarcoma, and Hodgkin's disease, and improving in many other solid tumors. It remains discouragingly unchanged in neuroblastoma.

Bibliography

D'Angio, G. J. Radiation Therapy for Solid Tumors. In K. J. Welch, et al. (eds.), *Pediatric Surgery.* Chicago: Year Book, 1986. P. 249.

D'Angio, G. J., et al. Decreased risk of radiation-associated second malignant neoplasms in actinomycin D–treated patients. *Cancer* 37[Suppl.]:1177, 1976.

D'Angio, G. J., et al. The treatment of Wilms' tumor: Results of the Second National Wilms' Tumor Study. *Cancer* 47:2302, 1981.

Gale, G. B., et al. Cancer in neonates: The experience at the Children's Hospital of Philadelphia. *Pediatrics* 70:409, 1982.

Hutchinson, G. B. Late neoplastic changes following medical irradiation. *Cancer* 37[Suppl.]:1102, 1976.

Jaffe, N. Cancer Chemotherapy. In K. J. Welch, et al. (eds.), *Pediatric Surgery.* Chicago: Year Book, 1986. P. 241.

Jaffe, N., et al. Rhabdomyosarcoma in children: Improved outlook with a multidisciplinary approach. *Am. J. Surg.* 125:482, 1973.

Lansky, S. B., and Cairns, N. U. Cancer: The Patient and the Family. In T. M. Holder and K. W. Ashcraft (eds.), *Pediatric Surgery.* Philadelphia: Saunders, 1980. P. 923.

Mike, V., et al. Incidence of second malignant neoplasms in children: Results of an international study. *Lancet* 2:1326, 1982.

Pearson, D., and D'Angio G. J. Radiation Therapy. In H. J. G. Bloom, et al. (eds.), *Cancer in Children: Clinical Management.* Berlin: Springer, 1975. P. 29.

Schabel, F. M., Jr. Concepts for systemic treatment of micrometastases. *Cancer* 35:15, 1975.

Tefft, M., et al. Acute and late effects on normal tissues following combined chemo- and radiotherapy for childhood rhabdomyosarcoma and Ewing's sarcoma. *Cancer* 37[Suppl.]:1201, 1976.

Trillin, A. S. Of dragons and garden peas. *N. Engl. J. Med.* 304:699, 1981.

Wilcox, W. S. The last surviving cancer cell: The chances of killing it. *Cancer Chemother. Rep.* 50:541, 1966.

83. Wilms' Tumor

Definition. *Wilms' tumor* (nephroblastoma) is a congenital tumor of the kidney, occurring in 8 of 100,000 children/year (Fig. 83-1). It is the **most common abdominal tumor of childhood** and the **most highly curable**. The median age of presentation is 3 years, but one-third of patients are under the age of 2 at diagnosis. There is no predilection for race or gender.

Pathophysiology

A. Histologically, Wilms' tumors demonstrate an unusual **diversity** of cellular patterns, usually a mix of mesenchymal and epithelial elements in differing stages of maturation. Renal blastema cells are seen, as well as glomeruli and tubules.

B. **Anaplastic or sarcomatous** patterns occur in 10% and are associated with a **much poorer outcome.**

C. Neoplastic growth replaces and **distorts** normal renal tissue but usually does not cause obstruction, bleeding, or pain; therefore, the tumor can grow to a huge size before it is detected. In most patients, the tumor is **"silent" for a long time.**

Clinical presentation

A. A **mass in the abdomen** is the common presenting finding. Symptoms may be totally absent. Typically, the mass is felt by the parent or pediatrician on a routine physical examination. Abdominal pain or vague complaints of weakness, anorexia, or weight loss are sometimes present. **Hematuria** occurs in about 20%.

B. **Physical examination** reveals a firm, immobile abdominal or flank mass in the retroperitoneum that does not move with respiration. Hypertension may be present.

C. **Associated anomalies** are present in about **15%** of children with Wilms' tumor. **Hypospadias, duplications** of the urinary tract, **hemihypertrophy**, and **aniridia** are the most common.

D. **Pulmonary metastases** are present in 5–7% of patients preoperatively. Another 7% are found to have intraabdominal metastases at operation.

Diagnosis

A. **Computerized tomography (CT)** is the preferred diagnostic study for suspected Wilms' tumor, for it most accurately differentiates it from neuroblastoma or other lesions. It also gives valuable information concerning intraabdominal spread, lymph-node involvement, and invasion of the tumor into adjacent organs or the vena cava. Intravenous pyelography (IVP) is inadequate for these purposes.

B. **Arteriography and venography** are **not indicated** unless it is not clear from CT whether the tumor arises in the kidney or liver.

C. **Unusual presentations. Nephroblastomatosis**—bilateral diffuse renal enlargement; **nonfunctioning kidney** (caused by vascular or ureteral obstruction); **extrarenal Wilms'** tumor—in the mediastinum, pelvis, or inguinal canal.

D. *Mesoblastic nephroma* is a benign renal tumor of neonates that is grossly similar to Wilms' tumor but histologically different. Surgical removal is curative.

Problems

A. **Differential diagnosis**

1. **Hydronephrosis.** Secondary to ureterovesical (UV) or ureteropelvic (UP) obstruction.

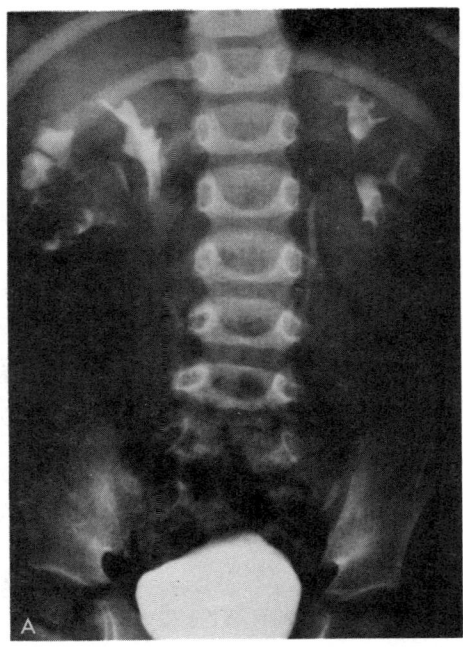

Fig. 83-1. Wilms' tumor. Excretory urogram demonstrates the intrarenal displacement and distortion of the collecting system typical of Wilms' tumor. (From L. L. Leape, Diagnosis and Management of Wilms' Tumor. In D. G. Skinner and J. B. De Kernion (Eds.), *Genitourinary Cancer*. Philadelphia: Saunders, 1978.

2. **Neuroblastoma.** Most commonly confused with Wilms' tumor; tends to be more central; extrarenal on x-ray; more likely to be calcified.
3. **Multicystic kidney.** Nonfunctional, cystic mass.
4. **Other renal or retroperitoneal tumors.**

B. **Errors in diagnosis are common:** 5% either way. Neuroblastoma is the major problem; both need operation. Ruptured Wilms' tumor may be mistaken for other conditions that cause peritoneal irritation, such as ruptured spleen or liver or appendicitis.

C. **Bilateral Wilms' tumor** is not as ominous a finding as might be supposed. The overall cure rate is the same as in unilateral tumor and is related to the stage and histologic findings. Treatment is focal resection of nodules and chemotherapy.

VI. **Treatment**

A. **The conquest of Wilms' tumor is a modern cancer success story.** The development of progressively more sophisticated treatment as the result of the National Wilms' Tumor Study has been a model for cancer therapy.

B. **Multidisciplinary care** has been the secret to success: appropriate use of surgical extirpation, chemotherapy, and radiation according to the nature of the tumor. A knowledgeable close-working team of oncologists, surgeons, pathologists, and radiation therapists is essential.

C. Staging of Wilms' tumor

Stage I: localized tumor, completely excised
Stage II: local invasion or spill, completely excised
Stage III: incomplete excision, massive spillage of tumor, or positive regional lymph nodes
Stage IV: metastatic disease (lung or liver)

D. Surgical removal of the tumor is necessary in all patients, and is usually the first step in treatment. The operative findings also determine the **stage.** If the tumor is **unresectable,** only biopsy and staging are performed. Chemotherapy is given to shrink the tumor, and a second attempt at extirpation is made 6–10 weeks later.

E. Chemotherapy is given to virtually all patients. Wilms' tumor is amazingly responsive to actinomycin D and vincristine. Doxorubicin (Adriamycin) is added in those with metastatic disease and in the 10% with unfavorable histologic findings, regardless of stage.

F. Radiation therapy is given if there is gross residual tumor after surgical excision, and if there are unfavorable histologic findings, regardless of stage. Radiation may also cure pulmonary metastases in some patients.

Preoperative preparation

A. Chest x-ray should be obtained to demonstrate gross metastases, but a more extensive evaluation for metastatic spread is deferred until the tumor diagnosis has been confirmed operatively.

B. Urine should be obtained for vanillylmandelic acid **(VMA)** determination in case the tumor turns out to be a neuroblastoma.

C. Blood should be available for intraoperative transfusion as necessary.

Operative care

A. A **generous transverse transabdominal incision** is used to permit thorough evaluation of the opposite kidney, as well as all of the abdomen, for possible spread of tumor.

B. Heroic efforts to remove all the tumor by resecting parts of adjacent organs **are not appropriate** or beneficial. If the tumor cannot be resected without damage to other organs, only biopsy and staging should be done. Chemotherapy is then given. The tumor can usually be resected at a second operation 6–10 weeks later.

C. Care is taken **not** to **rupture** the tumor (which may be friable). It is usually necessary to remove the adrenal gland with the kidney.

Postoperative care. No special measures are required unless there have been intraoperative complications.

Complications

A. Operative complications may result from the distortion of anatomy by the tumor.

1. **Damage to the blood supply of the opposite kidney** may result unless the artery and vein to both kidneys are identified before dividing those to the tumor.
2. **Tumor invasion** can lead to **inadvertent injury** of adjacent organs, particularly of the pancreas, spleen, liver, and intestine.
3. **Rupture of the tumor** may occur during removal.

B. Chemotherapy complications include infection, hair loss, immunodepression, leukopenia, and thrombocytopenia. Cardiotoxicity is seen with Adriamycin.

C. **Radiation therapy** complications result from damage to nearby normal tissue: spine (scoliosis), liver (atrophy), lungs (pulmonary insufficiency). Second malignancies have been reported in patients receiving high-dose radiation therapy and chemotherapy.

XI. **Prognosis.** The outcome in Wilms' tumor depends on multiple factors.
   A. **Stage** (the extent of spread). Distant metastases, breach of the capsule, and lymph-node involvement are unfavorable findings.
   B. **Histologic findings** (unfavorable versus favorable).
   C. **Size** of the tumor. Patients with large tumors do significantly worse.
   D. **Age** of the patient. Young children do much better.

XII. **Outcome.** The improvements in outcome after treatment for Wilms' tumor reflect advances in surgery, anesthesia, radiation therapy, and chemotherapy. In the past decade, specific tailoring of therapy to individuals according to stage and histologic findings has led to dramatic improvements in outcome. Current disease-free survival rates are as follows:

Stage I:	95%
Stages II, III:	85%
Stage IV:	75–80%
Unfavorable histology	25–50%

Bibliography

Beckwith, J. B. Wilms' tumor and other renal tumors of childhood: A selective review from the National Wilms' Tumor Study Pathology Center. *Hum. Pathol* 14:481, 1983.

Beckwith, J. B., and Palmer, N. F. Histopathology and prognosis of Wilms' tumor Results of the First National Wilms' Tumor Study. *Cancer* 41:1937, 1978.

Bishop, H. C., et al. Survival in bilateral Wilms' tumor. *J. Pediatr. Surg.* 12:631 1977.

D'Angio, G. J., et al. The treatment of Wilms' tumor: Results of the National Wilms Tumor Study. *Cancer* 38:633, 1976.

D'Angio, G. J., et al. The treatment of Wilms' tumor: Results of the Second National Wilms' Tumor Study. *Cancer* 47:2302, 1981.

D'Angio, G. J., et al. Results of the Third National Wilms' Tumor Study (NWTS-3) A preliminary report. Proceedings of the American Association for Cancer Research, Vol. 25, 1984.

Howell, C. G., et al. Therapy and outcome in 51 children with mesoblastic nephroma: A report of the National Wilms' Tumor Study. *J. Pediatr. Surg.* 6:826 1982.

Johnson, D. G. Wilms' Tumor. In T. M. Holder and K. W. Ashcraft (eds.), *Pediatric Surgery*. Philadelphia: Saunders, 1980. P. 932.

Leape, L. L. Diagnosis and Management of Wilms' Tumors and Neuroblastomas. In D. G. Skinner and J. B. De Kernion (eds.), *Genitourinary Cancer*. Philadelphia Saunders, 1978. PP. 179–199.

Leape, L. L., Breslow, N. E., and Bishop, H. C. The surgical treatment of Wilms tumor: Results of the National Wilms' Tumor Study. *Ann. Surg.* 187:351, 1978.

Mitus, A., Tefft, M., and Fellers, F. X. Long-term follow-up of renal functions of 10 children who underwent nephrectomy for malignant disease. *Pediatrics* 44:91, 1969.

Othersen, H. B., Jr. Wilms' Tumor. In K. J. Welch, et al. (eds.), *Pediatric Surgery* Chicago: Year Book, 1986. P. 293.

Thomas, P. R., et al. Late effects of treatment for Wilms' tumor. *Int. J. Radic Oncol. Biol. Phys.* 9:651, 1983.

Thomas, P. R., et al. Relapse patterns in irradiated Second National Wilms' Tumor Study (NWTS-2) Patients. *Proc. Am. Soc. Clin. Oncol.* 2:69, 1983.

84 Neuroblastoma

- **Definition.** *Neuroblastoma* is the most common solid tumor of childhood. It arises from the neural crest tissue along the sympathetic ganglion chain and in the adrenal medulla. Tumors arise in the abdomen (75%), posterior mediastinum (20%), neck, and organ of Zuckerkandl. Fifty percent develop in the adrenal medulla. The incidence is approximately 1 in 10,000. A rare multifocal familial form has been described.

- **Pathophysiology**
  - A. **Neuroblastoma has the unique capacity to undergo maturation to a benign form, ganglioneuroma, and to disappear.** Presumably this accounts for the finding that tiny neuroblastomas are found in stillborn infants at 100 times the incidence of the tumor in later life. This change to a benign form rarely happens after a tumor is clinically manifest, but if a tumor has mature elements in it, the prognosis is improved.
  - B. **Catecholamines** and their breakdown products are excreted by 90% of children with neuroblastoma: adrenalin, noradrenalin, DOPA, metanephrine, homovanillic acid, vanillylmandelic acid, and vanillylglycolic acid. These markers are useful for detecting recurrence after surgical removal of the tumor.
  - C. **Metastatic spread** occurs relatively early in neuroblastoma and accounts for the poor outlook in most children. Bone marrow, liver, lymph nodes, bone cortex, and lung are common sites. Subcutaneous tumor nodules sometimes occur.

Clinical presentation

  A. Neuroblastoma is a **tumor of young children:** half the patients present before the age of 2 years, 90% by the age of 8.

  B. An **abdominal mass** is the presenting finding in 75% of children.

  C. **Weight loss,** abdominal pain, distention, fever, anemia, and failure to thrive are associated symptoms. Hypertension is present in 25%, the result of catecholamine production by the tumor.

  D. Tumors arising in the **mediastinum** are frequently asymptomatic unless the stellate ganglion is involved, producing **Horner's syndrome.** Respiratory distress or dysphagia is rarely seen from compression of the bronchi or esophagus.

  E. **Proptosis** and **periorbital ecchymoses** may be the first sign of orbital metastases from neuroblastoma.

  F. **Paraplegia** may result from spinal-cord compression by tumor.

  G. **Flushing,** sweating, and irritability are occasionally caused by the catecholamines.

  H. **Cerebellar ataxia,** opsomyoclonus, and nystagmus are sometimes seen. The cause is unknown.

  I. **Intractable diarrhea** may occur from tumor production of vasoactive intestinal peptide (VIP) by a neuroblastoma.

Diagnosis

  A. **CT scan and MRI** are the preferred methods of diagnosing and evaluating neuroblastoma. Eighty percent will be found to have a fine stippled calcification. Involvement of the major vessels and extension into the liver, kidneys, or other

organs can usually be determined by the scan. Liver and lung metastases are readily detected by CT or MRI.
- B. **Wilms' tumor** can usually be differentiated from neuroblastoma by its intrarenal origin and lack of calcification, but if either tumor is large and is invading surrounding structures, preoperative distinction may be impossible.
- C. **Mediastinal neuroblastoma** is posterior in location and almost always causes erosion of the foramen of the spinal nerve and erosion and separation of the posterior segment of the ribs.
- D. **Bone-marrow metastases** are frequently evident on bone-marrow aspirate.
- E. **Bone isotope scan** and skeletal survey are performed to detect bony metastases.
- F. **Myelography** should be performed to look for "dumbbell" extension of mediastinal tumor if there are neurologic signs of spinal compression.

V. Treatment
- A. **Surgical removal** of the primary tumor is the preferred treatment for neuroblastoma and the only established method of cure at present. The need for chemotherapy and radiotherapy and the ultimate prognosis are dependent on **surgical staging.**
- B. **Staging of neuroblastoma**

    Stage I: tumor confined to a single organ, completely resected
    Stage II: tumor extending beyond the organ but not crossing the midline
    Stage III: large tumor extending beyond the midline and often unresectable, leaving gross residual disease
    Stage IV: distant metastases to bone and other organs
    Stage IV-S: stage IV tumor in a patient under the age of 1 year with metastases limited to liver, skin, or marrow

- C. **Chemotherapy** has been disappointing in the treatment of neuroblastoma. Tumor shrinkage can be obtained with either drug treatment or radiation therapy, but the cure rate is not demonstrably improved.
- D. Experiments with **total body irradiation** and bone-marrow transplantation have been carried out in desperation but without great success.
- E. **Immunologic characteristics** of neuroblastoma are interesting in view of demonstrated spontaneous regression and the fact that lymphocytes will inhibit tumor growth in tissue culture. So far, no mechanism of immunotherapy has been devised to use this characteristic to eradicate tumor.
- F. **Treatment protocols**

    Stage I: Surgical resection alone.
    Stage II: Surgical resection plus radiation (1200–2000 rad) if over 1 year of age.
    Stage III: Surgical resection of as much tumor as can be safely removed. Chemotherapy and radiation are given in maximal doses. A second-look procedure is carried out later, after maximal response to therapy.
    Stage IV: Chemotherapy is given after proof of the diagnosis is obtained by biopsy. Surgical resection of the tumor may later be possible. Occasional cures are obtained this way.
    Stage IV-S: Surgical resection alone. Chemotherapy is highly toxic in infants and of dubious value. Metastatic disease will usually disappear once the primary tumor is removed. If it does not, chemotherapy is indicated.

VI. Preoperative preparation
- A. **Catecholamines** are measured in a 24-hour urine collection preoperatively, so postoperative assay can be used to recognize recurrent disease.

B. Laminectomy is performed before thoracotomy if there is evidence of spinal-cord compression by a mediastinal neuroblastoma. Sometimes the operations can be combined.

Operative care

A. Large intravenous lines should be placed in the **upper extremities** for the rapid administration of blood if necessary.

B. Total excision of the tumor without spillage of cells is the desired surgical objective. Resection of adjacent organs does not enhance the chance of cure and should not be undertaken.

C. If the tumor is **unresectable,** or resection would expose the patient to life-threatening hazard, biopsy or partial excision is all that is performed.

D. A **second-look** procedure is carried out after maximal response to chemotherapy in patients with incompletely resected tumor and in those with stage IV disease who respond to chemotherapy.

Postoperative care.
Routine. Careful attention to restoration of blood volume and replacement of "third space" fluid loss is needed, but most children tolerate tumor surgery well.

Prognosis.
Outcome following treatment of neuroblastoma depends on age, stage, site, and degree of maturation of the tumor. Overall, the picture is gloomy, with a combined disease-free survival rate of only 37%.

A. Young patients do better. Survival is 75% in infants, 50% between ages 1 and 2, and only 20% in children over 2 years.

B. Stage has a significant effect on the disease-free survival rate:

Stage I:	90–100%
Stage II:	80%
Stage III:	35–50%
Stage IV:	10–20%
Stage IV–S:	80%

C. Abdominal tumors are the most lethal; fewer than a third of patients survive. Patients with mediastinal and cervical neuroblastomas have a very high survival rate (80–100%).

D. Infants who present with **opsomyoclonus** or **VIP diarrhea** do well, with disease-free survival rates greater than 80%.

Bibliography

Altman, A., and Baehner, R. L. Favorable prognosis for survival in children with coincident opsomyoclonus and neuroblastoma. *Cancer* 37:846, 1976.

Coldman, A. J., et al. Neuroblastoma: Influence of age at diagnosis, stage, site, and sex on prognosis. *Cancer* 46:1896, 1980.

El-Shafie, M., et al. Intractable diarrhea in children with VIP-secreting ganglioneuroblastoma. *J. Pediatr. Surg.* 18:34, 1983.

Evans, A. E., D'Angio, G. J., and Koop, C. E. The role of multimodal therapy in patients with local and regional neuroblastoma. *J. Pediatr. Surg.* 19:77, 1984.

Evans, A. E., Gerson, J., and Schnaufer, L. Spontaneous regression of neuroblastoma. *Natl. Cancer Inst. Monogr.* 44:49, 1976.

Filler, R. M., et al. Favorable outlook for children with mediastinal neuroblastoma. *J. Pediatr. Surg.* 7:136, 1972.

Grosfeld, J. L. Neuroblastoma. In K. J. Welch, et al. (eds.), *Pediatric Surgery.* Chicago: Year Book, 1986. P. 283.

Grosfeld, J. L., et al. Metastatic neuroblastoma: Factors influencing survival. *J. Pediatr. Surg.* 13:59, 1978.

Hayes, F. A., et al. Surgicopathologic staging of neuroblastoma: Prognostic significance of regional lymph node metastases. *J. Pediatr.* 102:59, 1983.

Holgerson, L. O., et al. Neuroblastoma with intraspinal (dumbbell) extension. *J. Pediatr. Surg.* 18:406, 1983.

Koop, C. E., and Schnaufer, L. Neuroblastoma. In T. M. Holder and K. W. Ashcraft (eds.), *Pediatric Surgery.* Philadelphia: Saunders, 1980. P. 944.

Laug, W. E., Siegel, S. E., and Shaw, K. N. F. Initial urinary catecholamine metabolite concentrations and prognosis in neuroblastoma. *Pediatrics* 62:77, 1978.

Leape, L. L., Lowman, J. T., and Loveland, G. C. Multifocal nondisseminated neuroblastoma. *J. Pediatr.* 92:75, 1978.

Voute, P. A. Neuroblastoma. In W. Sutow, D. Fernbach, and T. Vietti (eds.), *Clinical Pediatric Oncology.* St. Louis: Mosby, 1984. P. 559.

Young, D. G. Thoracic neuroblastoma/ganglioneuroma. *J. Pediatr. Surg.* 18:37, 1983.

85

Teratoma

I. **Definition.** A *teratoma* is a tumor of multiple tissues foreign to the organ in which it arises. The classic requirement that it contain derivatives from all three germ layers is not essential. Teratomas may arise at any age and may be either benign or malignant. Common sites are the sacrococcygeal region, ovary, testis, and retroperitoneum. Teratomas are also found in the brain, mouth, neck, stomach, mediastinum, and heart.

II. **Pathophysiology**

  A. Teratomas arise from **germ cells** and thus are most common in gonads and the sacrococcygeal area.

  B. **Benign** teratomas cause symptoms by compressing adjacent organs or by twisting, while **malignant** teratomas may invade or metastasize.

  C. **Functioning endocrine** tissue is occasionally found in a teratoma and may be responsible for symptoms. Insulin and gonadotropin secretion have been described.

III. **Clinical presentation** depends on the site and size of the teratoma.

IV. **Ovarian teratoma.** The ovary is the most common site of teratomas, which comprise 70% of ovarian tumors. Ovarian teratoma is discussed in detail in Chap. 90, Ovarian Tumors.

V. **Sacrococcygeal teratoma**

  A. **Clinical picture.** Sacrococcygeal teratoma is almost always present at birth. It varies greatly in size from a barely noticeable lump to a huge mass causing dystocia. Three-fourths of the patients are girls.

   1. The **mass** develops between the anus and the coccyx and is usually covered with skin. It may be diffuse or pedunculated, soft or firm, cystic or solid.

   2. The teratoma may extend internally through the pelvis and be palpable as a **suprapubic mass.** Tumors with a large intrapelvic extension are more likely to be malignant.

  B. **Diagnosis**

   1. The tumor is usually obvious on physical examination, but if it is small it may be missed and not discovered until months or years later, when it grows larger.

   2. **Rectal examination** demonstrates a posterior mass. No x-rays or special studies are needed in the typical case. The sacrum is normal.

   3. Differentiation from **myelomeningocele** may be difficult. In addition to having no intrarectal extension, myelomeningocele is more cephalad and covered with a serous membrane. It is usually associated with muscular weakness of the limbs or perineum, and x-rays of the sacrum show dysraphism.

   4. A **lipomeningocele** is even more difficult to distinguish, but it, too, has no extension inside the rectum, and it tends to overlie the sacrum rather than extend below the coccyx.

  C. **Treatment** is complete excision of the teratoma, separating its attachments by removal of the coccyx and division of the middle sacral artery branches. An abominal incision is sometimes needed if there is a large intrapelvic extension of the tumor.

D. **Prognosis** in sacrococcygeal teratoma is closely related to **age** at the time of operation. Ninety percent of neonatal sacrococcygeal teratomas are benign, whereas 90% of tumors removed after the age of 2 months are malignant.

1. If the tumor is **benign,** no further therapy is needed. The rare recurrence probably arises from retained bits of tumor and can be successfully treated by reexcision.
2. If the tumor is **malignant** (embryonal carcinoma, yolk sac carcinoma, germinoma), excision is frequently curative if the tumor can be completely removed. If the tumor recurs, the outlook is poor. Highly aggressive chemotherapy using VAC, doxorubicin (Adriamycin), bleomycin, and BCNU has resulted in some long-term disease-free survivors.

VI. **Presacral teratoma.** A special variant of sacrococcygeal teratoma is diagnosed by rectal examination as a mass in the presacral space.

A. **Clinical picture**
1. Presacral teratoma is **inherited,** transmitted as a Mendelian dominant trait.
2. Associated findings include **anal stenosis,** bony defect of the sacrum, dimpling of the sacral skin, and invasion of the rectal wall. The tumor may be attached to the meninges. Lower urinary tract anomalies are frequently present.
3. The tumor has been **benign** in 95% of patients described.
4. **Constipation** because of the anal stenosis is the most common presenting symptom. Urinary obstruction or infection with meningitis may be seen.

B. **Diagnosis** is by rectal examination after dilatation of the anal stenosis. Presacral meningocele can be differentiated by CT or MRI.

C. **Treatment** is excision of the tumor, which requires resection of part of the rectal wall, and correction of associated urinary tract anomalies.

VII. **Retroperitoneal teratoma**

A. **Clinical picture**
1. An **abdominal mass** of increasing girth is the presenting finding in most children. The tumor may be huge.
2. Vomiting, intestinal obstruction, and pain can result from compression of the intestine, but these symptoms are uncommon.
3. The tumor may arise within the kidney and may be indistinguishable from Wilms' tumor.

B. **Diagnosis** is suspected from plain abdominal x-rays, which may show calcification and even teeth. CT image will usually be characteristic, showing fat and calcium.

C. **Treatment** is excision of the tumor. Up to 10% of retroperitoneal teratomas are malignant. Aggressive chemotherapy is indicated in these patients.

VIII. **Gastric teratoma.** In contrast to retroperitoneal teratoma, teratoma arising in the stomach is always benign. Victims are almost exclusively male.

A. **Clinical picture.** A mass is noted by the parent, patient, or doctor. Hematemesis or anemia may be present.

B. **Diagnosis.** Barium study, CT, or MRI demonstrates a mass.

C. **Treatment** is excision with partial gastrectomy. Recurrence is rare.

IX. Mediastinal and cardiac teratoma. Teratoma in the mediastinum may occur in three locations: attached to the thymus in the anterior mediastinum, in the pericardium, or in the myocardium (intracardiac). Intracardiac teratoma is malignant in 25% of cases, but only 13% of mediastinal teratomas are malignant.

  A. Clinical picture

   1. **Mediastinal teratoma.** Respiratory symptoms predominate: wheezing, dyspnea, and cyanosis; the symptoms often improve if the patient lies prone. Chest x-ray may show what appears to be a huge heart shadow.
   2. **Pericardial teratoma.** Cardiac tamponade is the usual presenting symptom.
   3. **Myocardial teratoma.** Heart failure develops in a previously asymptomatic patient.

  B. Diagnosis is by CT, MRI, or cardiac catheterization studies performed for unexplained heart failure. Calcification by chest x-ray may be a clue.

  C. Treatment is excision of the tumor. Cardiac bypass is needed for removal of an intracardiac teratoma.

X. Cervicofacial teratoma. Teratomas of the neck or roof of the mouth may be huge and grotesque, causing distortion of the maxilla and jaw and producing airway obstruction.

  A. *Epignathus* is the term given to a teratoma arising from the base of the skull in the nasopharynx. Intracranial extension of the tumor may be extensive, making it difficult or impossible to remove. Fortunately, these are rare lesions.

  B. Cervical teratomas are usually associated with the thyroid gland but are rarely malignant. Flattening and distortion of the trachea may require long-term intubation after resection of the tumor.

Bibliography

Abeley, G. I. Alpha-fetoprotein in ontogenesis and its association with malignant tumors. *Adv. Cancer Res.* 14:295, 1971.
Altman, R. P., Randolph, J. G., and Lilly, J. R. Sacrococcygeal teratoma: American Academy of Pediatrics Surgical Section Survey, 1973. *J. Pediatr. Surg.* 9:389, 1974.
Ashcraft, K. W., and Holder, T. M. Hereditary presacral teratoma. *J. Pediatr. Surg.* 9:691, 1974.
Engel, R. M., Elkins, R. C., and Fletcher, B. D. Retroperitoneal teratoma: Review of literature and presentation of an unusual case. *Cancer* 22:1068, 1968.
Grosfeld, J. L., et al. Benign and malignant teratomas in children: Analysis of 85 patients. *Surgery* 80:297, 1976.
Gross, R. E., Clatworthy, H. W., Jr., and Meeker, I. A., Jr. Sacrococcygeal teratomas in infants and children: A report of 40 cases. *Surg. Gynecol. Obstet.* 92:341, 1951.
Mahour, G. H., Landing, B. H., and Woolley, M. M. Teratomas in children: Clinicopathologic studies in 133 patients. *Z. Kinderchir.* 23:365, 1978.
Noseworthy, J., et al. Sacrococcygeal germ cell tumors in childhood. *J. Pediatr. Surg.* 16:358, 1981.
Tapper, D., and Lack, E. E. Teratomas in infancy and childhood: A 54-year experience at the Children's Hospital Medical Center. *Ann. Surg.* 198:398, 1983.
Woolley, M. M. Teratoma. In T. M. Holder and K. W. Ashcraft (eds.), *Pediatric Surgery*. Philadelphia: Saunders, 1980. P. 960.
Woolley, M. M. Teratoma. In K. J. Welch, et al. (eds.), *Pediatric Surgery*. Chicago: Year Book, 1986. P. 265.

86 Rhabdomyosarcoma

Definition. Rhabdomyosarcoma accounts for 10% of malignant solid tumors in childhood. There are two tissue types: **embryonal** and **alveolar,** with very different outcomes and sites of predilection. *Sarcoma botryoides* is a polypoid embryonal rhabdomyosarcoma that occurs in visceral cavities such as the bladder or vagina.

Pathophysiology

A. Rhabdomyosarcoma arises from primitive **mesenchymal** cells anywhere in the body (except the brain), but it is not necessarily related to striated muscle.

B. The **alveolar** type is most commonly found in striated muscle of the trunk and limbs, and it is rarely seen in the orbit or genitourinary tract. It is associated with a **higher mortality:** 60% 5-year survival rate with present multimodal therapy.

C. **Embryonal** rhabdomyosarcoma is typically found in the genitourinary tract, orbit, head and neck, and retroperitoneum. It is more susceptible than the alveolar type to chemotherapy and radiation therapy, with current 5-year disease-free survival rates of nearly 85%.

D. Rhabdomyosarcomas may be **mixed** in type. The prognosis and treatment protocols are governed by the predominant pattern.

E. **Electron microscopy** may be needed for diagnosis of poorly differentiated rhabdomyosarcoma. **Z bands** are the characteristic finding. Immunochemical demonstration of **myosin** is also confirmatory.

F. In most patients the tumor is grossly well-localized at the time of diagnosis, but tumor may be microscopically disseminated in neighboring tissues or regional lymph nodes.

G. **Metastases** occur to **lung, bone, bone marrow,** and regional **lymph nodes.**

General principles

A. **Site.** Rhabdomyosarcoma can occur virtually anywhere in the body. Approximately one-fourth of instances occur in each of three areas: **head and neck, extremities,** and the **genitourinary tract.**

B. **Outcome** is related to **age, site, and tissue type.**

   1. Rhabdomyosarcoma of the **genitourinary tract** and **head and neck** is typically found in **infancy** and early childhood. Ninety percent or more are of the **embryonal** type and have a good prognosis.

   2. Tumors of the **trunk** and **abdominal** organs and paratesticular rhabdomyosarcoma are found in **older children** and are usually **alveolar.** The survival rate is considerably lower.

   3. **Orbital** (95% embryonal) and **limb** (45% alveolar) rhabdomyosarcomas occur at any age with excellent and poor prognoses, respectively.

C. **Metastatic survey** must be carried out in every patient with rhabdomyosarcoma. CT or MRI scan of the abdomen and chest is routine, as well as bone scan and bone-marrow aspiration. No chemical markers have been identified so far.

D. **Treatment** has been significantly improved in the past decade as a result of the Intergroup Rhabdomyosarcoma Study (IRS). Several general principles have emerged as guides to optimal therapy.

1. **Multimodal therapy** is required for all patients with rhabdomyosarcoma. Few patients are cured by surgery alone.
2. **Chemotherapy** can control micrometastatic disease, particularly in lymph nodes, but it is most effective when the tumor burden is low.
3. **Site and histologic type** are major determinants of therapy. Alveolar rhabdomyosarcoma requires much more aggressive therapy to achieve an optimal outcome.
4. **Chemotherapy and radiation alone work well in genitourinary and orbital rhabdomyosarcoma,** but not in other sites.
5. **Localized relapse** of tumor should be treated aggressively by operation, chemotherapy, and radiation.

IV. **Genitourinary rhabdomyosarcoma**
   A. **Clinical characteristics.** Rhabdomyosarcoma arising from the bladder, prostate, or vagina commonly presents with symptoms of **urinary obstruction, vaginal discharge,** or **bleeding.** Occasionally a **polypoid mass (sarcoma botryoides)** protrudes from the vagina or urethra. A suprapubic **mass** may be the presenting complaint.
   B. **Diagnosis** is by **biopsy,** directly or endoscopically. A mass in the prostate or base of the bladder can undergo biopsy by a needle introduced through the rectum.
   C. **Treatment**
      1. **Primary treatment** of genitourinary rhabdomyosarcoma is now **chemotherapy** (pulse VAC) with addition of radiation if the tumor is not completely eradicated by the drugs.
      2. **Partial cystectomy or anterior exenteration** is carried out if the tumor is not completely eradicated (20%). Exploratory laparotomy may be necessary to determine if there is residual gross disease to be removed.
   D. **Problems**
      1. Relief of **urinary obstruction** by catheter, suprapubic cystostomy, or nephrostomies may be required initially.
      2. **Intestinal obstruction** due to compression of the rectum is seldom complete. Use of a nasogastric tube and parenteral nutrition for a week or two during the initial phase of chemotherapy will usually obviate the need for colostomy.
      3. **Radiation** therapy results in **sterility** in a high percentage of girls treated for genitourinary rhabdomyosarcoma.
   E. **Prognosis** for disease-free survival after treatment of genitourinary rhabdomyosarcoma is good. **Overall, 75%** of patients appear to be cured.
      1. **Thirty percent** are apparently cured by **chemotherapy and radiation alone.**
      2. **Fifty percent** have an excellent response to chemotherapy and radiation, but have residual gross tumor. Ninety percent of these can be cured by **subsequent surgery.**
      3. **Twenty percent respond poorly** to adjuvant therapy and remain inoperable.

V. **Rhabdomyosarcoma of the extremities**
   A. **Clinical characteristics.** An **asymptomatic mass** in the arm or leg is the presenting finding in most children with rhabdomyosarcoma of the extremities. The tumor progresses slowly and is often present for many months before diagnosis and treatment, perhaps accounting for the poor results in many of these patients.

Table 86-1. Results of therapy of extremity rhabdomyosarcoma

Group	Definition	Five-year survival (%)
I	Localized disease Completely resected No lymph nodes	78
II	Localized disease Completely resected Microscopic residual or positive nodes (resected)	68
III	Incomplete resection Residual disease or nodes	52
IV	Metastatic disease	20

Source: From D. M. Hays, E. H. Soule, and W. Lawrence, Jr. Extremity lesions in the Intergroup Rhabdomyosarcoma Study (IRS-1): A preliminary report. *Cancer* 48:1, 1982.

- **B. Treatment.** Surgical excision is performed first, followed by chemotherapy and radiation therapy.
    1. **Wide local excision** is preferred to amputation. Inguinofemoral or axillary **lymph-node dissection** is carried out at the time of the initial operation. Retroperitoneal lymphadenectomy is performed later if the groin nodes are positive.
    2. **Chemotherapy:** pulse VAC, doxorubicin (Adriamycin), cisplatin.
    3. **Radiotherapy:** 4500 rad in 5 weeks.
- **C. Prognosis** is mixed in extremity rhabdomyosarcoma because of the high percentage of patients with alveolar tissue type (Table 86-1).

I. Head and neck rhabdomyosarcoma

- **A.** Two groups of patients with rhabdomyosarcoma of the head and neck have very different outlooks.
    1. **Tumors of the scalp, superficial face, parotid, and subtemporal** region can usually be grossly completely excised. A **90% survival** rate can be expected with current multimodal therapy.
    2. **Tumors of the nasopharynx, inner ear, paranasal sinuses, and pterygoid fossa** rarely lend themselves to complete excision. Cure is possible in fewer than **50%** of cases.
- **B. Rhabdomyosarcoma of the orbit** has the **most favorable prognosis of all rhabdomyosarcomas.** Chemotherapy and radiation therapy are sufficient in most cases. Long-term survival rates exceed **90%** for localized disease.

I. Miscellaneous rhabdomyosarcoma.
Rhabdomyosarcomas of the **biliary tract, retroperitoneum, perineum,** and **perianal** regions have a **poorer outlook** than others. They are more likely to be the alveolar type, and the diagnosis is often delayed, permitting metastatic spread. Overall survival at present is less than 20%.

Bibliography

Ariel, I. M., and Brinceno, M. Rhabdomyosarcoma of the extremities and trunk: Analysis of 150 patients treated by surgical resection. *J. Surg. Oncol.* 7:269, 1975.

Donaldson, S. S., et al. Rhabdomyosarcoma of head and neck in children. *Cancer* 31:26, 1973.

Fleming, I. D., et al. The role of surgical resection when combined with chemotherapy and radiation in the management of pelvic rhabdomyosarcoma. *Ann. Surg.* 199:509, 1984.

Gaiger, A. M., Soule, E. H., and Newton, W. A., Jr. Pathology of rhabdomyosarcoma: Experience of the Intergroup Rhabdomyosarcoma Study, 1972–78. *Natl. Cancer Inst. Monogr.* 56:19, 1981.

Gehan, E. A., et al. Prognostic factors in children with rhabdomyosarcoma. *Natl. Cancer Inst. Monogr.* 56:83, 1981.

Grosfeld, J. L. Rhabdomyosarcoma. In T. M. Holder and K. W. Ashcraft (eds.), *Pediatric Surgery*. Philadelphia: Saunders, 1980. P. 985.

Grosfeld, J. L., Clatworthy, H. W., Jr., and Newton, W. A., Jr. Combined therapy in childhood rhabdomyosarcoma: An analysis of 42 cases. *J. Pediatr. Surg.* 4:637, 1969.

Grosfeld, J. L., et al. Rhabdomyosarcoma in childhood: Analysis of survival in 98 cases. *J. Pediatr. Surg.* 18:141, 1983.

Hays, D. M., Soule, E. H., and Lawrence, W., Jr. Extremity lesions in The Intergroup Rhabdomyosarcoma Study (IRS-1): A preliminary report. *Cancer* 48:1, 1982.

Hays, D. M. Pelvic rhabdomyosarcomas in childhood: Diagnosis and concepts of management reviewed. *Cancer* 45:76, 1980.

Hays, D. M. Rhabdomyosarcoma. In K. J. Welch, et al. (eds.), *Pediatric Surgery*. Chicago: Year Book, 1986. P. 276.

Hays, D. M., et al. Primary chemotherapy in the treatment of children with bladder-prostate tumors in the intergroup rhabdomyosarcoma study (IRS-IL). *J. Pediatr. Surg.* 17:812, 1982.

Jaffe, N., et al. Rhabdomyosarcoma in children. *Am. J. Surg.* 125:482, 1973.

Maurer, H. M. Rhabdomyosarcoma in childhood and adolescence. *Curr. Probl. Cancer* 2:1, 1978.

87 Hodgkin's Disease

I. **Definition.** *Hodgkin's disease* is cancer of the lymphoid tissue. It is distinguished from non-Hodgkin's lymphoma by its characteristic location in lymph nodes and by the presence of the **Reed-Sternberg cell**. It accounts for 5% of childhood malignancies. Hodgkin's disease is rare before the age of 5 years but has a peak incidence in the second decade of life. Boys are more frequently affected than girls.

II. **Pathophysiology.** In most patients, enlargement of the affected lymph nodes causes little impairment of function. Massive mediastinal lymphadenopathy can produce tracheal compression with respiratory distress or the superior mediastinal syndrome from compression of the great veins. Disseminated disease may produce fever, weight loss, and malaise.

III. **Clinical presentation**

  A. **Painless enlargement** of cervical lymph nodes is the most common presenting complaint. The glands typically enlarge slowly but relentlessly. They are firm and rubbery to palpation, but nontender.

  B. **Mediastinal lymphadenopathy** is present in 50% of patients at the time of diagnosis.

  C. **Axillary, inguinal,** and **supraclavicular** lymph nodes can be involved either primarily or in addition to the cervical node disease. The liver and spleen are palpable in advanced disease.

  D. **Fever, weight loss, anorexia, and malaise** are present in approximately 30% of patients at the time of the diagnosis.

IV. **Diagnosis**

  A. **Chest x-ray** is obtained to demonstrate mediastinal disease and for follow-up of treatment.

  B. **CT or MRI** scan of the chest and abdomen may reveal involvement of other nodes or the liver or spleen.

  C. **Lymphangiography** has been used to define intraabdominal nodal disease, but its high error rate, difficulty of performance in young children, and significant complication rate have led most physicians to abandon it.

  D. **Lymph node biopsy** confirms the diagnosis. In addition to the typical histologic pattern, the pathologist must demonstrate the presence of the **Reed-Sternberg cell**.

  E. **Histologic classification** (Rye) is of prognostic value and determines the nature of treatment. In order of decreasing survival rates, the histologic types are:

    1. Lymphocytic predominant
    2. Nodular sclerosis
    3. Mixed cellularity
    4. Lymphocytic depletion (rarely seen in children)

  F. **Staging,** the determination of the extent of tumor spread, is the other factor in predicting outcome and determining treatment. The Ann Arbor classification is most widely used. Subscripts are used to indicate extralymphatic disease (e) or the absence (A) or presence (B) of systemic symptoms.

  Stage I: Single lymph node region involved

Stage II: Two or more lymph node regions involved on the same side of the diaphragm

Stage III: Disease on both sides of the diaphragm

Stage IV: Diffuse or disseminated involvement of one or more extralymphatic organs

G. **Staging laparotomy,** with splenectomy, biopsy of the liver, and sampling of intraabdominal lymph nodes, is performed in apparent stage I or II cervicomediastinal Hodgkin's disease and in patients with presumed stage III disease without histologic proof. The clinical stage (and thus the treatment) will be **changed in as many as 40%** of patients by the findings at laparotomy.

V. Treatment

A. **Radiation therapy** is the primary form of treatment for most patients with Hodgkin's disease. An extended field encompassing the affected nodes and adjacent regions is used for stage I or II disease, a "mantle" for cervical and mediastinal disease, and an inverted "Y" for abdominal and groin disease. Total nodal irradiation is used for stage III disease.

B. **Chemotherapy** is the primary therapy for disseminated disease, stage IV, but is added to radiation therapy for patients with systemic symptoms (B) or extranodal stage III disease. MOPP (mechlorethamine [*M*ustargen], vincristine [*O*ncovin], *p*rocarbazine, and *p*rednisone) has been the standard combination used, but there are many variations.

C. **Surgical excision is inadequate** treatment for Hodgkin's disease, which is seldom limited to a single node group. The surgeon's role is to establish the stage for accurate therapy.

VI. Staging laparotomy

A. **Objective.** To determine the extent of the spread of disease as precisely as possible.

B. **Biopsy sites**

1. Spleen (Splenectomy)
2. Liver. Random needle from both lobes and wedge
3. Lymph nodes
    a. Any nodes that are suspicious on CT or MRI
    b. Splenic hilum
    c. Celiac axis
    d. Mesentery
    e. Paraaortic from renal arteries to bifurcation
    f. Common iliac
    g. External iliac
4. Bone-marrow

C. The **ovaries** are relocated out of the radiation field in the hope of preserving fertility.

VII. Postoperative care. Routine

VIII. Complications

A. **Staging laparotomy.** As many as 10% of patients will develop one or more of the following complications: intestinal obstruction, wound infection, pancreatitis, retroperitoneal hematoma, pleural effusion, subphrenic abscess, thrombotic episodes.

B. Postsplenectomy sepsis has a higher mortality in patients with Hodgkin's disease than in others, presumably because of the immunodepression associated with the disease and its treatment. Reported mortality is 2–4%.

C. Chemotherapy and Radiation Therapy (see Chap. 82).

X. Prognosis. Ninety percent of children with Hodgkin's disease survive 5 years or more.

Bibliography

Bayle-Weisgerber, C., et al. Hodgkin's disease in children: Results of therapy in a mixed group of 178 clinical and pathologically staged patients over 13 years. *Cancer* 54:215, 1984.

Chilcote, R. R., Baehner, R. L., and Hammond, D. Septicemia and meningitis in children splenectomized for Hodgkin's disease. *N. Engl. J. Med.* 295:798, 1976.

Donaldson, S. S., and Kaplan, H. S. Complications of treatment of Hodgkin's disease in children. *Cancer Treat. Rep.* 66:977, 1982.

Exelby, P. R. Lymphoma. In T. M. Holder and K. W. Ashcraft (eds.), *Pediatric Surgery*. Philadelphia: Saunders, 1980. P. 973.

Filler, R. M., et al. Experience with clinical and operative staging of Hodgkin's disease in Children. *J. Pediatr. Surg.* 10:321, 1975.

Green, D. M., et al. The incidence of postsplenectomy sepsis and herpes zoster in children and adolescents with Hodgkin's disease. *Med. Pediatr. Oncol.* 67:285, 1979.

Green, D. M., et al. Staging laparotomy with splenectomy in children and adolescents with Hodgkin's disease. *Cancer Treat. Rev.* 10:23, 1983.

Kaplan, H. S. Hodgkin's Disease (2nd ed.). Cambridge, Mass.: Harvard University Press, 1980. P. 287.

Sullivan, M. P., Fuller, L. M., and Butler, J. J. Hodgkin's Disease. In W. Sutow et al. (eds.), *Clinical Pediatric Oncology* (2nd ed.). St. Louis: Mosby, 1984. Pp. 416–451.

Ternberg, J. L. Hodgkin's and Non-Hodgkin's Lymphoma. In K. J. Welch, et al. (eds.), *Pediatric Surgery*. Chicago: Year Book, 1986. P. 256.

88 Non-Hodgkin's Lymphoma

I. **Definition.** *Non-Hodgkin's lymphoma* is a heterogeneous group of lymphoid malignancies that is differentiated from Hodgkin's disease by its different sites of origin, variety of cell types, more highly malignant behavior, and absence of the Reed-Sternberg cell. It is more common than Hodgkin's disease in childhood and tends to occur at an earlier age.

II. **Pathophysiology.** Non-Hodgkin's lymphoma (NHL) has many histologic forms and occurs in a variety of locations, causing diverse symptoms. The classification of types is still changing.

   A. *Lymphoblastic lymphoma* is a tumor of T-cell origin that typically occurs in the anterior mediastinum, where it causes compression of the airway or the superior mediastinal syndrome. Spread to supraclavicular and cervical nodes, bone marrow, and meninges may occur early.

   B. *Burkitt's lymphoma* is a B-cell tumor that is most commonly found in the abdomen involving the ileum, colon, ovary, kidney, retroperitoneum, or liver. The tumor is often well-localized and without metastases.

   C. *Non-Burkitt's lymphoma* is histologically similar to Burkitt's lymphoma but tends to occur in peripheral lymph nodes.

   D. *Histiocytic lymphoma* affects males 2.5:1; may contain B cells, T cells, or null cells; and typically arises in extranodal sites such as gonads, soft tissue, bone, or mediastinum but rarely in the gastrointestinal tract.

   E. Because **dissemination** of NHL occurs early, disease may be widespread at the time of diagnosis.

   F. **Half** of children with NHL will develop **lymphocytic leukemia.**

III. **Clinical presentation**

   A. **Anterior mediastinal NHL** causes respiratory symptoms first in most children: wheezing, dyspnea, cough. Postural dyspnea, in which the child must sit upright to breathe, is seen in the later stages, followed by signs of compression of the great veins: the **superior mediastinal syndrome** (Fig. 88-1). Death can occur quickly from rapid growth of the tumor.

   B. **Abdominal** NHL is most likely to present with abdominal pain or a mass. Gastrointestinal bleeding or symptoms of intestinal obstruction are other presenting signs. NHL may be a cause of **intussusception.**

   C. **Cervical lymphoma** may be indistinguishable from other types of lymphadenopathy, although growth may be more rapid.

   D. **Respiratory distress** may result from pleural effusion, anterior mediastinal tumor, or NHL arising in the tonsil or paranasal sinuses.

   E. **Complications from metastases** to the meninges, lungs, bone marrow, or other organs may produce the presenting symptoms. The primary tumor in such cases can be difficult to locate.

IV. **Diagnosis**

   A. **Diagnosis** of non-Hodgkin's lymphoma is made by **pathologic examination** of the tumor tissue after excision.

   B. In the case of a rapidly expanding, **life-threatening anterior mediastinal lym-**

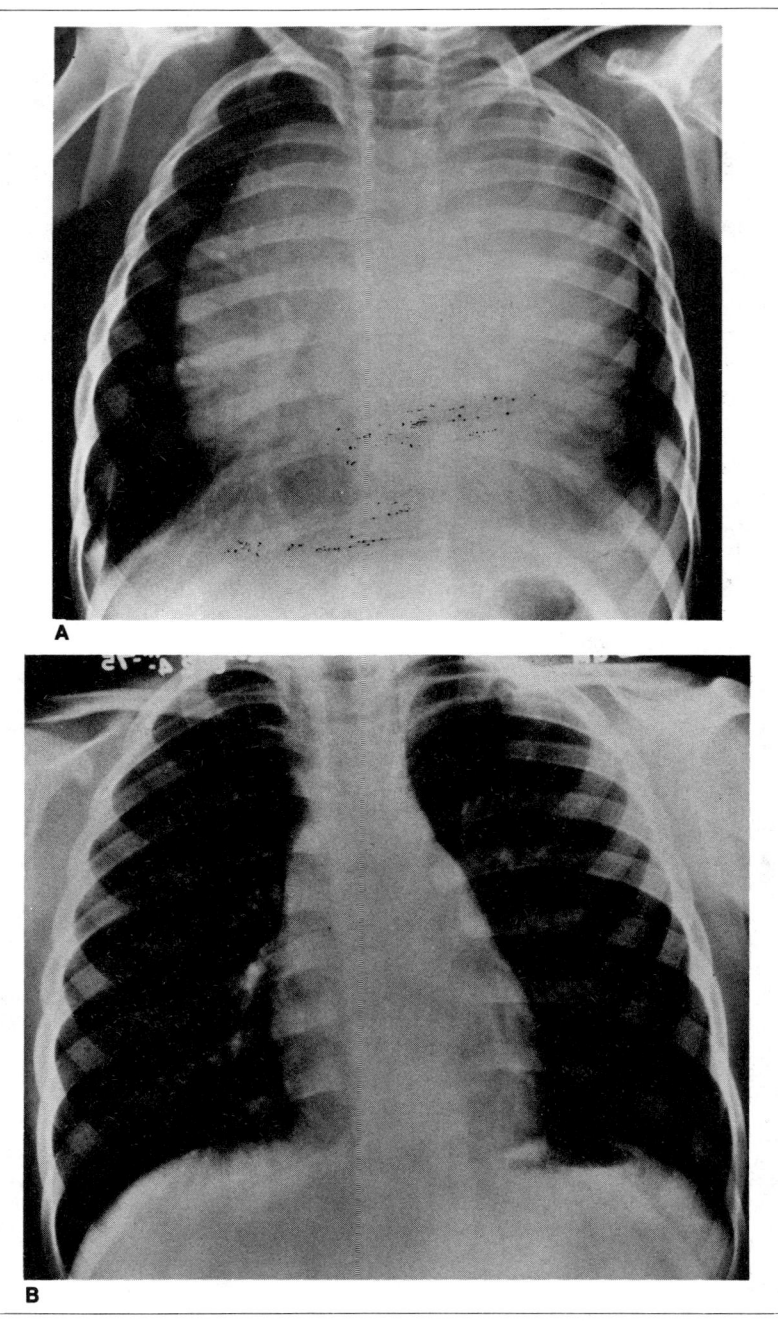

Fig. 88-1. Non-Hodgkin's lymphoma. A. Chest x-ray of a 9-year-old boy with severe respiratory distress demonstrates a huge mediastinal tumor. B. The same patient 5 days later after receiving radiation therapy and corticosteroids. Patient has remained free of disease for 11 years. (From L. L. Leape, Thoracic Surgical Problems in Infants and Children. In F. H. Ellis (Ed.), *Thoracic Surgery*. Philadelphia: Lippincott/Harper & Row, 1983.)

phoma, it may be necessary to treat with radiation or steroids to relieve airway pressure **before confirmation of the diagnosis histologically.**

C. **Bone-marrow** aspiration may provide the histologic diagnosis in confusing cases.

D. **Staging** of NHL is of limited value, since most patients have disseminated disease when diagnosed and require chemotherapy.

V. Problems. Because of the diversity of cell types and tissues of origin, non-Hodgkin's lymphoma can cause a wide variety of complications and problems in diagnosis and management.

A. **Superior mediastinal syndrome** from mediastinal lymphoma

B. **Optic nerve compression** from orbital tumor

C. **Meningeal erosion** from tumors of the paranasal sinuses.

D. **Airway obstruction** from tumor in the tonsil

E. **Respiratory distress** from **pleural effusion**

F. **Intestinal obstruction,** with or without intussusception

G. **Renal failure** from tumor infiltration

H. **Urinary obstruction** from retroperitoneal NHL

I. **Hyperuricemia** with development of urinary calculi during cytolytic therapy

J. **Spinal-cord compression** with weakness or paraplegia

Treatment

A. **Chemotherapy** is indicated for virtually every patient with non-Hodgkin's lymphoma since disseminated disease is almost always present and the risk of developing leukemia is high.

B. **Localized tumor** of the intestine is **resected** with wide margins and removal of the mesentery with its lymph nodes. If the disease is localized and radiation therapy and chemotherapy are given, reported cure rates are as high as 80%.

C. **Bulky abdominal disease** should be removed as completely as possible to enhance the effects of chemotherapy and radiation therapy.

D. **Mediastinal tumor** is treated with prednisone and radiation, often with rapid and dramatic response (Fig. 88-1).

E. **High fluid intake,** allopurinol, and alkalinization of the urine are given to prevent formation of uric acid stones resulting from rapid cell destruction when chemotherapy is given.

Prognosis. Aggressive chemotherapy with prophylactic treatment for lymphocytic leukemia has led to significant improvement in the outlook in this once nearly hopeless disease. A majority of patients can now expect long-term disease-free survival.

Bibliography

D'Angio, G. J., Mitus, A., and Evans, A. The superior mediastinal syndrome in children with cancer. *Am. J. Roentgenol.* 43:537, 1965.

Davenport, D., et al. Response of superior vena cava syndrome to radiation therapy. *Cancer* 38:157, 1976.

Exelby, P. R. Lymphoma. In T. M. Holder and K. W. Ashcraft (eds.), *Pediatric Surgery.* Philadelphia: Saunders, 1980. P. 973.

Goldman, A. The long-term outlook for children treated for non-Hodgkin's lymphoma: A report of the Children's Solid Tumor Group. *Br. J. Cancer* 44:872, 1981.

Jenkin, R. D., et al. Pediatric Non-Hodgkin's Lymphomas. In S. Rosenberg and H.

Kaplan (eds.), *Malignant Lymphomas: Etiology, Immunology, Pathology, Treatment.* New York: Academic, 1982. P. 591.

Jenkins, R. D. T., et al. Primary gastrointestinal tract lymphoma in childhood. *Radiology* 92:763, 1969.

Kemeny, M., Magrath, I., and Brennan, M. F. The role of surgery in the management of American Burkitt's lymphoma and its treatment. *Ann. Surg.* 196:82, 1982.

Malpas, J. S. Lymphomas in children. *Semin. Hematol.* 19:301, 1982.

Murphy, S. B. Childhood non-Hodgkin's lymphoma. *N. Engl. J. Med.* 299:1446, 1978.

Siegel, S. E., et al. Long-term Survival in Childhood Non-Hodgkin's Lymphoma. In J. H. Burchenal and H. F. Oettgen (eds.), *Cancer: Achievements, Challenges and Prospects for the 1980s.* New York: Grune & Stratton, 1981. Vol. 2, p. 225.

Ternberg, J. Hodgkin's and Non-Hodgkin's Lymphoma. In K. J. Welch, et al. (eds.), *Pediatric Surgery.* Chicago: Year Book, 1986. P. 256.

89 Liver Tumors

I. **Definition.** Three-fourths of tumors of the liver in children are malignant. But if the tumor is solitary and resectable, there is an excellent chance of cure. Benign tumors are more likely to be hemangiomas or other hamartomas.

II. **Pathophysiology**
   A. Liver tumors cause symptoms because of their **size,** abnormal blood flow, or platelet trapping.
   B. Infantile hemangioma of the liver may act as an **arteriovenous malformation** and cause congestive heart failure.
   C. **Platelet sequestration** in a hepatic hemangioma can cause a coagulopathy.
   D. **Spontaneous rupture** of a hepatic hemangioma may occur, with shock and death.
   E. Massive hepatomegaly can **compromise respiration** to the extent that ventilatory assistance is required.

III. **Clinical presentation**
   A. An **enlarged liver** is the first sign of a tumor in most children. It is noted by the parent or the physician at routine examination.
   B. Other symptoms include abdominal **pain,** loss of appetite, **weight loss,** and rarely, jaundice.
   C. The enlarged liver is usually **palpated** easily, but the tumor may or may not be obvious. If the tumor is huge, differentiating it from a renal tumor or neuroblastoma may be difficult.

IV. **Specific characteristics of benign hepatic tumors**
   A. *Hemangioendothelioma* is a tumor of infancy, usually presenting before 8 months of age.
      1. Tumors **vary** greatly in size and are usually **multiple.** Diffuse studding of the liver with hemangiomas is sometimes called hemangiomatosis. It grossly resembles metastatic disease.
      2. Forty percent of patients have **cutaneous hemangiomas** as well.
      3. **Heart failure** may be the presenting symptom in infants from this arteriovenous malformation.
      4. **Thrombocytopenia** may result from platelet trapping.
      5. Diagnosis is by CT, MRI, or radionuclide scan, which shows **multiple filling defects** throughout the liver.
      6. Because **spontaneous regression** occurs in most patients, no treatment is necessary if the infant is asymptomatic.
      7. **Prednisone,** 5 mg/kg/day, is given if there is severe coagulopathy from platelet trapping.
      8. **Heart failure** is treated with digitalis and diuretics. If it cannot be controlled, **embolization** or **ligation** of the hepatic artery should be carried out promptly because of the high mortality associated with this complication.
   B. **Cavernous hemangioma** is more common in older children, typically presenting as an asymptomatic hepatic mass.

1. Cutaneous hemangiomas are not usually present.
2. Heart failure and thrombocytopenia are much less commonly seen than in hemangioendothelioma of infancy.
3. Vascularity and vascular spaces can usually be seen on CT, MRI, or ultrasound, but an operation is often necessary to confirm the diagnosis.
4. Treatment is **controversial** since these growths neither regress nor undergo malignant change. Resection of large, well-localized lesions is desirable to prevent rupture or other complications.

C. **Hamartoma** of the liver presents in the first year of life in 80% of patients as a solitary asymptomatic mass, often quite large.
   1. CT or MRI reveals a mixed cystic and solid mass that cannot be differentiated from a malignant tumor.
   2. The tumor often is pedunculated or can be "shelled out," but lobar resection is sometimes required.

D. **Adenoma** and **focal nodular hyperplasia** are rare lesions found in older children. They are solid, solitary, often large, and usually asymptomatic. Because they cannot be differentiated from malignant liver tumors preoperatively, resection is indicated.

V. Specific characteristics of malignant hepatic tumors

A. **Hepatoblastoma** is the **most common liver tumor** of childhood. It occurs in infancy, rarely beyond 3 years of age, and affects boys twice as often as girls.
   1. A large **mass** in the liver is the usual presenting complaint. Nausea, vomiting, and distention may be present.
   2. CT or MRI shows a **solid** mass that is typically well-circumscribed and may show **calcifications.** Most are solitary.
   3. **Alpha fetoprotein** levels are elevated in 90% of patients.
   4. **Excision** of the tumor offers the only hope of cure but is possible in only 50% of patients.
   5. In **unresectable** tumors, biopsy is performed and **chemotherapy** (VAC, fluorouracil [5-FU]) given to shrink the tumor. Resection may be possible subsequently, with a significant chance of cure.
   6. The overall cure rate in hepatoblastoma is less than **50%.**

B. **Hepatocellular carcinoma** is second only to hepatoblastoma in frequency, but it carries a much more dismal prognosis.
   1. **Predisposing factors.** Biliary atresia, hepatitis B, cirrhosis, glycogen storage disease, Beckwith-Wiedemann syndrome, hemihypertrophy.
   2. Most children with hepatocellular carcinoma are found to have **unresectable** multicentric or invasive disease.
   3. Treatment is the same as for hepatoblastoma. Overall survival is only **12%.**

C. **Sarcomas** of the liver also have a dismal outlook, with few cures.

VI. Diagnosis

A. **CT or MRI scan** gives the most useful information. With contrast enhancement, the vascularity of the tumor can be assessed. Scan should include the **chest,** for pulmonary metastases are common in malignant liver tumors.

B. **Angiography** seldom contributes additional information of value in diagnosis or management and is not recommended as a routine.

C. **Alpha fetoprotein** determination should be made in every patient with a liver tumor. If elevated, malignancy is likely. It also serves as a marker for postoperative follow-up.

II. Indications for operation

A. **Operative biopsy or resection is necessary in almost all patients with solitary resectable liver tumors.**

B. With the exception of **infantile hemangiomatosis,** it is not possible to determine reliably with current imaging techniques whether a solid tumor of the liver is benign or malignant.

C. **Cure depends on resectability,** since chemotherapy alone is ineffective. Multifocal or diffuse tumors and those with metastases have little chance.

III. Preoperative preparation

A. Correct **coagulopathy.**

B. **Type and cross-match** at least one blood volume of blood.

C. Establish reliable venous access with **two large intravenous lines in the upper extremities** and a central venous catheter.

IV. Operative care

A. **Anatomic resection** along lobar planes is safest and most likely to leave adequate margin around a tumor.

B. **Control** of the vessels at the **porta** and the cava is established prior to resection. The arterial anatomy must be completely delineated.

C. Use of the **ultrasonic scalpel** has dramatically reduced the risk of hepatic resection as well as drastically decreasing blood loss.

V. Postoperative care

A. **Intensive care** and monitoring are essential after liver resection. Ventilatory assistance may be required.

B. **Volume replacement** is guided by central venous pressure, urine output, pulse, and hematocrit.

C. **Ten percent glucose** is given until the patient is taking food by mouth.

D. **Albumin** or fresh frozen plasma may be needed daily until liver synthesis is reestablished.

E. **Vitamin K** supplementation is advisable.

F. **Drains** are left in until drainage stops, often 2 or 3 weeks after major hepatic resection.

G. **Antibiotics** are given prophylactically for 24 hours.

H. **Chemotherapy** should be delayed until return of normal liver function in order not to inhibit regeneration.

Complications

A. **Subphrenic abscess** or collection of fluid (often sterile) in the operative site

B. **Bile leak** if bile duct tributaries have not been securely ligated

C. **Hemorrhage**

D. **Intestinal obstruction**

Prognosis. The overall cure rate for malignant liver tumors is less than 25%, but if the tumor is completely resectable, the outlook is considerably improved—probably 50–70% for hepatoblastoma.

Bibliography

Baggenstoss, A. H. Pathology of Tumors of Liver in Infancy and Childhood. In G. T. Pack and A. H. Islami (eds.), *Tumors of the Liver*. New York: Springer, 1970.

Braun, P., et al. Hemangiomatosis of the liver in infants. *J. Pediatr. Surg.* 10:121, 1975.

Brown, S. H., Neerhout, R. C., and Fonkalsrud, E. W. Prednisone therapy in the management of large hemangiomas of infants and children. *Surgery* 71:168, 1972.

Dehner, L. P. Hepatic tumors in the pediatric age group: A distinctive clinicopathologic spectrum. *Perspect. Pediatr. Pathol.* 4:217, 1978.

de Lorimier, A. A., et al. Hepatic artery ligation for hepatic hemangiomatosis. *N. Engl. J. Med.* 277, 1967.

Ehren, H., Mahour, G. H., and Isaacs, H., Jr. Benign liver tumors in infancy and childhood: Report of 48 cases. *Am. J. Surg.* 14:325, 1983.

Exelby, P. R., Filler, R. M., and Grosfeld, J. L. Liver tumors in children in particular reference to hepatoblastoma and hepatocellular carcinoma: American Academy of Pediatrics Surgical Section Survey, 1974. *J. Pediatr. Surg.* 10:329, 1975.

Filler, R. M. Liver Tumors. In T. M. Holder and K. W. Ashcraft (eds.), *Pediatric Surgery*. Philadelphia: Saunders, 1980. P. 953.

Hodgson, W. J. B., and DelGuercio, L. R. M. Preliminary experience in liver surgery using the ultrasonic scalpel. *Surgery* 95:230, 1984.

Lack, E. E., Neave, C., and Vawter, G. F. Hepatoblastoma: A clinical and pathologic study of 54 cases. *Am. J. Surg. Pathol.* 6:693, 1982.

Mattioli, L., Lee, K. R., and Holder, T. M. Hepatic artery ligation for cardiac failure due to hepatic hemangioma in the newborn. *J. Pediatr. Surg.* 9:859, 1974.

Nguyen, L., et al. Hepatic hemangioma in childhood: Medical management or surgical management? *J. Pediatr. Surg.* 17:576, 1982.

Randolph, J. G., and Guzzetta, P. C. Tumors of the Liver. In K. J. Welch, et al. (eds.), *Pediatric Surgery*. Chicago: Year Book, 1986. P. 302.

Rotman, M., et al. Radiation treatment of pediatric hepatic hemangiomatosis and coexisting cardiac failure. *N. Engl. J. Med.* 302:852, 1980.

Touloukian, R. J. Nonmalignant Liver Tumors and Hepatic Infections. In K. J. Welch, et al. (eds.), *Pediatric Surgery*. Chicago: Year Book, 1986. P. 1067.

Trastek, V. F., et al. Cavernous hemangiomas of the liver: Resect or observe? *Am. J. Surg.* 145:49, 1983.

90 Ovarian Tumors

Definition. Ovarian tumors constitute less than 2% of childhood neoplasms. They may occur at any age but are most common at puberty. Germ cell tumors account for 75% of ovarian tumors in children. Types of ovarian tumors are as follows:

A. Epithelial tumors
1. Serous
2. Mucinous
3. Endometrioid
4. Clear cell
5. Brenner
6. Mixed
7. Undifferentiated

B. Sex cord-stromal tumors
1. Granulosa-theca-cell
2. Androblastoma
3. Gynandroblastoma

C. Lipoid cell tumors

D. Germ cell tumors
1. Dysgerminoma
2. Endodermal sinus tumor
3. Embryonal carcinoma
4. Polyembryoma
5. Choriocarcinoma
6. Teratoma
7. Mixed

E. Gonadoblastoma
F. Soft-tissue tumors
G. Unclassified tumors
H. Metastatic tumors

Clinical presentation

A. Sexual precocity may result from hormone-secreting ovarian tumors, principally granulosa-theca cell tumors, embryonal carcinomas, or choriocarcinomas. These account for fewer than 5% of ovarian tumors in childhood and fewer than 10% of cases of isosexual precocity. The rare androblastoma will cause virilization.

B. Mass effects are the cause of symptoms from most ovarian tumors: vague abdominal pain, fullness, or distention. Torsion of an ovary and cyst may cause acute abdominal pain and tenderness indistinguishable from acute appendicitis.

C. **A palpable mass** is present by abdominal or rectal examination in most patients with an ovarian tumor.

III. **Diagnosis.** Ovarian tumors are easily recognized by ultrasound or CT or MRI scan. The presence of calcification or "teeth" identifies a teratoma, but in most cases the histologic nature cannot be predicted by the imaging findings. Full endocrinologic evaluation is indicated preoperatively in any girl with a functioning tumor.

IV. **Teratoma.** Nearly three-fourths of ovarian tumors in childhood are teratomas. Most are "dermoid" cysts with a risk of malignancy of less than 1%.

A. **Clinical features.** An asymptomatic **mass** or expanding girth is noted by the patient or doctor in most cases. Torsion of an ovarian teratoma may produce intermittent or constant **pelvic pain.** Teratomas may occur at any age but are more common between 8 and 12 years.

B. **Diagnosis.** Plain x-rays often show calcification, sometimes even a tooth. CT or MRI will demonstrate a well-circumscribed tumor of mixed densities, usually containing fat.

C. **Treatment.** Surgical excision is indicated for all teratomas.

1. **Benign teratoma (dermoid),** well-differentiated (75% of ovarian teratomas). Excision of the tumor and ovary alone is all that is necessary, preserving the tube if possible. The other ovary is inspected for tumor, and biopsy is performed if suspicious.

2. **Malignant teratoma** contains embryonal tissue as well as well-differentiated elements.

    a. Survival is related to the **grade:**

Grade	Embryonal tissue	Survival (%)
I	Minor amount	82
II	Moderate amount	62
III	Large quantity	30

    b. If tumor is confined to **one ovary,** salpingo-oophorectomy is followed by chemotherapy and a second-look procedure, with excision of any residual or recurrent disease.

    c. If there is **bilateral** disease, bilateral salpingo-oophorectomy and hysterectomy are performed, with chemotherapy and a second-look procedure.

    d. Intraabdominal **metastases** should be resected. Long-term disease-free survival has been reported after removal of bulk disease and aggressive chemotherapy.

V. **Dysgerminoma**

A. **Clinical features.** Dysgerminoma is the second most frequent ovarian tumor of childhood, but it is the tumor most likely to be malignant. It is histologically indistinguishable from seminoma. Twenty percent are bilateral. Symptoms are nonspecific: pain, torsion, hemorrhage, a mass.

B. **Diagnosis.** There are no specific tests to identify this tumor preoperatively. The diagnosis of dysgerminoma may be suspected at the time of operation if it is a bulky, solid, encapsulated, yellowish tumor.

C. **Treatment.** Salpingo-oophorectomy is performed with bisection and biopsy of the opposite ovary. If there is extension of tumor beyond one ovary, or if there is ascites, total abdominal hysterectomy with bilateral salpingo-oophorectomy is performed, with excision of suspicious paraaortic lymph nodes. Radiotherapy is given. Chemotherapy is of little value.

VI. Endodermal sinus tumor

A. Clinical features. Endodermal sinus tumors are highly malignant tumors that grow rapidly and spread readily, both within the abdomen and in distant metastases.

B. Diagnosis. Endodermal sinus tumors secrete alpha fetoprotein (AFP), which serves as a useful marker after removal to detect recurrence.

C. Treatment. Salpingo-oophorectomy is adequate surgical treatment for localized disease, but panhysterectomy and bilateral salpingo-oophorectomy are indicated for extensive disease. Whereas just a few years ago 90% of children with endodermal sinus tumors died, intensive chemotherapy with multiple agents has significantly improved results.

VII. Embryonal carcinoma

A. Clinical features. Like the endodermal sinus tumor, embryonal carcinoma is an aggressive tumor that often secretes AFP. In addition, it may secrete chorionic gonadotropin, producing precocious puberty.

B. Diagnosis. AFP and human chorionic gonadotropin (HCG) elevations indicate embryonal carcinoma. The mass may be huge.

C. Treatment. Surgical and adjuvant therapy programs are similar to those for endodermal sinus tumor, but in addition embryonal carcinoma is radiosensitive.

VIII. Granulosa-theca-cell tumor

A. Clinical features. Sexual precocity is the predominant presenting symptom in the majority of girls with granulosa-theca-cell ovarian tumors. Virilization has also been described. The tumor is bilateral in 10% of patients.

B. Diagnosis. The presence of a mass on physical examination or by CT or MRI aids in differentiating a functioning ovarian tumor from true sexual precocity, feminizing adrenal tumors, or tumors secreting gonadotropin.

C. Treatment. Since most granulosa-theca-cell tumors are benign or confined to one ovary, unilateral salpingo-oophorectomy is usually the operation of choice. More advanced disease requires more radical excision and radiation therapy. There is no effective chemotherapy. Overall mortality is less than 10%.

Bibliography

Adelman, S., Benson, C. D., and Hertzler, J. H. Surgical lesions of the ovary in infancy and childhood. *Surg. Gynecol. Obstet.* 141:219, 1975.

Brodeur, G. M., et al. Malignant germ cell tumors in 57 children and adolescents. *Cancer* 48:1890, 1981.

King, D. R. Ovarian Cysts and Tumors. In K. J. Welch, et al. (eds.), *Pediatric Surgery.* Chicago: Year Book, 1986. P. 1341.

Kosloske, A. M., et al. Management of immature teratoma of the ovary in children by conservative resection and chemotherapy. *J. Pediatr. Surg.* 11:839, 1976.

Scully, R. E. Ovarian tumors: A review. *Am. J. Pathol.* 87:686, 1977.

Talbert, J. L. Miscellaneous Childhood Tumors. In T. M. Holder and K. W. Ashcraft (eds.), *Pediatric Surgery.* Philadelphia: Saunders, 1980. P. 1007.

Tapper, D., and Lack, E. E. Teratomas in infancy and childhood. *Ann. Surg.* 198:398, 1983.

Towne, B. H., et al. Ovarian cysts and tumors in infancy and childhood. *J. Pediatr. Surg.* 10:311, 1975.

Wollner, N., et al. Malignant ovarian tumors in childhood. *Cancer* 37:1953, 1976.

91 Adrenal Tumors

Cushing's syndrome

A. Definition. Signs and symptoms of *Cushing's syndrome* include adiposity, amenorrhea, hypertrichosis, purple striae, hypertension, polyphagia, polydipsia, and polycythemia. It results from an excess of adrenal cortical hormones, principally cortisol.

1. **Pituitary hypersecretion of ACTH** causing adrenal hyperplasia **(Cushing's disease)** is the most common cause of Cushing's syndrome in adults, but in children adrenal cortical adenoma or carcinoma is more common. **Cortical carcinoma** accounts for over half the cases in children. Nonpituitary ACTH-secreting tumors can also cause Cushing's syndrome.

2. **Iatrogenic** Cushing's syndrome is a frequent complication of steroid medication.

B. Clinical presentation

1. **Obesity,** truncal and facial, with "moon facies" and a "buffalo hump" is the most obvious and common manifestation. Hypertension, peripheral edema, and pathologic fractures may occur.

2. Rapid **increase in weight** and height is found in young children and growth retardation in older children.

3. **Hirsutism,** amenorrhea, and acne result from the virilizing effects of excess androgen production.

C. Diagnosis of Cushing's syndrome is made by demonstration of excess production of **cortisol.**

1. **Suppression** of cortisol excretion by dexamethasone indicates excess pituitary ACTH is the cause. Failure of dexamethasone suppression with low plasma ACTH indicates an adrenal tumor; failure with a high plasma ACTH level suggests ectopic ACTH syndrome.

2. X-rays of the **sella turcica** may demonstrate widening suggestive of a pituitary tumor.

3. **CT or MRI** scan is used to identify the adrenal tumor.

D. Operative care

1. **Cushing's disease** is usually treated by transsphenoidal **hypophysectomy** or irradiation. Bilateral adrenalectomy has been abandoned in favor of the direct approach.

2. **Adrenalectomy** is the procedure of choice for adrenal tumor, benign or malignant. Wide local excision and excision of metastases are needed for carcinoma.

E. Postoperative care

1. **Corticosteroids,** prednisone or hydrocortisone, are given during the operation and in the postoperative period, with gradual weaning over a period of months.

2. **Chemotherapy is ineffective** for adrenal carcinoma, but ortho, para-DDD may block hormone secretion and its unpleasant effects. Radiotherapy is of no value in the treatment of adrenal tumors.

II. Virilizing adrenal cortical tumors

A. **Definition.** Premature puberty in a boy or virilization in a girl may result from an androgen-secreting tumor of the adrenal gland or gonad. While benign adenoma can be the cause, most of these functional tumors are carcinomas, with a high mortality.

B. **Clinical presentation.** Development of facial and pubic hair, acne, and in boys, growth of the genitalia, signify excessive androgens. The tumor is usually palpable.

C. **Diagnosis.** Excess androgens, principally **17-ketosteroids,** can be detected in the blood and urine. CT or MRI scan will demonstrate the tumor. The gonads are the other primary suspect and must also be evaluated.

D. **Operative care.** Transabdominal total adrenalectomy is required. The kidney may have to be removed as well if it is invaded by tumor.

E. **Postoperative care.** Adrenal hormone replacement is not necessary if only one adrenal gland is removed. These tumors are relatively resistant to radiation, but show some response to chemotherapy. Hormonal secretion by metastatic or recurrent disease can be blocked by ortho, para-DDD. Pulmonary metastases can be resected, sometimes with cure.

III. Pheochromocytoma

A. **Definition.** *Pheochromocytoma* is a tumor of the adrenal **medulla** that secretes epinephrine, norepinephrine, and dopamine. Approximately 6% of cases are malignant. In 10% of cases, pheochromocytoma is familial, part of the syndrome of multiple endocrine adenomas (MEA).

B. **Clinical presentation.** Hypertension, headaches, and sweating are the most common symptoms. Nausea and vomiting, weight loss, abdominal pain, visual disturbances, polyuria, and polydipsia are frequently seen. Emotional disturbances are frequently suspected because of anxiety and nervousness caused by the hormones. Convulsions and coma may result from hypertensive encephalopathy.

C. **Diagnosis**

1. **Elevated catecholamines** and their metabolites in the blood and urine establish the diagnosis of pheochromocytoma. In addition to epinephrine and norepinephrine, VMA and metanephrine are measured.

2. **CT or MRI** scan will usually localize the tumor, which may also be evident on plain film of the abdomen because of calcifications. In difficult cases arteriography or selective venous sampling from the vena cava may be necessary.

D. **Preoperative preparation** is of critical importance in pheochromocytoma because of the risk of severe complications from hypertension.

1. **Phenoxybenzamine,** an alpha-adrenergic-blocking agent, is given as soon as the diagnosis is made and for 1–2 weeks preoperatively. If an urgent operation is required, phentolamine is used.

2. **Propranolol,** a beta-adrenergic blocker, is given immediately preoperatively and during the operation to control tachycardia and prevent arrhythmia from the alpha-blockade.

E. **Operative care**

1. **Anesthetic management is difficult** and critical. Hypertension must be controlled during surgical excision of the tumor; hypotension from sudden decrease in catecholamines must be combated after the tumor has been removed. Patients with pheochromocytoma have a contracted blood volume which must be rapidly expanded as the tumor is removed. Anesthetic agents that stimulate the release of catecholamines or histamine must be avoided

Arterial, venous, and urinary catheters and continuous monitoring of the ECG are essential.

2. **Surgical resection** is through a generous transverse incision permitting examination of the entire abdomen and the opposite adrenal gland. Gentle mobilization and excision of the tumor with minimal manipulation will decrease the release of catecholamines, but a radical resection must be carried out to ensure that no tumor is left behind.

F. Postoperative care

1. **Norepinephrine infusion** may be required to maintain the blood pressure postoperatively for several days. Blood volume is expanded as indicated.

2. **Failure** of hypertension **to subside** within a few weeks after the operation, or its recurrence later, usually signifies the presence of a **second tumor.**

Bibliography

Altman, A. J., and Schwartz, A. D. (eds.). Tumors of the Sympathetic Nervous System. In *Malignant Diseases of Infancy, Childhood and Adolescence.* Philadelphia: Saunders, 1978. P. 326.

Burrington, J. D., and Stephens, C. A. Virilizing tumors of the adrenal gland in childhood: Report of eight cases. *J. Pediatr. Surg.* 4:291, 1969.

Bloom, D. A., and Fonkalsrud, E. W. Surgical management of pheochromocytoma in children. *J. Pediatr. Surg.* 9:179, 1974.

Ellis, D., and Gartner, J. C. The intraoperative medical management of childhood pheochromocytoma. *J. Pediatr. Surg.* 15:655, 1980.

Fonkalsrud, E. W. The Adrenal Glands. In K. J. Welch, et al. (eds.), *Pediatric Surgery.* Chicago: Year Book, 1986. P. 1113.

Gold, E. M. The Cushing's syndrome: Changing views of diagnosis and treatment. *Ann. Intern. Med.* 90:829, 1979.

Kaufman, B. H., et al. Pheochromocytoma in the pediatric age group: Current status. *J. Pediatr. Surg.* 18:879, 1983.

Styne, D. M., et al. Treatment of Cushing's disease in childhood and adolescence by transsphenoidal microadenomectomy. *N. Engl. J. Med.* 310:889, 1984.

Talbert, J. L. Miscellaneous Childhood Tumors. In T. M. Holder and K. W. Ashcraft (eds.), *Pediatric Surgery.* Philadelphia: Saunders, 1980. P. 1007.

VIII Trauma

92

Trauma: General Principles

I. **Incidence**

  A. **Trauma is the leading cause of death in childhood** at all ages after the first year of life. **Each year:**

  1. **More than 12,000 children die from trauma**—more than die from all other causes combined.

  2. **One child in five is injured** sufficiently to come to a hospital emergency room for treatment.

  3. **One child in 100 is hospitalized for trauma.**

  B. **For each death** from trauma, there are **four or five children who are seriously and permanently disabled**—about 50,000 per year. Trauma is the number one health problem in pediatrics.

II. **Causes of injury**

  A. **The automobile** is the major cause of childhood injury and death, accounting for approximately **half of the deaths** and nearly **two-thirds of hospital admissions for serious injury. Unlike adults** who are usually injured as drivers or passengers, children are much more likely to be **pedestrian** or **cyclist** victims.

  B. **Falls** from a height and playtime accidents are second in frequency.

  C. **Child abuse** has emerged as an important cause of major injury in children, especially the very young.

  D. In **urban** areas, **gunshot** wounds and **stabbings** are significant problems in teenagers.

III. **Blunt trauma.** Ninety percent of serious injuries in children are the result of blunt trauma. **Common characteristics** are as follows:

  A. **Multiple injuries.** In a typical automobile-pedestrian accident, the leg is struck by the bumper, the chest or abdomen collides with the grille and hood, and the child is propelled through space to land on his head. **Two-thirds of children with life-threatening injuries have three systems or more involved.**

  B. **Occult injury.** Internal injuries are often much worse than they appear from initial examination.

  C. **Head injury.** Eighty percent of children with major trauma have severe brain injury, and many are in coma. Coma confounds diagnosis, requiring reliance on x-rays and laboratory tests.

  D. **Progressive injury.** Edema formation, bleeding into the tissues, and peritoneal irritation from spilled intestinal contents all become worse with time, extending the injury.

  E. **Secondary effects. Hemorrhage** and **hypoxia** may be more hazardous to the patient than the primary injury. Reduced blood volume results in poor tissue perfusion with tissue hypoxia and acidosis. This can cause serious or fatal damage to the heart, brain, or lungs even when these organs are unaffected by the primary injury.

Objectives of initial treatment of major trauma

  A. **Restoration of function** of damaged organs, such as by insertion of a chest tube to inflate a collapsed lung

B. **Compensation for reduced function,** such as by ventilatory assistance
C. **Prevention of progression** of the primary injury, such as by prevention of brain swelling
D. **Prevention of secondary organ damage,** such as from uncontrolled bleeding or hypoxia

V. **Initial care of the severely injured patient.** The initial care received by the seriously injured child often determines the outcome. Life-threatening injuries can rapidly become fatal if not promptly and properly diagnosed and treated. (See the section Trauma Checklists in Appendix C.)

   A. **Organization.** Successful treatment requires a calm and **well-organized** approach, **preplanned** to ensure that the **personnel** and **resources** are available for the trauma patient when he arrives, often with little warning.
   B. **Teamwork** is the essence of efficient trauma resuscitation. Delegation of responsibility permits simultaneous performance of essential tasks and rapid assessment and treatment.
      1. One member assesses the injuries and attends to the **airway** and **ventilation.**
      2. A second member establishes an **intravenous** line and administers fluids.
      3. A third member attends to **supportive** and routine **diagnostic** procedures such as placement of ECG leads; sending blood samples; and placement of a nasogastric tube, Foley catheter, and temperature probe.
   C. **Priorities.** The **first priority is to maintain the function of the heart and lungs while preventing progressive brain damage** from either a head injury or poor perfusion. Initial attention is directed to ventilation and circulation.
   D. **Procedures.** The **neck is immobilized** and all clothing is removed. The patient is rapidly examined (60 seconds) to assess the major obvious injuries. The "**ABCs**" are applicable:
      1. **Airway** patency is the **first priority.** The mouth is cleared of blood or secretions. If the patient is unconscious, it may be necessary to lift the chin or hold the mandible forward to permit ventilation. If this does not work, endotracheal intubation is necessary.

         Note: Hyperextension of the neck for intubation can result in spinal-cord damage and quadriplegia if there is an unrecognized cervical-spine fracture. The neck must be immobilized with a collar and intubation deferred if possible until cervical x-rays are taken and found to be normal.

      2. **Breathing** must be supported by hand or mechanical ventilation if the patient is not ventilating adequately.
      3. **Circulation** is maintained by restoring circulating blood volume, which has been depleted by hemorrhage. A large-bore catheter is inserted into an antecubital vein if it can be easily and rapidly done, or a cutdown is performed in the saphenous vein at the ankle.
         a. **Volume restoration** can be adequately accomplished in most patients by the rapid infusion of **Ringer's lactate** solution, **3 ml** for each **1 ml** of estimated **blood loss.**
         b. **If the patient is hypotensive, the volume of blood lost is at least 25%** of the estimated circulating blood volume. **This amount is given as rapidly as possible** to restore circulation. A second bolus is given if there is little or poor response to the first.
         c. **Blood volume** can be calculated as **8% of estimated body weight** (BW) in children at all ages. Estimated blood volume **[EBV] in milliliters = 40 × BW in pounds.)**

d. **Failure to respond to two boluses of 25% EBV** indicates continuing serious blood loss. Immediate operation is needed to control hemorrhage.

4. While the preceding procedures are being carried out, insertion of a **nasogastric tube, Foley catheter,** and **temperature probe** and placement of **ECG leads** are performed by another team member.

5. **Venipuncture** (femoral vein if patient is unstable) is performed and specimens are sent for **CBC, type and crossmatch,** and **amylase** level. Other studies are seldom indicated. Electrolytes, calcium, and BUN are unchanged immediately after injury and do not need to be measured.

6. **Additional intravenous lines** are inserted as necessary. If there is severe abdominal trauma, these lines must be placed in the **upper extremity** so that blood may be transfused even if operative clamping of the inferior vena cava is necessary.

7. **Cervical-spine x-rays** are taken. If all seven vertebrae are identified without fracture or malalignment, the collar may be removed.

8. **Complete physical examination** is now performed, including a **rectal** examination and inspection of the **back** and head of the patient.

9. A **history** of the circumstances of the injury and the past medical history of the patient are obtained.

10. **Open wounds** are dressed.

11. **X-rays** are obtained as indicated by physical findings. Chest and abdominal films are taken routinely.

VI. Assessment and therapy. Once the initial examination and stabilization is completed, it is time to sit down, evaluate the findings, and plan further studies and treatment.

A. **List positive findings** and preliminary **diagnoses.** Calculate **trauma score** and **Glasgow coma score** (see Appendix C).

B. **Institute emergency treatment.**

1. Serious **head injury with coma** requires immediate **hyperventilation** to decrease the development of cerebral edema. Head CT is performed to identify intracranial bleeding.

2. **Poor response** to fluid resuscitation is an indication for **peritoneal tap or lavage** to identify intraperitoneal bleeding, which requires immediate operative treatment (see Chap. 109).

3. If the patient responds well, but there is evidence of **continuing bleeding** and the source is not obvious, **CT scan** of the abdomen should be obtained.

C. **Perform diagnostic studies** as indicated by clinical findings.

VII. Monitoring the trauma patient. If immediate operative treatment is not required, the patient is transferred to the **intensive care unit** for treatment and **monitoring.**

A. **Neurologic.** Brain injury is the most important threat to life and useful recovery in the severely injured child. Aggressive treatment and monitoring are essential. **Intracranial pressure** (bolt) monitoring is sometimes advisable. The following are noted frequently:

1. **State of consciousness, response to stimuli**

2. **Pupil size, equality, reactivity**

3. **Pulse, blood pressure, respirations**

B. **Hemodynamic.** Adequacy of peripheral perfusion must be continuously assessed both to guide fluid therapy and to detect continued bleeding.
  1. **Pulse, blood pressure.**
  2. **Skin color, temperature, capillary refill.**
  3. **Urine output, osmolality.**
  4. **Central venous pressure** if large-volume transfusions are necessary or the patient is unstable.
  5. **Arterial blood gases.** An indwelling arterial catheter facilitates repeated studies as well as drawing of blood.
C. **Ventilatory.** If assisted respiration is required.

VIII. **Emotional care.** Major trauma usually strikes a normal child without warning. The child and the family need care and understanding by doctors and nurses who are experienced in dealing with sick children.
  A. **Parents** are frequently **overwhelmed** and justifiably **frightened.**
    1. The responsible **physician must keep parents informed** and provide as much reassurance as possible.
    2. **Seeing the child** is important for the parent and must be provided for as soon as the child is stabilized.
    3. **Someone other than the physician** (who is usually too busy) must provide initial **counsel and support.** This can be a nurse, social worker, or trained layperson, but it is very important, particularly if the child later dies.
  B. The **child** will be **terrified** if awake (or upon wakening).
    1. Amidst the tumult of the evaluation and resuscitation, **someone must tell the child what is going on** and warn him of painful maneuvers.
    2. It is important that the child be **told that he is not going to die**—even when that possibility has not even occurred to those caring for him.
    3. **Psychiatric care** is frequently needed after physical recovery.

Bibliography

Accident Facts. Chicago: National Safety Council, 1982.
Bruce, D. A., et al. Diffuse cerebral swelling following head injuries in children: The syndrome of malignant brain edema. *J. Neurosurg.* 54:170, 1981.
Burrington, J. D. Childhood Trauma. In T. M. Holder and K. W. Ashcraft (eds.): *Pediatric Surgery.* Philadelphia: Saunders, 1980. P. 138.
Eichelberger, M. R., and Randolph, J. G. Pediatric trauma: An algorithm for diagnosis and therapy. *J. Trauma* 23:91, 1983.
Haller, J. A. Pediatric trauma. *J.A.M.A.* 249:47, 1983.
Kettrick R. G., and Ludwig, S. Resuscitation: Pediatric Basic and Advanced Life Support. In G. Fleisher and S. Ludwig (eds.), *Textbook of Pediatric Emergency Medicine.* Baltimore: Williams & Wilkins, 1983. P. 1.
Mayer, T., et al. The modified injury severity scale in pediatric multiple trauma patients. *J. Pediatr. Surg.* 15:719, 1980.
Mayer, T., et al. Causes of morbidity and mortality in severe pediatric trauma. *J.A.M.A.* 245:719, 1981.
O'Neill, J. A., Jr. Emergency Management of the Injured Child. In K. J. Welch, et al. (eds.), *Pediatric Surgery.* Chicago: Year Book, 1986. P. 135.
O'Neill, J. A., Jr. Infants and Children as Accident Victims. In K. J. Welch, et al. (eds.), *Pediatric Surgery.* Chicago: Year Book, 1986. P. 133.

93

Head Injuries

(Also see Chap. 92, Trauma: General Principles.)

I. **Definition.** Injury to the brain is the leading cause of traumatic death in childhood and the major unsolved problem in management of the severely injured child. Seventy percent of motor vehicle accident victims have a head injury. Cranial trauma is more common in children than in adults because of childrens' thinner skulls and their greater likelihood of being thrown.

   A. Head injury should be suspected in every child who is struck by an automobile and in any who are unconscious for even a short period of time, however mild the accident may seem.

   B. **Scalp lacerations** and linear **skull fractures** are common in children and may or may not be associated with serious intracranial injury.

   C. **Life-threatening cranial injuries**
   1. Open skull fracture
   2. Diffuse brain swelling
   3. Brain contusion
   4. Subdural hematoma
   5. Epidural hematoma
   6. Intracerebral hematoma
   7. CSF leak

II. **Clinical presentation**

   A. **Coma** frequently accompanies other severe injuries and requires prompt evaluation and treatment.

   B. **Restlessness** and combativeness may be signs of either cerebral injury or hypoxia.

   C. **Intracranial injury does not cause tachycardia and hypotension.** Look for evidence of blood loss elsewhere, particularly in the abdomen. A large scalp laceration in a small child can also result in significant blood loss and hypotension.

   D. **Bradycardia** and **hypertension** are signs of increased intracranial pressure and require prompt evaluation.

III. **Diagnosis**

   A. **History** of the accident is important. How was the child struck? Was he unconscious when discovered? Was there a lucid interval followed by deterioration?

   B. **Level of consciousness is the most important parameter** to assess and follow in the diagnosis and management of a child with a head injury. The Glasgow coma scale is an objective and reproducible measure (Table 93-1).

   C. **Neurologic examination** is completed, with particular attention to:
   1. **Cranial nerves,** especially **pupil size** and reactivity, and **eye movements.** Ocular deviation or pupil inequality may indicate tentorial herniation. Facial pain or sensitivity and the corneal reflex are tested.
   2. **Lateralizing motor responses.** Response to pain, spontaneous movements, hemiparesis.

Table 93-1. Glasgow Coma Scale

Eye opening	Spontaneous	4
	To voice	3
	To pain	2
	None	1
Verbal response	Oriented	5
	Confused	4
	Inappropriate words	3
	Incomprehensible sounds	2
	None	1
Best motor response	Obeys commands	6
	Localizes pain	5
	Withdraws (pain)	4
	Flexion (pain)	3
	Extension (pain)	2
	None	1

   3. **Posturing.** Decerebrate or decorticate.
   4. **Funduscopic** examination is not necessary initially, for it takes time for papilledema to develop.
   D. The **head** is examined for scalp lacerations, hematoma, and fractures. Open wounds are probed for fracture. Ears and nose are searched for blood or CSF.
   E. **Skull x-rays** are routinely obtained to look for fractures, but in most patients they contribute little to treatment. Accordingly, they are not performed until the patient is stabilized.
   F. **CT or MRI** is the most reliable method of evaluating intracranial injury and bleeding. A scan should be obtained promptly in every child with a severe head injury, particularly those with coma, lateralizing signs, or deteriorating level of consciousness.

IV. **Treatment**
   A. **First, follow the "ABCs" of resuscitation** (see Chap. 92). Life-threatening injuries of other organs may be present. The first priorities are to secure the airway, ensure adequate ventilation, and restore perfusion. **Hypoxia and hypotension are far greater immediate threats to the brain than intracranial hemorrhage in most patients.**
   B. **Monitor neurologic signs.** Glasgow coma scale, pupil size and reactivity, motor responses, vital signs. Start a flow sheet.
   C. **Treat increased intracranial pressure.**
      1. **IVs are isosmolar** (not 5% D/W) given at normal rates to avoid increasing brain swelling.
      2. Give **mannitol** (20%, 1–2 gm/kg IV) rapidly if the patient shows neurologic deterioration. It should not be given prophylactically since it may increase bleeding by rapid shrinkage of the brain. Insert a urinary catheter first.
      3. The use of dexamethasone **(Decadron)** is debatable, as is the prophylactic use of anticonvulsants.
      4. **Hyperventilate** to produce hypocapnia, which inhibits brain swelling. The patient is intubated and artificially ventilated.
   D. **Intracranial pressure monitoring** (bolt transducer) is often useful in the management of brain edema.

E. Give **antibiotics** if there is an open fracture, particularly of the base of the skull associated with CSF leak.

F. **Mild head injuries** are a common problem in pediatric practice. If the child was not rendered unconscious and the neurologic examination is normal, he is reexamined after several hours. If the examination is normal, it is safe to send the child home with instructions to return if he demonstrates:

1. Unusual behavior
2. Difficulty in arousing
3. Gait disturbance
4. Severe headache
5. Bleeding from the nose or ears
6. Sleepiness
7. Unusual eye movements
8. Vomiting
9. Fever or chills

Indications for operation

A. **Tentorial herniation** of the brain. A single fixed, dilated pupil or deviation of eyes. Emergency craniotomy is necessary without taking time for CT or other studies.

B. **CT scan findings of intracranial hematoma**—subdural, epidural, or intracerebral.

C. **Compound (open) skull fracture.**

D. **Depressed skull fracture** (not an emergency if the patient is neurologically intact).

Operative care.
With improved imaging techniques (CT and MRI), precise localization of the hematoma is usually possible, so that exploratory burr holes are seldom needed. Craniotomy permits more adequate removal of clot.

Complications.
Severe, permanent neurologic deficit is a tragic and all-too-common outcome of serious head injuries. Long-term institutional care is frequently necessary.

Prognosis.
The outlook depends on whether the injury is reparable and whether it is properly treated in time.

Bibliography

Bruce, D. A. Outcome Following Head Trauma in Childhood. In K. Shapiro (ed.), *Pediatric Head Trauma*. Mount Kisco, N.Y.: Futura, 1983. Pp. 213–222.

Bruce, D. A. Central Nervous System Injuries. In K. J. Welch, et al. (eds.), *Pediatric Surgery*. Chicago: Year Book, 1986. P. 209.

Bruce, D. A., et al. The pathophysiology, treatment and outcome following severe head injury in children. *Childs Brain* 5:174, 1979.

Gennarelli, T. A., et al. Influence of the type of intracranial lesion on outcome from severe head injury. *J. Neurosurg.* 52:26, 1982.

Mayer, T., et al. Effect of multiple trauma on outcome of pediatric patients with neurological injuries. *Childs Brain* 8:189, 1981.

94 Chest Injuries

I. **Definition.** Injuries to the chest account for 25% of fatalities after blunt trauma in children, second only to head injuries. Airway obstruction or a crushed chest injury can be rapidly fatal yet can often be treated successfully by simple measures if treatment is given promptly.

   A. Significant chest injury is suspected whenever a child has received a severe blow to the chest, such as being struck or run over by a car, thrown against the dashboard, or crushed under a falling object, even if symptoms are mild. **Every severely injured child should receive a chest x-ray.**

   B. **Maintaining the airway and ventilation is the first priority** in resuscitation, without awaiting blood gas determination. If the child is in respiratory distress intubate and ventilate. Insert a chest tube if tension pneumothorax is present.

   C. **Central injuries** are more likely to be lethal than are lateral ones because of the position of the heart or great vessels.

   D. Because of the **elasticity** of the child's chest wall, blunt trauma can result in severe injury to the thoracic viscera without fractures or even apparent deformity.

   E. **Immediately life-threatening injuries** include airway obstruction, flail chest, open or tension pneumothorax, hemothorax, and cardiac tamponade.

   F. **Potentially lethal injuries** include rupture of the trachea, bronchus, great vessels, or diaphragm; pulmonary contusion; myocardial contusion; and perforation of the esophagus.

II. **Airway obstruction**

   A. **Facial injuries,** foreign bodies, fractured larynx, blood, and secretions can obstruct the airway.

   B. **Stridor, crowing, or inability** of the patient **to ventilate** is obvious on examination. Complete obstruction is rapidly fatal.

   C. **Treatment.** Remove any foreign body, suction blood and secretions, and pull the tongue forward. Laryngoscopy may be necessary. Insert an endotracheal tube if other measures fail. Tracheostomy is rarely necessary acutely.

III. **Tracheobronchial rupture**

   A. Rupture of the tracheobronchial tree releases **air under pressure** into the subcutaneous space, the mediastinum, and often the pleural cavity, causing pneumothorax.

   B. **Respiratory distress** may be caused by airway obstruction or tension pneumothorax.

   C. **Diagnosis** of tracheal rupture is suggested by the finding of subcutaneous emphysema or mediastinal air. Lower tracheal or bronchial rupture results in **massive air leak,** which continues after insertion of a chest tube (Fig. 94-1). Bronchial rupture may seal promptly, becoming evident days or weeks later as stricture formation causes refractory lung collapse.

   D. **Treatment.** Tracheal rupture is treated by passage of an endotracheal tube to establish ventilation. Pneumothorax requires insertion of a chest tube. Prompt thoracotomy and repair of a tracheal or bronchial rupture is necessary if the air leak is massive.

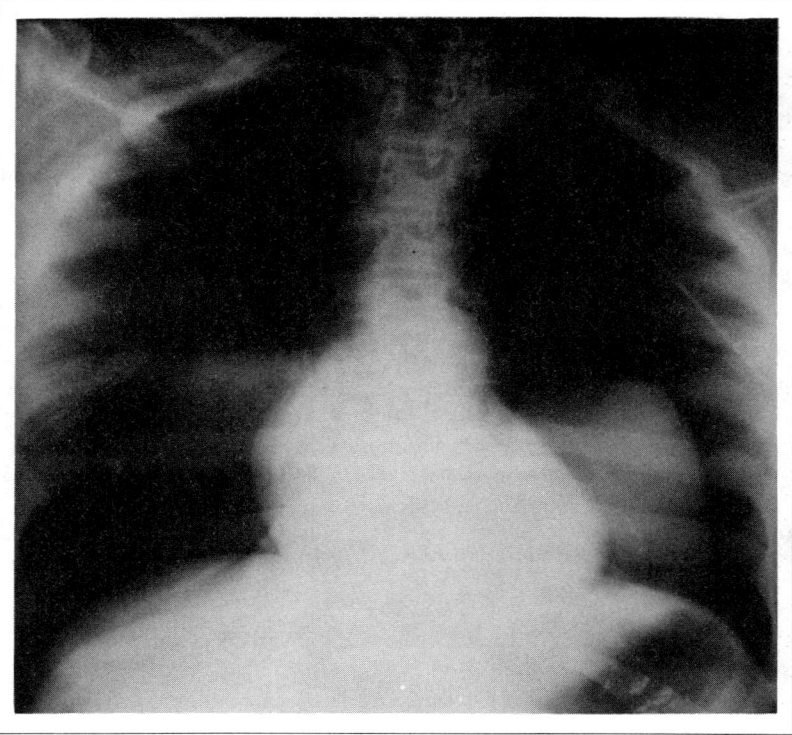

Fig. 94-1. Bronchial avulsion. Admission chest x-ray of 14-year-old girl who developed bilateral pneumothorax after massive trauma. Left bronchus was completely avulsed. Operative repair was followed by complete recovery. (From L. L. Leape, Bronchial avulsion. *J. Thorac. Cardiovasc. Surg.* 62:470–472, 1971.)

IV. Open pneumothorax

A. An opening in the chest wall exposes the lung to atmospheric pressure, causing collapse and respiratory distress.

B. Treatment. The opening is closed with a petroleum jelly gauze dressing, sealing the pleural space. A chest tube is inserted to reexpand the lung.

V. Tension pneumothorax

A. Parenchymal lung lacerations and some chest-wall injuries permit air to enter the pleural space but not exit. Accumulation of air under pressure collapses the lung and shifts the mediastinum toward the opposite side. The contralateral lung is compressed and the cavae are angulated, interfering with venous return.

B. Respiratory distress is severe and progressive. Death may rapidly ensue. Breath sounds are absent on the affected side, which is usually hyperresonant as well.

C. Diagnosis is by **chest x-ray.**

D. Treatment. Immediate insertion of a chest tube (see Chap. 108).

VI. Flail chest

A. Mobility of part of the chest wall secondary to multiple rib fractures prevents

development of the negative pressure necessary for ventilation. Respiratory distress develops from paradoxical movement.
B. **Treatment.** Intubate and give positive pressure ventilation to stabilize the chest and ventilate the lungs. Later internal operative fixation may shorten the time of ventilator dependence in severe cases.

Hemothorax
A. **Rupture of** large vessels causing massive hemothorax is usually rapidly fatal; treatable cases of hemothorax typically result from laceration of the **intercostal or mammary arteries.** Bleeding is seldom from the lung because of the low pressure in the pulmonary artery.
B. **Chest x-ray** reveals the diagnosis. **Pneumothorax** is usually present as well. Massive hemothorax causes hypovolemic shock.
C. **Treatment.** Chest-tube drainage is established, blood is replaced, and the rate of bleeding is carefully monitored. Most (80%) bleeding stops spontaneously. Continuing severe bleeding is an indication for thoracotomy.

Pulmonary contusion
A. **Crush injury** of the lung may not be obvious on initial appraisal. Signs develop as edema and hemorrhage into the parenchyma interfere with gas exchange.
B. A history of **massive chest injury,** such as being run over, alerts the clinician to the possibility of significant lung contusion. Respiratory distress, often absent at first, gradually develops and inexorably worsens.
C. **Serial chest x-rays** show development of diffuse parenchymal densities, which progress to opacification—a **"white lung."**
D. **Treatment.** Ventilatory support (intubation and respirator). It is doubtful that any medications are of benefit. Mortality is high.

Diaphragmatic rupture
A. **Rupture of the diaphragm** impairs the bellows function of the muscle, exposes the pleural space to the higher intraabdominal pressure, and permits herniation of abdominal viscera into the chest. It is more likely to occur on the left side.
B. **Increasing respiratory distress** is the usual symptom, but many patients are asymptomatic, at least initially.
C. Diagnosis is by **chest x-ray,** showing blurred diaphragmatic shadow, elevation, poor motion, and sometimes, herniation.
D. **Treatment.** Operative repair of the diaphragm when the patient is stabilized. Ventilatory support may be necessary beforehand if other, more serious injuries mandate delay in repair.

Cardiac tamponade
A. Because of the unyielding nature of the pericardium, accumulation of even small amounts of blood in the pericardial space compresses the heart and inhibits venous return. Bleeding is usually from small pericardial or epicardial veins.
B. **Increasing central venous pressure,** falling blood pressure, and distended neck veins are typical findings. If bleeding continues, tamponade is rapidly fatal.
C. **Diagnosis.** Pulsus paradoxus and the finding of a widened mediastinal shadow on chest x-ray. Ultrasound, if there is time, shows decreased amplitude of cardiac contractions. Pericardial tap demonstrates blood and temporarily brings dramatic relief of symptoms.
D. **Treatment.** Thoracotomy with pericardial "window" decompression. Pericardiocentesis is inadequate treatment.

XI. Myocardial contusion

A. Myocardial injury occurs to some degree in **every crush injury** of the chest but is seldom clinically apparent.

B. Arrhythmias are seen immediately after injury and may be life-threatening. Heart failure may develop later.

C. Diagnosis is by electrocardiographic evidence of rhythm disturbance and ST changes. Myocardial enzymes are elevated.

D. Treatment. Arrhythmias are treated with procainamide or lidocaine. Inotropic support may be needed.

XII. Great vessel rupture

A. Deceleration injuries may produce rupture of the thoracic aorta at the point of fixation by the ligamentum arteriosum. The injury is fatal at the scene of accident in 80% of patients. Bleeding from small lacerations is sometimes stopped by hematoma tamponade, but 80% of these patients bleed again within 24 hours. Penetrating trauma can injure the cavae or pulmonary vessels as well as the aorta.

B. Aortic rupture should be suspected if chest x-ray shows a **widened mediastinal shadow,** displacement of the trachea or esophagus, multiple rib fractures, fractures of the posterior portions of the upper ribs, or fractures of the scapula.

C. Diagnosis is by aortogram, which should be performed immediately.

D. Treatment. Immediate surgical repair.

XIII. Esophageal perforation

A. Injury to the esophagus by either blunt or penetrating trauma **is rare.** Most esophageal injuries are iatrogenic, caused by instrumentation or operation, or self-induced, from swallowing a foreign body or caustic. Mediastinitis results from bacterial and chemical contamination and is rapidly progressive.

B. Fever, chest pain, and difficulty swallowing are the usual symptoms. Chest x-ray shows mediastinal widening, pleural effusion, and pneumomediastinum.

C. Diagnosis is by **contrast swallow** x-ray.

D. Treatment. Repair and drainage.

Bibliography

Bellinger, S. B. Penetrating chest injuries in children. *Ann. Thorac. Surg.* 14:635, 1972.

Eichelberger, M. R., and Randolph, J. G. Thoracic trauma in children. *Surg. Clin. North Am.* 61:1181, 1981.

Golladay, E. S., Donahoo, J. S., and Haller, J. A. Special problems of cardiac injuries in infants and children. *J. Trauma* 19:526, 1979.

Haller, J. A., Jr. Thoracic Injuries. In K. J. Welch, et al. (eds.), *Pediatric Surgery.* Chicago: Year Book, 1986. P. 143.

Haller, J. A., and Shermeta, D. W. Major thoracic trauma in children. *Pediatr. Clin. North Am.* 22:341, 1975.

Kirsh, M. M., and Sloan, H. *Blunt Chest Trauma: General Principles of Management.* Boston: Little, Brown, 1977.

Leape, L. L. Bronchial avulsion: Successful repair after bilateral pneumothorax. *J. Thorac. Cardiovasc. Surg.* 62:470, 1971.

Meller, J. L., Little, A. G., and Shermeta, D. W. Thoracic trauma in children. *Pediatrics* 74:813, 1984.

Myers, W. O., Leape, L. L., and Holder, T. M. Bronchial rupture in a child with subsequent stenosis, resection, and anastomosis. *Ann. Thorac. Surg.* 12:442, 1971.

Simpson, J. S. Thoracic Injuries. In R. Touloukian (ed.), *Care of the Injured Child.* Baltimore: Waverly Press, 1975. Pp. 132–142.

95 Abdominal Trauma

Also see Chap. 92, Trauma: General Principles.

I. **Definition.** Ninety percent of serious abdominal injuries in children are the result of **blunt trauma.** Motor vehicle accidents are the leading cause, followed by falls and child abuse.
   A. **Children are at greater risk** of serious injury than adults, because their less well-developed abdominal muscles give poorer protection and their small size makes them more vulnerable to being thrown within a car or when struck.
   B. **The spleen** is the organ **most likely to be damaged,** followed by the liver, kidney, pancreas, intestine, and bladder.

II. **Pathophysiology.** Blunt trauma of the abdomen causes crushing, deceleration, and occasionally, shear injuries.
   A. **Crushing** results in predictable patterns of injury.
      1. **Encapsulated parenchymatous organs** (spleen, liver, kidney) are subject to a **bursting** force, which results in injuries that vary from a minor capsular tear to total disruption.
      2. The **pancreas** and **duodenum** are particularly vulnerable to crushing where they overlie the **spine.** Traumatic intramural hematoma of the duodenum is typically a pediatric injury.
      3. **Mesenteric tears** and **intestinal perforations** also result from impalement against the spine.
   B. **Deceleration injuries** result from movement of an organ next to a fixed point, such as the liver at the hepatic veins.

Clinical presentation. Serious intraabdominal trauma must be suspected in any patient who **(1)** has been **struck by an automobile, (2)** has **fallen from a considerable height,** or **(3) is unconscious.** The symptoms vary widely.
   A. **Life-threatening internal hemorrhage** may require immediate laparotomy.
   B. Other patients have **no signs** or symptoms initially but gradually show evidence of intraperitoneal bleeding or contamination.
   C. Diagnosis of an intraabdominal injury is often complicated by the presence of **coma** from an associated head injury.
   D. **Tire marks,** abrasions, and bruises on the abdomen are important clues to the possibility of serious intraabdominal trauma.
   E. Undiagnosed, **uncontrolled bleeding** must be presumed to be **intraabdominal** in origin until ruled out.

Diagnosis

   A. In the **conscious** patient, **physical examination** is the primary method of diagnosis. Repeated examinations are necessary to detect evolving signs of bleeding or peritoneal contamination. Tenderness, guarding, or palpable masses or organs are indications for further studies.
   B. In the **unconscious** patient, **CT imaging** of the abdomen should be performed. If CT is not available, peritoneal lavage should be carried out.

- **C. Peritoneal lavage** is quicker than CT and thus should be performed if uncontrolled intraabdominal bleeding is suspected, or if there are progressive peritoneal signs (see Chap. 109).
- **D. CT** imaging is preferred for diagnosis of injuries of the solid organs: **liver, spleen, kidneys, and pancreas.** If it is not available, nuclear scans, ultrasound, and contrast studies are helpful.
- **E. Plain x-rays** of the abdomen are of **limited value** but may show free air or disturbed gas patterns.
- **F.** If **bladder rupture** is suspected, **cystogram** is performed.
- **G. Retrograde urethrogram** should be performed for suspected urethral injuries **prior to insertion of a catheter** if there is passage of blood.
- **H. Arteriography** may be necessary in cases of questionable viability of the kidney.

V. Indications for operation
- **A. Immediate**
    1. **Uncontrolled, life-threatening bleeding**
    2. **Grossly bloody peritoneal lavage**
- **B. Urgent**
    1. **Positive lavage** (greater than 50,000 RBC/mm^3, bile or intestinal contents)
    2. **Free air** on abdominal x-ray
    3. **Progressive peritoneal signs**
    4. **Severe damage of the liver, spleen, or kidney** with devascularized tissue
    5. **Arteriographic** evidence of interruption of the blood supply of the **kidney**
- **C. Later**
    1. **Continued bleeding** from ruptured spleen, liver, or kidney
    2. **Extravasation of urine**
    3. Evidence of **peritoneal irritation** suggesting intestinal perforation

VI. Nonoperative care. Many abdominal injuries are best treated without an operation. Most lacerations of the liver and spleen stop bleeding spontaneously and heal without suture. Nonoperative care is appropriate if bleeding has stopped and there is no peritoneal contamination. A prerequisite is precise diagnosis, i.e., demonstration of the lesion on CT or nuclear scan. (See specific organ discussions, following, for details.)

VII. Preoperative preparation
- **A. Resuscitation** should be accomplished **before induction of anesthesia** unless the patient is in extremis. Two large-bore catheters should be inserted into upper extremity veins to permit rapid resuscitation and transfusion of large volumes of blood if necessary during the operation. The blood volume should be restored to normal before induction of anesthesia (see Chap. 92).
- **B.** Except when exsanguination is threatened, preoperative **diagnostic studies** are performed to define the injury accurately. "Exploratory" surgery is seldom appropriate.
- **C. Priority of care** requires judgment based on experience with children with multiple severe injuries. Immediately life-threatening conditions obviously take precedence. Treatment of a serious head injury takes precedence over nonexsanguinating abdominal trauma. Treatment of major vascular injuries of the

extremities takes precedence over nonexsanguinating intrathoracic or intraabdominal injuries.

D. **Adequate amounts of blood** must be cross-matched for patients with severe intraabdominal injury. In general, this means an amount at least equal to the estimated blood volume.

VIII. **Operative care.** A transverse incision placed appropriately for the anticipated operation is used unless the patient is in extremis, in which case a midline full-length incision is used (see the chapters on specific organs, following, for details).

IX. **Postoperative care.** Postoperative care consists of continuation of the preoperative resuscitation and stabilization measures, frequently complicated by associated injuries, particularly of the brain. Intensive care support is necessary if the injuries are severe.

A. The child in **coma** requires close monitoring to detect evidence of intracranial bleeding or increasing pressure.

B. **Ventilatory support** is usually required (see Chap. 7).

C. **Adequacy of circulation** and blood volume is closely monitored by frequent readings of vital signs, urine output, central venous pressure, hematocrit, and arterial blood gases.

X. **Complications.** Complications are common in the patient with multiple injuries. They must be constantly suspected and promptly detected and treated.

A. **Bleeding.**

B. **Infection** may result from retained devitalized tissue or blood, or from inadequately drained sites of continuing leakage of intestinal or pancreatic juices. Wound infections are common.

C. **Overlooked associated injuries** may produce complications hours or days after the injury.

XI. **Prognosis.** The prognosis following major abdominal trauma depends on the extent of the injuries and their reparability. In most patients with severe intraabdominal trauma, the ultimate outcome is determined by the severity of the head injury.

Bibliography

Barlow, B., Niemirska M., and Gandhi, R. Ten years' experience with pediatric gunshot wounds. *J. Pediatr. Surg.* 17:927, 1982.

Barlow, B., Niemirska, M., and Gandhi, R. P. Stab wounds in children. *J. Pediatr. Surg.* 18:926, 1983.

Burrington, J. C. Childhood Trauma. In T. M. Holder and K. W. Ashcraft (eds.), *Pediatric Surgery*. Philadelphia: Saunders, 1980. P. 138.

DuPriest, R. W., Jr., Rodriguez, A., and Shatney, C. H. Peritoneal lavage in children and adolescents with blunt abdominal trauma. *Am. Surg.* 48:460, 1982.

Eichelberger, M. R., and Randolph, J. G. Abdominal Trauma. In K. J. Welch, et al. (eds.), *Pediatric Surgery*. Chicago: Year Book, 1986. P. 154.

Karp, M. P., et al. The role of computed tomography in the evaluation of blunt abdominal trauma in children. *J. Pediatr. Surg.* 16:316, 1981.

Nance, F. C., and Cohn, I., Jr. Surgical judgment in the management of stab wounds of the abdomen: A retrospective and prospective analysis based on a study of 600 stabbed patients. *Ann. Surg.* 170:569, 1969.

Powell, R. W., et al. Peritoneal lavage in children with blunt abdominal trauma. *J. Pediatr. Surg.* 11:973, 1976.

Shaftan, G. W. Indication for operation in abdominal trauma. *Am. J. Surg.* 99:657, 1960.

96

Spleen Injuries

Also see Chap. 92, Trauma: General Principles, and Chap. 95, Abdominal Trauma.

- **Definition.** The spleen is the organ **most likely to be injured** in a child. Serious damage may result from apparently minor impact. **Suspect** splenic injury in any child with a left upper quadrant or lower chest injury, however trivial, and in all motor vehicle accident victims.
- **Clinical presentation**
  - **A. Signs and symptoms** of splenic injury vary widely. If the child is seen shortly after injury, or if the rate of blood loss is slow, there may be no signs or symptoms. Conversely, patients with major splenic injury may be in shock from blood loss. **An initial negative examination does not eliminate the possibility of splenic injury.**
  - **B. Left upper quadrant abrasions,** tire marks, or other local evidence of trauma should alert the physician to the possibility of splenic injury. **Rib fractures are uncommon** in children with splenic trauma.
  - **C. Typical signs and symptoms** of splenic injury:
    1. **Left-upper-quadrant pain and tenderness**
    2. **A palpable spleen**
    3. **Left shoulder pain,** caused by diaphragmatic irritation
  - **D. A falling hematocrit** in an asymptomatic patient may be the only clinical evidence of splenic injury.
  - **E. Signs of massive intraabdominal hemorrhage** with shock may also be seen if there is splenic avulsion or the spleen is pulverized.

Diagnosis

- **A. CT scan** is the preferred method of diagnosing splenic injuries since it provides detailed anatomic information about the spleen as well as the other abdominal organs.
- **B. Nuclear scan** with technetium 99 may also be used to assess splenic injury (Fig. 96-1). Anatomic detail is less precise than with CT scan, but evaluation of viability of the spleen may be better.
- **C. Plain x-rays** of the abdomen may show loss of splenic outline, increase in the size of the spleen, and indentation of the greater curvature of the stomach, but these signs are not reliable and are frequently absent. **Pleural effusion** may result from subphrenic hematoma from a ruptured spleen.
- **D. Laparoscopy** can be used to diagnose splenic injury, but it is invasive and requires general anesthesia in a child. Its major value is the assessment of the extent of splenic and other organ injuries when the indications for laparotomy are equivocal.

Nonoperative care

- **A. Most injuries of the spleen will heal without operation.** Nonoperative treatment consists of:
  1. **Bed rest for 1 week in the hospital.** The patient is carefully monitored and serial hematocrits are obtained to detect continued bleeding. Transfusion is given if needed.

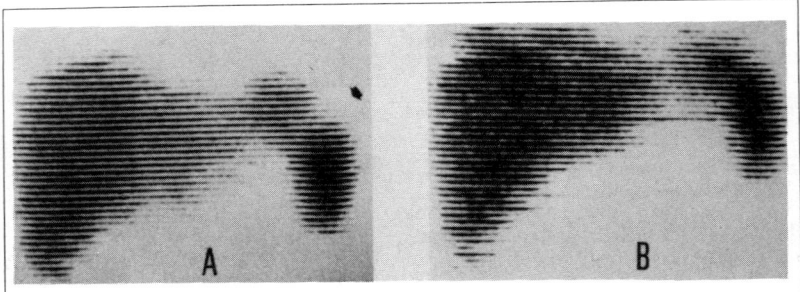

Fig. 96-1. Ruptured spleen. A. Scintigram showing defect in spleen consistent with laceration. B. Follow-up isotope study two months later shows healing of the spleen.

    2. **Restricted activity** (no athletics) for **3 months.**
    3. **Follow-up CT** or isotope scans at 6 and 12 weeks to document healing.
  B. Nonoperative care is **not appropriate** for splenic injuries with **extensive devascularization** or **uncontrolled bleeding.**

V. Indications for operation

  A. **Persistent bleeding,** manifested as continued hypotension despite transfusion or the loss of 40% or more of the estimated blood volume in a 24-hour period.
  B. **Devascularization** of the spleen.
  C. **Associated injuries.** If other organs are injured, laparotomy may be necessary to identify and correct the source of bleeding.
  D. **Operative evaluation and repair** is advocated for **all splenic injuries** by some surgeons to decrease the duration of restricted activity and to eliminate the possibility of delayed rupture.

VI. Operative care

  A. **Repair** of the injured spleen is usually possible.
    1. **The spleen is preserved if at all possible** because of the risk of **postsplenectomy sepsis** (see Chap. 76).
    2. **Minor lacerations** with arrested bleeding and good clot do not require suturing. The clot should not be disrupted.
    3. **Direct suture** with heavy absorbable material tied over polytef (Teflon) pledgets is used for most major lacerations. Use of **microcellular collagen** is sometimes helpful.
    4. A **devascularized segment** of the spleen is **resected.**
  B. **Splenectomy is sometimes unavoidable**
    1. If the spleen is **avulsed, pulverized,** or otherwise beyond repair.
    2. If the patient is **unstable** and has other more serious injuries.
    3. If the patient has **mononucleosis or hemophilia.**

VII. Complications

  A. **Bleeding.**
  B. **Infection** in the incision or in a hematoma at the operative site.

C. Overwhelming postsplenectomy sepsis, which may occur if the spleen has been removed. The mortality from severe infection is 50% in a splenectomized patient. Prophylactic antibiotics may lower the risk.

III. **Prognosis.** If even half of the spleen is retained, normal function is to be expected. After total splenectomy, the only significant handicap is susceptibility to infection.

Bibliography

Buntain, W. L., and Lynn, H. B. Splenorrhaphy: Changing concepts for the traumatized spleen. *Surgery* 86:748, 1979.

Cooney, D. R., et al. Comparative methods of splenic preservation. *J. Pediatr. Surg.* 16:327, 1981.

Douglas, G. L., and Simpson, J. S. The conservative management of splenic trauma. *J. Pediatr. Surg.* 6:565, 1971.

Eichelberger, M. R., and Randolph, J. G. Abdominal Trauma. In K. J. Welch, et al. (eds.), *Pediatric Surgery*. Chicago: Year Book, 1986. P. 154.

Leape, L. L., and Bordy, M. D. Neonatal rupture of the spleen. *Pediatrics* 47:101, 1971.

Wesson, D. E., et al. Ruptured spleen: When to operate? *J. Pediatr. Surg.* 16:324, 1981.

97 Liver Injuries

Also see Chap. 92, Trauma: General Principles, and Chap. 95, Abdominal Trauma

I. **Definition.** Rupture of the liver is responsible for more deaths than injury to any other abdominal organ. The right lobe is involved 4 times as frequently as the left. Blunt trauma usually results in a bursting injury, which may vary from a relatively minor capsular tear to pulverization of an entire lobe. **Suspect** liver injury in any patient with:
   A. **Severe abdominal impact** (direct blow)
   B. **Unexplained hypovolemia**
   C. **Intraperitoneal bleeding**

I. **Clinical presentation**
   A. **Evidence of severe upper abdominal trauma** (tire marks, major abrasions, or ecchymoses) should alert the physician to the possibility of significant liver injury.
   B. **Massive intraabdominal hemorrhage** with shock suggests injury to the liver. (Great-vessel injury can also cause exsanguinating hemorrhage but is much less common.)
   C. **Signs and symptoms** may be absent if the child is seen shortly after injury or if the bleeding is slow or has stopped.
   D. **Specific signs and symptoms** of liver injury:
      1. **Right-upper-quadrant pain and tenderness**
      2. **A palpable liver**
      3. **Right shoulder pain,** caused by diaphragmatic irritation
   E. **As with splenic injury, a falling hematocrit** may be the only clinical evidence of hepatic trauma in an asymptomatic patient.
   F. **Other major injuries** commonly accompany hepatic rupture and complicate evaluation of physical signs. Most common are injuries to the lower chest: **pulmonary contusion, hemothorax, diaphragmatic rupture,** and **renal trauma.**

Diagnosis
   A. **Peritoneal lavage** that is grossly positive (pure blood) in a patient with unstable hypovolemia usually indicates major liver or splenic injury. Emergency laparotomy should be performed immediately. Further diagnostic studies are not indicated.
   B. **CT** is the preferred method of diagnosing hepatic injuries in stable patients. It provides detailed anatomic information that permits rational decision making about the need for operation.
   C. **Nuclear scan** using technetium 99 may also be used to assess hepatic injury but is inferior in providing anatomic detail. Serial scans are a useful way to monitor hepatic healing.
   D. **Plain x-rays** of the abdomen are of little value in assessing liver injury.
   E. **Laparoscopy** has a limited role in the management of liver injuries. In a stable patient with minor or moderate blood loss, visualization of a minor liver laceration that does not require operative repair can avoid laparotomy.

IV. Nonoperative care.
Minor lacerations of the liver will heal spontaneously. The nonoperative treatment program is the same as for splenic injuries.
  - **A. Bed rest for 1 week in the hospital.** The patient is carefully monitored and serial hematocrits are obtained to detect continued bleeding. Transfusion is given if needed.
  - **B. Restricted activity** (no athletics) for **3 months.**
  - **C. Follow-up CT** or isotope scans at 6 and 12 weeks to document healing.

V. Indications for operation
  - **A. The unstable patient.** It may not be possible to resuscitate a child if there is massive liver injury. **Immediate laparotomy is necessary** to control the bleeding.
  - **B. Persistent bleeding,** manifested as continued hypotension despite transfusion or the loss of 40% or more of the estimated blood volume in a 24-hour period.
  - **C. Associated injuries.** If other abdominal organs are injured, it may not be possible to identify the source of bleeding without laparotomy.
  - **D. Operative evaluation and repair** is advocated by some surgeons for **all hepatic injuries** as the only sure way to determine the extent of injury.

VI. Operative care
  - **A. Minor lacerations** of the liver with arrested bleeding do not require suturing. The clot must not be disrupted.
  - **B. Direct suture** with heavy absorbable material (0 Vicryl) is appropriate for most major lacerations. Bleeding points and obvious biliary radicles should be ligated or clipped. Use of **microcellular collagen** is sometimes helpful.
  - **C. Resection** of part of the liver is necessary in about 10% of patients. Indications for resection are:
    1. **Injury to the hepatic veins** or other inaccessible major vessels
    2. **Dead or devitalized tissue**
    3. **Major bile duct injury deep within the liver**
  - **D. Packing** of bleeding areas that cannot be sutured can sometimes be accomplished, using omentum. In desperate situations with massive uncontrolled bleeding, the raw surface of the liver can be packed with laparotomy packs to tamponade the bleeding, followed by closing of the abdomen. Reoperation and control is done at 12–24 hours.
  - **E. Ligation** of the right or left **hepatic artery** can also be used in lieu of resection in difficult situations.
  - **F. Biliary intubation drainage** is **not necessary,** but the operative site must be well drained.

VII. Postoperative care
  - **A. Maintenance of blood volume and fluid balance** is the immediate postoperative challenge after liver resection. Hemodynamic monitoring and frequent measurement of the hematocrit are needed.
  - **B. Metabolic function** of the liver must be monitored and supported, particularly **glucose** metabolism and the production of serum **albumin.** Blood glucose should be checked every 4 hours in the immediate postoperative period. Albumin levels should be determined daily.
  - **C. Coagulation factors** may be disturbed by massive transfusions and must be monitored. Platelet and fresh plasma infusions are frequently necessary.

- **D. Ventilatory support** is frequently necessary in these patients with massive multiple injuries.
- **E. Parenteral nutrition** is advisable since most patients are unable to tolerate enteral nutrition.
- **F. Antibiotics** are given if there is peritoneal contamination from associated intestinal injuries or hypotension, but they are not given for liver injuries alone.

Complications

- **A. Bleeding** from the operative site is not uncommon and may require reoperation for control.
- **B. Infection** in the incision or in a hematoma at the operative site may occur if there is contamination or inadequate drainage. Subphrenic and subhepatic collections of bile or blood favor the development of abscesses.
- **C. Hemobilia** may result from a large hematoma or area of unresected pulverized tissue deep within the liver. **Hematemesis, melena, and biliary colic** are the usual signs. **Jaundice** frequently occurs. Spontaneous healing occurs in most cases. Transfusions may be necessary. If bleeding persists, selective arterial embolization may be effective. Reoperation with ligation of the vessels and packing or resection is occasionally necessary.

Prognosis. Following recovery from successful repair of liver injuries, including resection of 50% or more of the liver, full return of function can be expected.

Bibliography

Aaron, S., Fulton, R. L., and Mays, E. T. Selective ligation of the hepatic artery for trauma of the liver. *Surg. Gynecol. Obstet.* 141:187, 1975.

Canty, T. G., and Aaron, W. S. Hepatic artery ligation for exsanguinating liver injuries in children. *J. Pediatr. Surg.* 10:693, 1975.

Karp, M. P., et al. The nonoperative management of pediatric hepatic trauma. *J. Pediatr. Surg.* 18:512, 1983.

98 Pancreas Injuries

Also see Chap. 92, Trauma: General Principles, and Chap. 95, Abdominal Trauma.

I. Definition. Because of its location directly overlying the spine, the pancreas is easily crushed by a deep injury to the upper abdomen such as being run over by a car's tire, falling on a handlebar, or being kicked. **Suspect** pancreatic injury if:

   A. There is significant **upper abdominal trauma**
   B. There are **peritoneal signs** without evidence of bleeding
   C. The **peritoneal lavage** fluid has a **high amylase** content

Pathophysiology. Injury to the pancreas causes release of highly irritating pancreatic enzymes, which produce a severe inflammatory reaction.

   A. **Peritoneal contamination** results in chemical peritonitis, with edema, outpouring of fluid into the peritoneal space, and systemic signs of inflammation: fever and leukocytosis.
   B. **Autodigestion** occurs if the injury is confined to the pancreas itself. If the injury is mild, it may heal without residue. More extensive damage may go on to **pseudocyst** formation or rupture into the peritoneal cavity or lesser sac, causing peritonitis and **abscess** formation.

Clinical presentation

   A. Since most patients with pancreatic rupture have other serious injuries and may be in coma, evidence of pancreatic trauma **may not be obvious initially.**
   B. Severe upper **abdominal pain** usually develops quickly after pancreatic rupture.
   C. **Abdominal distention** and ileus ensue, followed by progressive signs of **peritonitis:** tenderness and spasm. Rigidity may be a late sign.
   D. **Fever** and **leukocytosis** will occur within a few hours.
   E. **Hypovolemic shock** develops as continuing spillage of pancreatic enzymes causes progression of the peritoneal "burn."
   F. **Delayed appearance** of symptoms and signs for days or weeks following pancreatic injury may occur if the posterior peritoneum is intact and disruption has not occurred.

Diagnosis

   A. A **high serum amylase** level (> 300 Somogyi units) may indicate pancreatic injury. Unfortunately, hyperamylasemia in injured patients is usually **not** caused by pancreatic injury, and about 20 percent of patients with a transected pancreas have normal serum amylase level. Because a **rising** amylase level is significant, amylase determinations should be made at 6-hour intervals in the immediate postinjury period.
   B. A high **amylase** level (> 1000 units/100 ml) in the **peritoneal lavage** is diagnostic of pancreatic injury.
   C. **CT scan** should be obtained if either serum or lavage amylase is elevated; it is the most reliable method of diagnosing the extent of pancreatic injury.

Nonoperative care

   A. **Crush** injuries of the pancreas not associated with severe intraperitoneal spillage of enzymes will usually **heal spontaneously** if treated with intestinal rest (nasogastric decompression and no feeding) for 1–2 weeks.

    B. **Fluid resuscitation** with saline and plasma is given in the first 23–48 hours.

    C. **Parenteral nutrition** should commence early since enteral nutrition will not be possible for 1–2 weeks.

    D. The patient must be **monitored** for development of a **pseudocyst.** Ultrasound or CT should be performed at 2 and 4 weeks for this purpose.

VI. **Indications for operation**

    A. **Pancreatic injuries are seldom isolated.** Frequently the patient is operated on for other injuries and a pancreatic injury is discovered as well.

    B. Pancreatic injury requires operative treatment when there is (1) **pancreatic disruption** via CT; (2) a high amylase level in the peritoneal lavage fluid; or (3) **progressive severe pancreatitis** with shock, peritonitis, and hyperamylasemia.

VII. **Operative care**

    A. **Debridement** of devitalized tissue, hemostasis, and **drainage** with large sump catheters is the appropriate treatment for most pancreatic injuries. Simple stab wounds are sutured and drained.

    B. **Resection** of the distal pancreas is performed for pancreatic transection. Intestinal drainage is not necessary. The **spleen** should be preserved if possible.

    C. **Pancreatoduodenal resection (Whipple procedure)** is indicated if there is destruction of the head of the pancreas, fortunately a rare occurrence.

VIII. **Postoperative care**

    A. **Intensive care** is usually required because of multiple organ injuries in these patients.

    B. **Antibiotics** are given because the chemical irritation of pancreatic enzymes favors peritoneal sepsis (cephazolin [Kefzol], 20 mg/kg q8h, and clindamycin, 10 mg/kg q8h).

    C. **Ventilatory support** is frequently necessary in patients with massive multiple injuries.

    D. **Parenteral nutrition** is started early postoperatively since enteral nutrition will not be possible for a week or more.

IX. **Complications.** Complications are common after pancreatic injury.

    A. **Infection** may result from retained devitalized tissue or blood, or from inadequate drainage of the operative site. Abscess may develop in the lesser sac or in the subphrenic or subhepatic spaces. Wound infections are common.

    B. **Pancreatic fistula** can occur, with drainage through an abdominal incision or into an abscess.

    C. **Pancreatic pseudocyst** may develop after pancreatic injury. Disruption of the pancreatic parenchyma with autodigestion is presumed to be the cause (see Chap. 99).

    D. **Chronic pancreatitis** may occur long after recovery from pancreatic injury or pseudocyst. It may indicate stricture of the pancreatic duct, which should be sought by retrograde catheterization studies and corrected surgically.

X. **Prognosis.** Following operative treatment of pancreatic injury or pancreatic pseudocyst, the outcome is largely determined by the incidence of complications. In all but a very few individuals, there is sufficient remaining functioning pancreas to support life and nutrition. Abscess formation, fistulization, and recurrence of cyst are all well-recognized complications.

Bibliography

Graham, J. M., et al. Surgical management of acute pancreatic injuries in children. *J. Pediatr. Surg.* 13:693, 1978.

Graham, J. M., et al. Combined pancreato-duodenal injuries. *J. Trauma* 19:340, 1979.

Jones, R. C. Management of pancreatic trauma. *Ann. Surg.* 187:555, 1978.

Robey, E., Mullen, J. T., and Schwab, C. W. Blunt transection of the pancreas treated by distal pancreatectomy, splenic salvage, and hyperalimentation. *Ann. Surg.* 196:695, 1982.

99 Pancreatic Pseudocyst

Definition. *Pancreatic pseudocyst* is an acquired collection of fluid in the pancreas as a result of injury or pancreatitis. Autodigestion by pancreatic enzymes is thought to be the cause.

Clinical picture. Pseudocysts are frequently asymptomatic. They should be suspected and looked for after every case of severe pancreatic trauma or pancreatitis. Sometimes the antecedent trauma is thought to be trivial.

A. The **time lag** from injury to the recognition of a pseudocyst varies from 2 weeks to 2 years. It averages 5 months.

B. **Symptoms** of pancreatic pseudocyst are pain and vomiting. Fever, leukocytosis, and elevated amylase are usually found also. A **mass** is sometimes palpable in the upper abdomen.

C. The **clinical course** of pancreatic pseudocyst is unpredictable.

1. **Spontaneous disappearance** may take place, especially if the cyst is small. Resolution will occur within 3 weeks if at all.
2. **Rupture** of a pancreatic pseudocyst can also occur. This is marked by a sudden worsening in the patient's condition, with pain, fever, leukocytosis to 25–30,000, distention, and ileus.
3. **Hemorrhage** may occur in the cyst itself or from erosion into the stomach or duodenum.
4. **Maturation** of the cyst is the hoped-for result in the absence of spontaneous resolution. Development of a thick wall makes it suitable for surgical drainage.

Diagnosis of pancreatic pseudocyst is by **ultrasound, CT, or MRI**, which will demonstrate a cyst when it is quite small, long before it is evident clinically. Routine monitoring by ultrasound should be carried out following pancreatic trauma or pancreatitis. Upper GI series will demonstrate extrinsic compression of the stomach or duodenum if the cyst is large.

Indications for operation.

- **Failure of spontaneous resolution.** If a pseudocyst is present for more than 3 weeks, resolution will not occur.
- **Development of a thick wall.** Internal drainage cannot be accomplished unless the cyst wall is thick enough to hold sutures—approximately 5 mm. Wall thickness can be determined by CT or ultrasound.
- **Failure to improve.** The child with a pancreatic pseudocyst who is acutely ill and not improving requires operative drainage.

Operative care

External drainage by catheter to the outside is necessary if the cyst wall is not thick enough for anastomosis to the gut. Because the failure rate, morbidity, complication rate, reoperation rate, and mortality are all higher following external drainage, internal drainage is much preferred.

Internal drainage may be accomplished by two methods.

1. **Roux-Y cyst-jejunostomy** entails dividing a loop of jejunum and anastomosing the end to the cyst wall. Jejunojejunostomy distally reestablishes gut continuity but prevents intestinal contents from reaching the cyst.

2. **Cyst-gastrostomy or cyst-duodenostomy** drains the cyst directly into the adjacent viscus. It is not easier to perform than cyst-jejunostomy and has the disadvantage of exposing the cyst to gastric or duodenal contents. However, it usually works well in spite of this.

VI. Complications

A. Recurrent pseudocyst
B. Chronic pancreatitis

Bibliography

Bradley, E. L. Spontaneous resolution of pancreatic pseudocysts. *Am. J. Surg.* 129:23, 1975.

Cooney, D. R., and Grosfeld, J. L. Operative management of pancreatic pseudocysts in infants and children. *Ann. Surg.* 182:590, 1975.

Dahman, B., and Stephens, C. A. Pseudocysts of the pancreas after blunt abdominal trauma in children. *J. Pediatr. Surg.* 16:17, 1981.

Garel, L., et al. Pseudocysts of the pancreas in children which require surgery. *Pediatr. Radiol.* 13:120, 1983.

Harkanyi, Z., et al. Gray-scale echography of traumatic pancreatic cysts in children. *Pediatr. Radiol.* 11:81, 1981.

Pokorny, W. J., et al. Pancreatic pseudocysts in children. *Surg. Gynecol. Obstet.* 151:182, 1980.

Shatney, C. H., and Lillehei, R. C. The timing of surgical treatment of pancreatic pseudocysts. *Surg. Gynecol. Obstet.* 152:809, 1981.

Windell, R. L. Needle aspiration and the treatment of pancreatic pseudocysts in childhood. *Ann. R. Coll. Surg. Engl.* 65:331, 1983.

100 Intestinal Injuries

Also see Chap. 92, Trauma: General Principles, and Chap. 95, Abdominal Trauma.

Definition. Because of its mobility, the intestine is less likely to be injured than the solid organs. Not surprisingly, intestinal injuries are most common in the segments that are fixed: the duodenum and the ascending and descending colon. In adults, penetrating trauma is the major cause of intestinal injuries, but in children, blunt trauma is the chief offender.

Pathophysiology

A. **Hematoma** in the intestinal wall may produce obstruction. If the blood supply is intact, the hematoma will gradually be absorbed, relieving the obstruction.

B. **Perforation** of the intestine leads to prompt peritoneal contamination with intestinal contents. In the upper intestine, the injury is largely chemical, and peritoneal irritation produces early symptoms. Stool extravasation from the colon, on the other hand, elicits a milder response until bacterial invasion and multiplication take place, which take hours.

C. **Devascularization** of the gut from injury to the mesentery results in segmental intestinal infarction, which also takes hours to become manifested.

Clinical presentation

A. **Duodenal injury. Intramural hematoma of the duodenum** is the most common intestinal injury in children. It results from compression of the duodenum against the spine. Duodenal injuries are more common in children than in adults because of their smaller size and weaker abdominal musculature. Even seemingly mild blunt trauma may cause a serious injury.

   1. **Suspect** duodenal injury in any child with focal blunt injury to the upper abdomen, such as handlebar injuries and kicks.

   2. **Signs and symptoms.** The extent of the obstruction may not be evident for several days after injury, when bilious **vomiting** occurs, as in high intestinal obstruction from any cause. There is **tenderness** to deep palpation in the epigastrium. Peritoneal signs are usually absent.

B. **Intestinal injuries** of the remaining small bowel are uncommon after blunt trauma but are not rare after penetrating trauma.

   1. **Suspect** intestinal injury in every patient with a penetrating injury to the abdomen, as well as in any child with increasing signs of peritoneal irritation after trauma.

   2. **Signs and symptoms.** Abdominal tenderness, distention, ileus; increasing peritoneal signs on physical examination.

C. **Colonic injuries** are almost always secondary to penetrating trauma, either transabdominal or transrectal.

   1. **Suspect** colon injury in any child with rectal trauma or with stab or gunshot wounds to the abdomen.

   2. **Signs and symptoms** develop slowly but are progressive. Look for tenderness and peritoneal signs, with ileus and abdominal distention. Vomiting is a late symptom. If the diagnosis is missed, signs of sepsis develop within 24–48 hours.

D. **Rectal injuries** may result from penetrating injuries of the anorectum or from a fractured pelvis.
   1. **Suspect** rectal injury in all patients with pelvic fracture, blood in the rectum, or air in the perirectal tissues by x-ray.
   2. **Signs and symptoms** are often absent until infection develops. Rectal bleeding may be the only early sign.

IV. **Diagnosis.** Worsening signs of peritonitis are sufficient indication for laparotomy without further diagnostic studies. In others, consider the following diagnostic signs:
   A. **Free air** on upright or decubitus film of the abdomen is diagnostic of perforation of the gastrointestinal tract. Similarly, air within the soft tissues of the pelvis indicates a rectal perforation.
   B. **Peritoneal lavage** revealing intestinal contents is also diagnostic of intestinal perforation.
   C. **Contrast x-rays (water soluble)** will demonstrate obstruction and the characteristic spiral pattern of **intramural hematoma of the duodenum.** Occult perforation of the bowel may be demonstrated by extravasation of the contrast material.
   D. **CT scan** of the abdomen may reveal hematoma or disruption of the intestine.
   E. **Sigmoidoscopy** may reveal a perforation and should be performed if there is blood in the rectum.

V. **Nonoperative care.** Traumatic intramural hematoma of the duodenum often can be treated nonoperatively. Nasogastric decompression and total parenteral nutrition may be necessary for several weeks, however, often producing more morbidity than operative care.

VI. **Indications for operation**
   A. **Perforation**
   B. **Infarction**
   C. **Obstruction** that does not resolve with decompressive treatment.

VII. **Operative care**
   A. **Small-bowel injuries** are usually easily repaired by direct suture after resection of devitalized tissue.
   B. **Intramural hematoma** of the duodenum is treated by evacuation of the clot and debridement of devitalized tissue.
   C. **Colon injuries** are closed directly if there is little or no spillage of fecal material. Severe injuries are exteriorized as a colostomy or resected with anastomosis and a protective proximal colostomy.
   D. **Rectal injuries** require a protective colostomy and external drainage as well as repair of the injury itself.

VIII. **Complications**
   A. **Abscesses** may develop from contamination of the peritoneal space by intestinal contents.
   B. **Intestinal obstruction** can result from stricture of the bowel at an anastomosis but more commonly results from adhesions.
   C. **Fistula** may develop if there is infection about the closure or anastomosis.
   D. **Stricture** may form after repair of an intestinal injury if the devascularized tissue is not adequately excised. Strictures are common after repair of rectal injuries.

E. **Incontinence** can occur if there is destruction of the anal sphincters and the puborectalis muscle.

IX. **Prognosis.** Almost all intestinal injuries can be repaired with excellent functional results. In most patients, outcome depends on recovery from associated injuries.

Bibliography

Black, C. T., et al. Anorectal trauma in children. *J. Pediatr. Surg.* 17:501, 1982.
Burrington, J. D. Childhood Trauma. In T. M. Holder and K. W. Ashcraft (eds.), *Pediatric Surgery.* Philadelphia: Saunders, 1980. P. 138.
Eichelberger, M. R., and Randolph, J. G. Abdominal Trauma. In K. J. Welch, et al. (eds.), *Pediatric Surgery.* Chicago: Year Book, 1986. P. 154.
Graham, J. M., et al. Combined pancreato-duodenal injuries. *J. Trauma* 19:340, 1979.
Grasberger, R. C., and Hirsch, E. F. Rectal trauma. *Am. J. Surg.* 145:795, 1983.
Holgersen, L. O., and Bishop, H. C. Nonoperative treatment of duodenal hematoma in childhood. *J. Pediatr. Surg.* 12:11, 1977.
Kakos, G. S., Grosfeld, J. L., and Morse, T. S. Small bowel injuries in children after blunt abdominal traum. *Ann. Surg.* 174:238, 1971.
Mahour, G. H., et al. Duodenal hematoma in infancy and childhood. *J. Pediatr. Surg.* 6:153, 1971.
Maull, K. I., Fallahzadeh, H., and Mays, E. T. Selective management of post-traumatic obstructing intramural hematoma of the duodenum. *Surg. Gynecol. Obstet.* 146:221, 1978.
Robertson, H. D., et al. Management of rectal trauma. *Surg. Gynecol. Obstet.* 154:161, 1982.
Slim, M. S., Makaroun, M., and Shammai, A. R. Primary repair of colorectal injuries in childhood. *J. Pediatr. Surg.* 16:1008, 1981.
Touloukian, R. J. Protocol for the nonoperative treatment of obstructing intramural duodenal hematoma during childhood. *Am. J. Surg.* 145:330, 1983.
Woolley, M. M., Mahour, G. H., and Sloan, T. Duodenal hematoma in infancy and childhood: Changing etiology and changing treatment. *Am. J. Surg.* 136:8, 1978.

101 Retroperitoneal Hematoma

Also see Chap. 92, Trauma: General Principles, and Chap. 95, Abdominal Trauma.

I. **Definition.** Hemorrhage in the retroperitoneal space may originate from laceration of either arteries or veins and results from either penetrating or blunt trauma. It is most commonly seen as a consequence of renal or pelvic injury.

II. **Pathophysiology.** Laceration of vessels in the retroperitoneal space without injury to the peritoneum leads to bleeding that is confined by the peritoneum, a relatively inelastic membrane.

   A. **Venous bleeding** behind the peritoneum is commonly associated with renal or pelvic injury. It will usually stop as pressure rises to exceed that in the veins.

   B. **Arterial bleeding** pressure stretches or ruptures the peritoneum, permitting continuing expansion of the hematoma.

III. **Clinical presentation**

   A. **Suspect** retroperitoneal hematoma in any patient with **pelvic** or **renal** trauma when there is evidence of considerable blood loss but the known amount is insufficient to account for the findings and peritoneal lavage is negative.

   B. **Signs and symptoms.** Hypovolemia, abdominal distention, swelling and bluish discoloration of the flanks or pelvis, elevation of the base of the bladder by rectal exam or x-ray.

IV. **Diagnosis**

   A. **CT** is the most reliable and least invasive method for diagnosing and quantitating the extent of retroperitoneal hematoma.

   B. **Angiography** is indicated for a midline posterior hematoma, which may be caused by an aortic rupture that can rapidly expand.

   C. **Abdominal exploration** for other injuries may reveal an unsuspected retroperitoneal hematoma.

V. **Nonoperative care**

   A. **Posterior lateral** and **pelvic** hematomas that are not expanding are best treated nonoperatively by bed rest and transfusion.

   B. **Arterial bleeding** may be controllable by angiographic embolization if it is not due to rupture of a major vessel.

VI. **Indications for operation**

   A. **Retroperitoneal hematoma** caused by a **penetrating** wound should be treated by operation since the source is usually single and easily controlled.

   B. **Expanding midline hematoma** indicates aortic rupture. Exploration is mandatory.

VII. **Operative care.** Identification and ligation of a bleeding artery is possible in most cases, but finding responsible bleeding veins in lacerations caused by blunt trauma is frequently impossible. For this reason, the tamponade provided by the **posterior peritoneum should not be disturbed unless the bleeding is uncontrolled and life-threatening.** Nonexpanding retroperitoneal hematoma found at exploration should not be disturbed.

VIII. Complications
A. Rebleeding may occur with ambulation. It is usually self-limited unless it is arterial, in which case an emergency operation may be required.

B. Infection is rare unless there is contamination by intestinal contents.

IX. Prognosis.
Uncomplicated retroperitoneal hematoma usually resolves and heals without long-term sequelae.

Bibliography
Eichelberger, M. R., and Randolph, J. G. In K. J. Welch, et al. (eds.), *Pediatric Surgery*. Chicago: Year Book, 1986. P. 154.

Reichard, S. A., et al. Pelvic fractures in children: Review of 120 patients with a new look at general management. *J. Pediatr. Surg.* 15:727, 1980.

102 Urinary Tract Injuries

Also see Chap. 92, Trauma: General Principles, and Chap. 95, Abdominal Trauma.

I. **Ureteral injuries.** The ureter is rarely injured by blunt or penetrating trauma. Iatrogenic injuries are more common.

   A. **Suspect** ureteral injury in gunshot wounds of the flank or if an injured child with a previously "normal" intravenous pyelogram (IVP) develops a collection of urine in the abdomen.

   B. **Clinical presentation.** Ureteral injuries are seldom evident clinically until a day or two after injury, when extravasation of urine is discovered. Fever, a flank mass, flank tenderness, abdominal distention, and urinary fistula to the skin or bowel are the usual modes of presentation.

   C. **Diagnosis.** "Double dose" infusion urogram may demonstrate the leak, but in most patients **retrograde ureterography** is necessary to confirm the diagnosis.

   D. **Treatment**

   1. **Nonoperative care** is appropriate for minor injuries, which usually heal without stricture if the ureter is splinted with a catheter for 5–7 days.

   2. **Operative repair** should be carried out promptly for ureteral transection or partial loss. If ureteral injury has been present for several days or more, primary repair is inadvisable. The urine collection is drained and urine flow is diverted by nephrostomy. Ureteral repair is carried out several months later.

   E. **Complications** include ureteral stricture, fistula, stone formation, and persistent infection.

   F. **Prognosis** is good for minor injuries, but major injuries may ultimately result in the need for nephrectomy.

II. **Bladder injuries.** Because of its abdominal location, a child's bladder is more likely to be injured than an adult's.

   A. **Suspect** bladder injury if there is a pelvic fracture, suprapubic bruising, or a penetrating wound of the pelvis. **Spontaneous rupture** of the bladder may occur if there is a neurogenic bladder or severe bladder-outlet obstruction.

   B. **Clinical presentation.** Retroperitoneal extravasation of urine results in **edema** of the suprapubic region or perineum. Intraperitoneal rupture of the bladder causes **urinary ascites,** with abdominal distention, ileus, fever, and elevation of the BUN and WBC. Hematuria is minor or absent in most bladder lacerations. If leakage is severe, the child stops voiding.

   C. **Diagnosis. Cystogram** with a large amount of contrast material will reveal the rupture. Urine or blood in the retroperitoneal space may compress the bladder from the sides, giving a "spinning top" appearance.

   D. **Treatment.** Bladder injuries require operative repair. A suprapubic cystostomy tube is placed for drainage until healing is complete. Antibiotics are given.

   E. **Complications.** Infection, fibrosis, bladder stones, and vesicocutaneous fistula may occur.

   F. **Prognosis** is good for most bladder injuries.

III. **Urethral injuries** are most likely to occur in the posterior urethra, where the organ is fixed by the urogenital diaphragm and easily torn by displacement of the pubic bones.

A. **Suspect** urethral injury if there is a pelvic fracture, urinary retention, or bleeding from the urethra with a normal IVP.

B. **Clinical presentation.** Urinary retention and hematuria are the most common complaints. **Blood at the meatus** is a typical finding of urethral injury. Rectal examination reveals a soft, fluctuant mass at the base of the bladder. Scrotal and perineal swelling may result from extravasated urine or blood. The patient may be unable to urinate.

C. **Diagnosis** is made by **urethrogram.** If a catheter can be passed, dye is instilled into the bladder for a voiding study. If the catheter will not pass, a retrograde study is obtained.

D. **Treatment**

1. **Nonoperative care** may be successful if a catheter can be passed through the urethra into the bladder. The catheter must not be placed on traction. It is left in place for 3 weeks and antibiotics are given.

2. **Operative treatment** is necessary if a catheter cannot be placed. The two ends of the urethra should be brought together and splinted with an indwelling catheter. This is sometimes a formidable task, requiring both transurethral and transcystic passage of instruments or open exposure. **Diversion** by means of suprapubic cystostomy is advisable. The extravasation and hamatoma are drained. Antibiotics are given.

E. **Complications are common** after urethral injury in boys. **Stricture** is present to some degree in all patients and requires aggressive treatment with dilatations. Later, operative urethroplasty may be required. Infection, incontinence, impotence, and infertility are possible late complications.

F. **Prognosis** depends on the severity of the injury. Total disruption of the urethra is accompanied by a high incidence of early and late complications.

IV. **Genital injuries** seldom result from major trauma, such as automobile accidents, but rather from straddle falls, minor household incidents such as catching the foreskin in a zipper, or exploratory genital play. **Complications of circumcision are by far the most common form of injury to the penis.** They include denudation of the shaft, amputation of the glans, bisection of the glans, and total loss of the organ. Testicular injuries are rare and usually result from contact sports or kicks.

A. **Suspect sexual abuse** if injuries to the penis or vulva are inconsistent with the history given.

B. **Clinical presentation** varies, but the nature of the injury is usually obvious on inspection.

C. **Diagnosis** is by examination in most children. In penile injuries, urethrogram may be indicated.

D. **Treatment** is surgical repair for all serious injuries of the genitalia.

1. Vulvar, penile, and scrotal **lacerations** are usually easily repaired and heal well because of their extensive blood supply. Skin flaps can be used to replace avulsed skin.

2. An **amputated penis** can sometimes be repaired if an operation is performed within 6 hours of injury.

3. **Testicular injury may result in torsion of the testis.** Exploration is advised if severe pain persists for more than a few hours. If torsion is not found, the tunica albuginea is incised to relieve pressure from hematoma.

E. **Complications** of penile injuries include urethral stricture, shortening, chordee, and impotence. Unilateral testicular loss results in no disability if the other testis is normal.

Bibliography

Bright, T. C., and Peters, P. C. Ureteral injuries due to external violence: 10-year experience with 59 cases. *J. Trauma* 17:616, 1977.

Cass, A. S. Immediate radiological evaluation and early surgical management of genitourinary injuries from external trauma. *J. Urol.* 122:772, 1979.

Cromie, W. J. Genitourinary injuries in the neonate. *Clin. Pediatr.* 18:292, 1979.

Ezell, W. W., et al. Mechanical traumatic injury to the genitalia in children. *J. Urol.* 102:788, 1969.

Flowerdrew, R., Fishman, I. J., and Churchill, B. M. Management of penile zipper injury. *J. Urol.* 117:671, 1977.

Hays, E. E., Sandler, C. M., and Corriere, J. N., Jr. Management of the ruptured bladder secondary to blunt abdominal trauma. *J. Urol.* 129:946, 1983.

Snyder, H. McC. III, and Caldamone, A. A. In K. J. Welch, et al. (eds.), *Pediatric Surgery*. Chicago: Year Book, 1986. P. 174.

103 Kidney Injuries

Also see Chap. 92, Trauma: General Principles, and Chap. 95, Abdominal Trauma.

I. **Definition.** The kidneys are more readily injured in children than in adults because they are less protected by the weaker rib cage and abdominal muscles. Most renal injuries result from blunt trauma. Congenital malformations or Wilms' tumor makes the kidney more vulnerable to injury.

   A. **Suspect** renal injury in every child with hematuria, as well as in those with fractures of the lower ribs or thoracolumbar vertebrae, or with an injured liver or spleen.

   B. **Types of injuries**
      1. **Parenchymal tear with subcapsular or retroperitoneal** bleeding. These patients may have no hematuria. Extravasation of urine is seldom a problem.
      2. **Parenchymal tear with rupture into the pelvis** or a **calix.** Hematuria is present and may be profuse, with accumulation of clots in the bladder. Extravasation of urine may be considerable.
      3. **Rupture of the renal pelvis** with massive urinary extravasation.
      4. **Severance or thrombosis of the blood supply.** Complete disruption can result in rapid massive blood loss.

II. **Clinical presentation**

   A. **Hematuria** may be the only sign of serious renal injury. Flank **hematoma, tenderness,** and abdominal muscle **spasm** in the region of the kidney are also suggestive.
   B. A **renal mass** may be palpable, especially in a small child.
   C. **Hypovolemic shock** may result from extensive blood loss from renal fracture.
   D. **Fever, leukocytosis,** and **elevated BUN** or creatinine are late findings of renal hematoma or urinary extravasation.

III. **Diagnosis**

   A. **Abdominal x-ray** may show absence of the psoas shadow and obliteration of the normal renal contour, curvature of the spine concave toward the injury, and vertebral fracture.
   B. **Infusion intravenous urogram** is the simplest way to define the presence and extent of renal injury.
   C. **CT** done in search of an abdominal injury will demonstrate renal fracture, but contrast enhancement must be performed to demonstrate renal function and anatomy.
   D. **Renal isotope scan** is the simple method of demonstrating that the blood supply to the kidney is intact.
   E. **Arteriography** is performed if the kidney is not visualized by contrast study or scan. Operative repair must be accomplished within a few hours after interruption of the blood supply if the kidney is to be salvaged.

IV. **Nonoperative care**

   A. The child with severe renal injury almost always has **associated major injuries** of other organs. Their treatment may take precedence.

B. **Most (80%) renal injuries do not require operative treatment.** The hematoma tamponades the bleeding parenchymal vessels and eventually is absorbed, with healing of the injury.

C. **Antibiotics, analgesics,** and **overhydration** to maintain high urine flow are the mainstays of treatment of renal injury.

V. **Indications for operation**

A. **Emergency operation** is indicated for:
1. Devascularization of all or a major segment of the kidney
2. Continued bleeding requiring repeated transfusion
3. Accumulation of clots in the bladder that cannot be managed by catheter irrigation

B. **Delayed operative treatment** is indicated for:
1. Continuing extravasation of urine
2. Recurrent renal bleeding
3. Calcified mass or abscess
4. Aneurysm of the renal artery
5. Hypertension caused by arterial stricture or contracted kidney

VI. **Operative care.** Although every effort is made to preserve as much renal substance as possible, children who require operative treatment are those with the most severe injuries. These may be irreparable and require nephrectomy.

A. **Transabdominal exposure** (not the flank nephrectomy incision) permits control of the vascular pedicle before Gerota's fascia is opened. This maneuver enhances the likelihood of salvage of at least part of a damaged kidney.

B. A **devascularized kidney** can occasionally be salvaged if there is a discrete vascular injury that can be repaired.

C. **Partial nephrectomy** is sometimes possible if only part of the kidney is devascularized.

VII. **Complications**

A. **Early complications**
1. Bleeding
2. Abscess
3. Renal failure
4. Urinary extravasation
5. Urinary ascites

B. **Late complications**
1. Hypertension
2. Calcified hematoma
3. Hydronephrosis
4. Stone formation
5. Renal pseudocyst
6. Arteriovenous fistula
7. Urothorax
8. Urointestinal fistula

III. Prognosis. Most injured kidneys recover completely.

Bibliography

Cass, A. S. Blunt renal trauma in children. *J. Trauma* 23:123, 1983.
Federle, M. P., et al. The role of computed tomography in renal trauma. *Radiology* 141:455, 1981.
Mandour, W. A., et al. Blunt renal trauma in the pediatric patient. *J. Pediatr. Surg.* 16:669, 1981.
Snyder, H. McC. III, and Caldamone, A. A. Genitourinary Injuries. In K. J. Welch, et al. (eds.), *Pediatric Surgery*. Chicago: Year Book, 1986. P. 174.
Thompson, I. M., et al. Results of nonoperative management of blunt renal trauma. *J. Urol.* 118:522, 1977.

104   Burns

I. **Definition.** Each year more than 100,000 children are hospitalized with and 2500–3000 die from burns. The vast majority of burns occur **in the home** and result from preventable accidents. Burns are a common form of **child abuse,** which should always be suspected if the circumstances of the burn incident seem incongruous with the findings. **Scalds** are the most common form of thermal injury under the age of 3, affecting boys twice as frequently as girls. Flame burns are more common after the age of 3 and affect girls and boys with equal frequency.

II. **Pathophysiology**

A. **Severity** of thermal injury is the product of temperature and duration of exposure. Very brief exposure to very high temperature may result in only superficial injury (e.g., flash burn from gasoline explosion), while prolonged immersion in relatively low-temperature hot water can produce a full-thickness burn. Full-thickness injury occurs more readily in young children because of their thinner skin.

B. **Classification** of burns

1. **First degree:** erythema
2. **Second degree:** partial-thickness necrosis
3. **Third degree:** full-thickness destruction of the skin and its appendages

C. **Capillary injury** from a deep second- or third-degree burn results in massive leakage of plasma into the tissues, with rapid formation of **tissue edema.** If the burn is extensive (20% or more), fluid loss depletes the circulating blood volume. **Hypovolemia** results in poor tissue perfusion, anaerobic metabolism, and acidosis.

D. Burn injury creates a **hypermetabolic state** with increased excretion of catecholamines, insulin, glucagon, and other mediators. Protein and caloric needs are increased.

E. **Eschar** formation from a full-thickness burn can limit tissue swelling and cause compression of major blood vessels with resultant **ischemia,** particularly in the extremities. Thoracic eschar can cause respiratory failure.

F. A burn destroys the normal **thermal and vapor barriers** of skin, increasing heat and water loss and causing hypothermia and dehydration.

G. **Dead skin** is a **culture medium** for bacteria, which rapidly multiply if antibiotic prophylaxis is not given.

H. **Immune mechanisms** are impaired by thermal injury. Decreased opsonization, chemotaxis, and neutrophil function increase the patient's susceptibility to infection.

I. **Young children** have special liabilities that make them more susceptible than adults to serious effects from a burn.

1. Body-surface-to-weight ratio (BSA:BW) is higher than in adults, increasing heat and water loss.
2. The lungs are less able to compensate for the markedly increased metabolic demands of injury. Ventilatory assistance may be required.
3. Limited renal capacity to handle osmotic load or large volumes of free water may cause fluid retention.

J. **Closed-space** fires may result in inhalation of hot gases causing airway burns. Products of combustion produce severe chemical injury to the bronchioles and lung.

K. **Electrical burns** produce destruction deep into the tissues with muscle necrosis in addition to skin loss, often much more extensive than initially apparent.

III. **Clinical presentation.** Burns vary tremendously in severity—from a trivial scald to a life-threatening full-thickness flame burn of more than half the body surface.

   A. **Sunburn** is usually a superficial (first-degree) injury, without significant fluid shift or metabolic effect.

   B. **Scalds** in children most commonly result from a toddler reaching up and tipping over a pot of hot liquid on the stove. The injury is typical: scalds of the face, anterior chest, and upper arm. The burn is usually a mix of first and second degree (erythema and blisters), but third-degree injury may occur if duration of contact with the hot liquid is extended by the presence of clothing.

   C. **Flame burns** usually have some areas of full-thickness injury. If the burn affects more than 10% of the body surface, fluid losses are significant and require intravenous replacement.

   D. **Burns of the face and neck** may be associated with inhalation of hot gases, which results in edema and **obstruction of the airway.** Endotracheal intubation may be necessary.

IV. **Diagnosis**

   A. **History** of the circumstances of the burn accident should include the time of injury, the burning substance, and if a flame burn, whether it occurred in a closed space.

Table 104-1. Estimation of percentage of burn by age

Area	< 1 year	1–4	5–9	10–14	15 +
Head	19	17	13	11	9
Neck	2	2	2	2	2
Anterior trunk	13	13	13	13	13
Posterior trunk	13	13	13	13	13
Right buttock	2.5	2.5	2.5	2.5	2.5
Left buttock	2.5	2.5	2.5	2.5	2.5
Genitalia	1	1	1	1	1
Right upper arm	4	4	4	4	4
Left upper arm	4	4	4	4	4
Right lower arm	3	3	3	3	3
Left lower arm	3	3	3	3	3
Right hand	2.5	2.5	2.5	2.5	2.5
Left hand	2.5	2.5	2.5	2.5	2.5
Right thigh	5.5	6.5	8	8.5	9
Left thigh	5.5	6.5	8	8.5	9
Right leg	5	5	5.5	6	6.5
Left leg	5	5	5.5	6	6.5
Right foot	3.5	3.5	3.5	3.5	3.5
Left foot	3.5	3.5	3.5	3.5	3.5

Table 104-2. Clinical diagnosis of burn depth

Depth	Color	Surface	Sensation	Healing	Cause
First degree	Bright red	Dry with focal exfoliation	Painful	3–6 days	Sunburn or flash
Second degree	Red and mottled	Blisters and exudate	Painful	10–21 days	Flash injury, spill scald
Deep second degree	Dark red or pale yellow to off-white	Denuded with minimal exudate	Dim pinprick; intact dermal sensation	More than 3 wk	Scald of long duration; flash of high intensity
Third degree	Very dark red, white, charred, translucent	Leathery, thrombosed dermal vessels	Anesthetic except for deep pressure	Grafting always required	Flame burns; strong chemicals, hot objects, prolonged scalds

B. The **extent** of the burn (%BSA) determines the need for fluid therapy and the risk to life of a full-thickness burn (Table 104-1).

C. The **depth** of the burn determines the risk of infection, the need for skin grafting, and the outcome and functional result (Table 104-2).

D. **First-degree** burns involve the superficial layers only. There is erythema and pain but no blisters. The burn is of little physiologic importance, and there is no need for fluid resuscitation or concern about infection. The child needs only symptomatic care.

E. **Second-degree** burns result from partial destruction of the skin. They may be red and wet, painful, and very sensitive to touch. Deep second-degree burns are less sensitive, and the skin may be pale and stiff. Distinction between deep second-degree and third-degree burns is difficult.

F. **Third-degree** burns result when all of the skin and dermal elements are destroyed. They are dry and leathery; black, brown, or white in color; and anesthetic. Thrombosed blood vessels may be visible through the parchment-like skin.

G. The **typical errors** in evaluation of a burn are overestimation of the extent of the burn and underestimation of its depth.

H. Injury to **other organs** must not be overlooked when evaluating a burn. The **lungs** in particular may be injured from inhalation of products of combustion, which can cause a fatal chemical tracheobronchitis.

V. **Problems**

A. Care of a major burn is a **therapeutic challenge** of considerable magnitude, requiring knowledge, skill, and the devotion of a great deal of time to the patient. The rewards are survival and rehabilitation to a useful life. Care naturally evolves in three stages, each with its special problems: resuscitation, excision and grafting, and rehabilitation.

B. **Resuscitation** requires intravenous replacement of fluids, ensuring an adequate airway, and prevention of ischemic limb damage from eschar compression.

C. **Excision** of the dead skin with replacement by grafting from areas of unburned skin is relatively simple in a small burn but highly complicated and difficult when much of the body surface is destroyed. The major therapeutic challenges during this period are prevention of infection, control of heat and water loss, and maintenance of nutrition.

D. **Rehabilitation** of the severely burned child may take months to years. Plastic revision of scars, regrafting, and mobilization of joints are difficult and time consuming.

VI. **Treatment of minor burns**

A. **Definition.** A partial-thickness burn of no more than 15% of body surface, or a full-thickness burn less than 2% of body surface, that does not involve the face, hands, feet, or perineum in a child over a year old. Scalds or flash burns are the usual causes.

B. **First aid.** Prompt application of cold water. If this is done instantly, many scalds and minor flame burns will result in first- or second-degree injury only.

C. **Treatment.** The burn is cleaned with soap or detergent and water and covered with a bland ointment and protective dressing. Silver sulfadiazine (Silvadene) is effective and prevents infection in deeper injuries. Analgesics are necessary for a few days. Hospitalization is not usually required. Closed treatment (dressing) is advisable in young children to prevent rubbing and contamination. It is sometimes impractical on the face or neck, which can be left exposed.

D. **Blisters** are left intact; they are debrided when they break.

E. **Dressings** are changed daily. The burn is washed gently with soap and warm water, followed by reapplication of silver sulfadiazine. If there is saturation of the dressing with exudate, twice-daily dressing changes may be needed.

F. The burn should be **reexamined** by the physician at 3, 7, and 14 days, by which time a partial-thickness injury should be healed.

G. **Antibiotics** are not needed unless infection develops as indicated by progressive erythema and tenderness extending out from the periphery of the burn.

H. Small areas of **full-thickness burn** are best treated by immediate excision and grafting.

VII. **Initial treatment of major burns**

A. **First aid.** Burning clothing is extinguished by covering the child with a blanket, towel, rug, or coat, or rolling him slowly on the ground. Immediate application of cold water will decrease the depth of the burn injury. No ointments should be applied. The burn is covered and the patient is transported to a center.

B. **Triage** of burns

1. **First-degree** burns seldom require hospitalization.
2. **Second-degree** burns:
   a. <10%: outpatient care
   b. 10–20%: general hospital
   c. >20%: burn center
3. **Third-degree** burns:
   a. <2%: outpatient care
   b. 2–10%: general hospital
   c. >10%: burn center
4. **Complicated burns:** burn center.
   a. Serious burns of hands, feet, face, perineum
   b. Inhalation injury
   c. Severe associated injury (e.g., fractures)
5. **Infants** require hospitalization for all but the smallest burns.

C. Initial assessment

1. **Strip patient** and examine every inch of the body surface.
2. **Evaluate airway.** Suspect airway injury if there is hoarseness, cough, or facial and neck burns, especially around the nose and lips, or if the burn occurred in a closed space.
3. **Evaluate for associated injuries.** They may take precedence.
4. **Start fluids** using a large-bore IV catheter, through burned skin if necessary.
5. **Weigh** child.
6. **Insert urinary catheter** if the burn is greater than 20% and intravenous fluids will be needed.
7. Obtain **chest x-ray** for baseline evaluation.

D. Estimate extent and depth of the burn.
The traditional "rule of nines" is not adequate for children (Table 104-2).

E. Give intravenous fluids
if the extent of the burn is more than 15% of body surface—less than 10% for infants.

1. **Objectives.** To restore blood volume to maintain perfusion.
2. **Crystalloid** (lactated Ringer's solution) works as well as plasma. No glucose is needed because of glucose mobilization due to stress of trauma.
3. **Calculate fluid** requirements by the modified Brooke Army Hospital formula using **entire extent** of burn, both second and third degree:
   a. 3 ml/kg/% burn in 24 hours.
   b. 4 ml/kg/% burn for children under 2.
   c. One-half is given in the first 8 hours, initially very rapidly.
   d. One-half is given in the next 16 hours.
4. **No potassium** is given because of the large amounts released from the injured tissue.
5. **Fluid formulas are first approximations.** Adjust volume according to physiologic response (urine output, pulse, blood pressure, central venous pressure, hematocrit).
6. **Second 24 hours.** Give plasma, since capillaries will now "hold" it and it will help mobilize tissue fluid.
   a. 0.3 ml/kg/% for 30–50% burn
   b. 0.4 ml/kg/% for 50–70% burn
   c. 0.5 ml/kg/% for over 70% burn
7. Give **maintenance** fluids, 5% D/.2NS for metabolic needs, at standard rates after the first day.
8. **Replace evaporative water loss,** 1–2 ml/kg/%/24 hours, also with 5% D/.2NS.
9. **Monitor electrolytes.** Hyponatremia may result from excess free water administration. Hypokalemia may occur during diuretic phase on second or third day.
10. **Transfuse** packed red cells to keep hematocrit above 35.

F. Miscellaneous support

1. **Nasogastric tube** is inserted if the burn is more than 20%, for all patients who have ileus. It can usually be removed at 48 hours.

2. **Cimetidine,** 10 mg/kg q4h, is given to reduce the risk of Curling's ulcer. Gastric acidity is measured q2h, and antacid, 30–60 ml, is given down the tube if pH is less than 5.0.
3. **Tetanus** prophylaxis with toxoid is given if the child has not been immunized in the past 5 years. Nonimmunized patients receive toxin-antitoxin (TAT) and immune globulin.
4. **Antibiotics** are not given unless evidence of cellulitis develops. This usually occurs after the third day and is caused by streptococcal infection, which responds to penicillin. The wound is cultured weekly, as are intravenous catheters, urine, and pulmonary secretions.
5. **Analgesia** is given intravenously as needed.
6. **Nutritional support** should begin on the second day, using tube feedings or TPN. The goal is for the child to maintain basal weight, which often requires more than the usual 100 cal/kg/day and 3 gm/kg/day of protein.

G. Wound care

1. The burn is gently **debrided** and washed with antibacterial detergent once the child is stabilized and fluid resuscitation has been started. Loose tissue and hair are removed. The patient is sedated with IV morphine or fentanyl.
2. **Silver sulfadiazine ointment** is applied, and covered with gauze dressings.
3. The entire burn must be **washed off and inspected daily** by the physician for evidence of sepsis and progress in healing.
4. Burned **hands** are elevated and active motion is carried out for 5 minutes every hour to reduce edema. Fingertips are left exposed to permit evaluation of the circulation.

H. Monitoring

1. **Vital signs.** Pulse, blood pressure, respirations, temperature.
2. **Peripheral circulation.**
3. **Mental state.**
4. **Urine output.** Urine flow should be approximately 1 ml/kg/hour. Higher values may indicate overresuscitation and cause pulmonary edema. Low output is an indication for more fluid, not diuretics.

    Exception: Extra fluid is given to produce a high urine output to facilitate excretion of myoglobin if there is muscle necrosis from deep burns, extensive crush, or electrical injuries.
5. **Hematocrit**
6. Central venous pressure **(CVP)** if burn is more than 50% or if the child's response is sluggish.
7. **Daily weights.** Expect 15–20% gain in the first 24 hours after a major burn. Diuresis begins on the second or third day.

I. Intubate if respiratory failure develops:

1. **Acute upper airway obstruction:** oral or laryngeal edema
2. **Inability to handle secretions** due to inhalation injury
3. Lower airway **inhalation injury** with respiratory failure

J. Treatment of inhalation injury

1. Warm, humidified **oxygen** to treat carbon monoxide inhalation and because of impaired alveolar function

2. **Coughing, suctioning** prn
3. **Bronchoscopy** to remove secretions
4. **Bronchodilators**
5. Intubation and **ventilatory assistance** when needed
6. **Antibiotics** for documented infection (not prophylactic)

K. **Escharotomy** is performed in the first 24 hours if circulation is impaired by the unyielding burned skin. The trunk and extremities are the critical areas.

1. **Cyanosis, delayed capillary refill,** paresthesias, and deep pain are signs of circulatory impairment.
2. Swelling and coolness are not reliable signs.
3. Use of the **Doppler** flowmeter is the best way to assess blood flow, once vascular volume has been restored.
4. Escharotomies are made along the lateral side of the extremity or chest, through the skin to the subcutaneous fat. Fasciotomies are not indicated.

L. **Complications of burns.** Few diseases or injuries are as susceptible to complications as a major burn.

A. **Pneumonia** is the most common cause of death in burned children.
B. **Burn-wound sepsis** may occur in spite of careful use of topical antibacterials. Systemic antibiotics are given according to wound culture results.
C. **Suppurative thrombophlebitis** is a common complication of the prolonged use of intravenous catheters. The usual organism is *Staphylococcus*. The treatment is immediate excision of the vein.
D. **Curlings's ulcer** still occurs in burn patients, although the incidence has been reduced significantly by the use of prophylactic cimetidine. It carries a high mortality from bleeding or perforation. Vagotomy and antrectomy may be necessary.
E. **Psychologic** complications are common because of the stress and pain of the prolonged illness of a major burn.

Coverage of the burn wound

A. **Partial-thickness** wounds heal within 2–3 weeks. Full-thickness eschar separation takes a little longer. Excision of eschar is carried out earlier if the lines of demarcation of a third-degree burn are clear.
B. **Repeated excisions** and skin grafting may take weeks to cover a major burn.
C. **Artificial skin** or heterografts (pigskin) are necessary for temporary coverage in very extensive burns.
D. **Prevention of sepsis** is necessary to prepare the wound for grafting and to maintain the graft afterward.
E. **Nutritional maintenance** is essential during this period—with tube feedings, elemental diets, or total parenteral nutrition (TPN).

Rehabilitation. Return to full function and normal activity may take many months. Experienced physical and occupational therapists and psychologic counselors are essential in this process.

Prognosis. The outlook for meaningful recovery after a major burn has never been better. There should be no mortality with burns of less than 30% of body surface at any age. Survival is often reported with burns of 80–90% of the body, so a full effort is almost always indicated.

Bibliography

Alexander, J. W., et al. Prophylactic antibiotics as an adjunct for skin grafting in clean reconstructive surgery following burn injury. *J. Trauma* 22:687, 1982.

Artz, C. P., Moncrief, J. A., and Pruitt, B. A. *Burns: A Team Approach.* Philadelphia: Saunders, 1979. P. 3.

Boykin, J. V., et al. Cold-water treatment of scald injury and inhibition of histamine mediated burn edema. *J. Surg. Res.* 31:111, 1981.

Bruck, H. M., Asch, M. J., and Pruitt, B. A. Burns in children: A 10-year experience with 412 patients. *J. Trauma* 10:658, 1970.

Charnock, E. L., and Meehan, J. J. Postburn respiratory injuries in children. *Pediatr. Clin. North Am.* 271:661, 1980.

Durtschi, M. B., et al. A prospective study of prophylactic penicillin in acutely burned hospitalized patients. *J. Trauma* 22:11, 1982.

Goodwin, C. W., et al. Randomized trial of efficacy of crystalloid and colloid resuscitation on hemodynamic response and lung water following thermal injury. *Ann. Surg.* 196:520, 1983.

Larson, D., et al. Contracture and scar formation in the burn patient. *Clin. Plast. Surg.* 1:653, 1974.

Leape, L. L. Initial changes in burns. I. Tissue changes in burned and unburned skin of rhesus monkeys. *J. Trauma* 10:488, 1970.

Leape, L. L. Urgency of fluid administration in burn resuscitation. *J. Surg. Res.* 11:513, 1971.

Moncrief, J. A., and Mason, A. D. Evaporative water loss in the burned patient. *J. Trauma* 4:180, 1964.

O'Neill, J. A., Jr. Burns. In T. M. Holder and K. W. Ashcraft (eds.), *Pediatric Surgery.* Philadelphia: Saunders, 1980. P. 123.

O'Neill, J. A. Fluid resuscitation in the burned child: A reappraisal. *J. Pediatr. Surg.* 17:604, 1982.

O'Neill, J. A., Jr. Burns. In K. J. Welch, et al. (eds.), *Pediatric Surgery.* Chicago: Year Book, 1986. P. 220.

Pruitt, B. A., Dowling, J. A., and Moncrief, J. A. Escharotomy in early burn care. *Arch. Surg.* 96:502, 1968.

Pruitt, B. A., O'Neill, J. A., and Moncrief, J. A. Successful control of burn wound sepsis. *J.A.M.A.* 203:1054, 1968.

Raine, P. A., and Azmy, A. A review of thermal injuries in young children. *J. Pediatr. Surg.* 18:21, 1983.

105 Child Abuse

I. **Definition.** Intentional injury of children is a serious societal problem, one that seems to be increasing in frequency.

   A. In addition to receiving deliberate **physical injuries,** children are also victims of **psychologic abuse, nutritional neglect, hygienic neglect,** and deprivation or **delay in medical treatment** for illness. **Sexual abuse** has become a problem of incredible magnitude.

   B. The **incidence** of child abuse is unknown, but the problem clearly afflicts millions of children annually in the United States. It is estimated that 5% of all admissions to emergency rooms result from inflicted injuries.

II. **Social characteristics**

   A. **Most children are injured at home by a family member** or caretaker. A parent is responsible 75% of the time.

   B. **Social and economic stresses** on the parents are key factors in child abuse. It is much more common in lower socioeconomic groups.

   C. **Immature parents** are at high risk of victimizing their children when stressed. Young, single mothers are particularly vulnerable.

   D. **Parents** of abused children frequently have severe **personality disorders** and frequently have been victims themselves.

   E. **Victims** are commonly under the age of **2 years,** although child abuse is seen at every age. Boys are more likely to be victims of physical trauma, girls of sexual abuse.

III. **Clinical presentation**

   A. **An endless variety of symptoms and signs** may be the presenting findings in child abuse. Virtually every kind of disease may be mimicked. Since the history of injury is usually not given, the clinician may not think of inflicted injury as a possible cause.

   B. **Evidence of prior injury** is found in most cases, particularly old cutaneous bruises or abrasions and fractures of the skull and long bones.

   C. **Soft-tissue injuries, fractures, and head injuries are most common,** in that order. Combined injuries are the rule.

   D. **Soft-tissue injuries**

   1. **Ecchymoses, hematomas, abrasions, and burns** are the typical injuries of child abuse. Lacerations are seldom inflicted injuries.

   2. **The pattern is characteristic:** lesions over the cheeks, trunk, genitalia, and upper legs. Orbital hemorrhage may result from blows to the head. Patterns of beating with a coat hanger, belt, or whip may be discernible. Lesions are typically **multiple** and in various stages of healing.

   3. **Burns** are usually from **contact** with a hot object, such as a cigarette or iron, or from immersion in hot water. The pattern may be obviously inconsistent with the story given. Many "accidental" burns represent child abuse in the form of neglect.

   E. **Fractures**

   1. The **association** of **long-bone fractures** and **skull fractures** has long been considered a pathognomonic finding of the "battered child syndrome."

2. The **majority** of abused children with fractures will have old or new **soft-tissue injuries as well.** In suspected abuse, skeletal survey x-rays may uncover old, unreported healed fractures.

3. The **pathology reflects the mechanism of injury:** The child is suddenly twisted, thrown, struck, or violently shaken by the limbs. Epiphyseal separations, metaphyseal fractures, and subperiosteal hemorrhage result. The extent of the injury is out of proportion to the history given.

4. **Multiple lesions** of differing ages are typically found. Big bones are most commonly broken. The order of frequency of bones fractured is humerus, femur, tibia, ulna, radius, vertebrae, fibula, clavicle, scapula, facial bones, ribs.

F. **Head injuries** cause the most deaths and permanent disability.

1. Head injury must always be **suspected** when **soft-tissue injuries** or **fractures** suggestive of child abuse are found.

2. **External findings may be minimal** or those of soft blunt trauma such as hematoma on the side of the head inflicted by a blow of the hand.

3. **Coma** may be the presenting symptom of intracranial hemorrhage caused by shaking, with no evidence of external trauma and no skull fracture. If extradural hematoma is present, the child can deteriorate rapidly.

G. **Visceral trauma** is present in about 15% of hospitalized abused children; it carries a high mortality since it is frequently neglected and treatment delayed.

1. Common **abdominal injuries** are liver and kidney fractures, intramural hematoma of the duodenum, ruptured pancreas, perforations of the bowel, and mesenteric tears.

2. **Thoracic injuries** include lung contusion and pneumothorax.

IV. Diagnosis

A. **Child abuse** should be suspected in any child with trauma in whom the **history** is **inconsistent** with the physical findings. Discovery of old injuries for which there are inadequate explanations is a suspicious finding.

B. **Association** of **soft-tissue injuries** and multiple **fractures** is highly suggestive of child abuse, particularly if the lesions are of **different ages** or there are prior injuries.

C. **Skull and skeletal survey x-rays** are obtained if the pattern of injury is consistent with child abuse.

D. **Suspicious findings** require further investigation of the past history of injuries and an evaluation of the **home situation.**

E. **Physical findings must be carefully documented.** In addition to obvious injuries, there may be evidence of physical neglect, e.g., the child is dirty and malnourished.

F. **Abnormal parental behavior** is strong evidence for child abuse. Apparent detachment or inappropriate overreaction, reluctance to provide information, refusal to consent to diagnostic studies, and hostility to the physician are highly suggestive characteristics. The parents may complain about irrelevant problems or blame the injury on a sibling of the patient. They may be difficult to find after the child is hospitalized.

G. **Behavior of the victim** may also be a clue to child abuse. The child may be unusually fearful or display no emotion at all.

H. **Radiographic features** of inflicted trauma

1. Multiple fractures of different ages

2. Exaggerated periosteal reaction
3. Metaphyseal fragmentation and epiphyseal separation
4. Fractures associated with violent twists, jerks, or shakes
5. Unexplained skeletal fractures associated with skull fractures or subdural hematomas

Treatment

A. **Suspected child abuse** must, by law, be reported to the proper state or municipal authorities. It is essential that even unproved cases be referred for further investigation since the natural history of child abuse is that it recurs. The physician is protected from suit for false accusation in every state.

B. The **child should be admitted** to the hospital for protection during the investigation. This often can be done for the purpose of care without officially taking custody.

C. The **natural reaction** of physicians and nurses to child abuse is anger at the parents and the desire to protect the child by taking him away from them. This is sometimes necessary but often nonproductive, since it seldom alters parental behavior, and the child will amost always ultimately be returned to the home.

D. **Counseling, support,** and correction of difficult social and economic conditions is more likely to change behavior. The physician should not be judgmental, but helpful. Abusing parents need help and most are anxious to receive it.

Bibliography

Caffey, J. Multiple fractures in the long bones of infants suffering from chronic subdural hematoma. *Am. J. Roentgenol.* 56:167, 1946.

Caffey, J. The whiplash shaken infant syndrome: Manual shaking of the extremities with whiplash-induced intracranial and intraocular bleedings, linked with residual permanent brain damage and mental retardation. *Pediatrics* 54:396, 1974.

DeJong, A. R., Emmett, G. A., and Hervada, A. R. Sexual abuse of children. *Am. J. Dis. Child.* 136:129, 1982.

Hebeler, J. R. The Abused Child. In T. M. Holder and K. W. Ashcraft (eds.), *Pediatric Surgery*. Philadelphia: Saunders, 1980. P. 94.

Kempe, C. H., et al. The battered child syndrome. *J.A.M.A.* 181:17, 1962.

Kempe, C. H., and Helfer, R. E. *Helping the Battered Child and His Family*. Philadelphia: Lippincott, 1972.

O'Neill, J. A., Jr. Child Abuse. In K. J. Welch, et al. (eds.), *Pediatric Surgery*. Chicago: Year Book, 1986. P. 138.

O'Neill, J. A., et al. Patterns of injury in the battered child syndrome. *J. Trauma* 13:332, 1973.

Touloukian, R. J. Abdominal visceral injuries in battered children. *Pediatrics* 42:642, 1968.

IX
Common Procedures

Vascular Access

I. Umbilical artery catheterization

A. Indications. Umbilical artery access is indicated in the critically ill neonate who requires continuous or frequent monitoring of arterial blood gases or arterial pressure. Because of the risk of complications, it should not be used for more than a week, nor for fluid infusion except in an emergency.

B. Technique

1. Equipment
   a. Cutdown set: 4 fine hemostats, scalpel with No. 15 blade, scissors, fine-toothed and plain forceps, needle holder, probe, 3-ml syringes, sponges, sterile towels
   b. Umbilical tape or heavy (0) ligature
   c. Umbilical artery catheter, size 3½F or 5F
2. Use the distance from the shoulder to the umbilicus as a rough guide to the length of catheter to be inserted so that the tip of the catheter is in the desired position just above the diaphragm. Place a tie around the catheter to mark the length.
3. Prepare the cord and abdomen with antiseptic solution and drape with sterile towels.
4. Place an umbilical tape around the base of the cord and tie it loosely.
5. Amputate the cord with a scalpel 1 cm from the skin.
6. Identify the two arteries and gently introduce a probe into one to dilate it. Leave it in for one minute.
7. Insert the saline-filled catheter and advance it the predetermined distance. If the catheter will not pass into the aorta or if the leg turns blue, remove the catheter and try the other artery.
8. Tie down the tape or ligature, then fix the catheter in place with a separate suture into the skin and around the catheter.
9. Apply antibiotic ointment and secure catheter with tape to skin.
10. Connect the catheter to a continuous infusion of heparinized saline (1 U/ml).
11. Verify via x-ray that the catheter tip is above the diaphragm.

C. Complications

1. **Thromboembolism.** Thrombosis of the iliac artery can result in loss of a leg or paraplegia. Thrombosis in the aorta can cause hypertension, renal failure, or mesenteric ischemia.
2. **Perforation** of the umbilical or iliac artery.
3. **Necrotizing enterocolitis** from spasm or thrombosis of the aorta or mesenteric arteries.
4. **Hemorrhage** from accidental dislodgment or disconnection of the catheter.
5. **Omphalitis** from infection at the catheter site. Extension into the umbilical vein can cause portal vein thrombosis.

II. Radial artery cutdown

A. Indications. An arterial cutdown is necessary when frequent arterial blood sampling is required and neither an umbilical catheter nor percutaneous puncture can be used.

1. Patients receiving ventilatory assistance, especially when beginning ventilation and when weaning
2. Critically ill patients requiring constant monitoring of arterial pressure, frequent blood sampling, and repeated arterial blood gas determinations

B. Technique

1. Equipment
   a. Cutdown set: 4 fine hemostats, scalpel with No. 15 blade, scissors, fine-toothed and plain forceps, needle holder, 3-ml syringes, sponges, sterile towels
   b. Sutures and ligatures of 4-0 absorbable material (Vicryl or polyglycolic acid [Dexon])
   c. Angiocath or similar needle-catheter, size 20 or 22, with stopcock and heparinized saline solution
2. Tape the baby's hand to a padded armboard with the wrist hyperextended over a gauze roll.
3. Prepare the skin with antibacterial solution and drape with sterile towels.
4. Locate the artery by palpation of the pulse in the groove just medial to the radial styloid. If the pulse cannot be palpated, use a Doppler pulse detector or transillumination.
5. Infiltrate 1% lidocaine into the overlying skin.
6. Prepare the ligatures, suture, and needle-catheter. Attach the stopcock to the needle, fill it with heparinized saline, and leave the syringe attached.
7. Make a small transverse incision in the skin crease overlying the artery.
8. Expose the artery by blunt dissection of the soft tissues with a hemostat opening it parallel to the artery.
9. Pass a ligature around the artery and secure it with a hemostat. Do not tie it.
10. Holding the ligature on traction, puncture the artery with the needle catheter, bevel down, and thread the catheter into the artery for 1–2 cm. Good pulsatile flow of red blood should be obtained. Remove the needle.
11. Flush the catheter and attached stopcock with heparin-saline and close the stopcock.
12. Unless there is leakage around the catheter, remove the traction ligature.
13. Close the wound with several simple sutures.
14. Apply antibiotic ointment and a sterile dressing to the exit site of the catheter.
15. Tape the dressing and the catheter in place before connecting to monitoring tubing to avoid accidental dislodgment.
16. Connect to continuous-infusion transducer tubing.

C. Complications

1. **Ischemia of the hand** may occur from vasospasm or from thrombosis secondary to the placement of the catheter. If the ulnar artery is small, occl-

sion of the radial artery may not permit sufficient blood supply to the hand. The catheter must be removed.

2. **Accidental dislodgment** or disconnection is more hazardous with an arterial line than a venous one since severe hemorrhage can occur. The patient should not be left unattended, and the catheter should be removed once frequent sampling is no longer needed.

3. The arterial line should not be used to infuse fluids, drugs, or blood products because of the hazard of permanent arterial damage and ischemia.

Venous cutdown

A. Indications. Insertion of a catheter in a vein by surgical exposure is indicated when percutaneous puncture has failed and in emergency situations when prompt venous access is required.

B. Technique

1. Equipment

   a. Cutdown set: 4 fine hemostats, scalpel with No. 15 blade, scissors, fine-toothed and plain forceps, needle holder, 3-ml syringes, sponges, sterile towels.

   b. Sutures and ligatures of 4-0 absorbable material (Vicryl or polyglycolic acid).

   c. Intravenous catheter of appropriate size. A large catheter is less likely to kink off or plug (size 20 for a newborn).

2. Sites

   a. Saphenous vein at the ankle—lateral to the medial malleolus, between it and the extensor tendons.

   b. Cephalic vein at the elbow—in the antecubital space.

3. Position the extremity and tape it to a padded board.
4. Prepare the skin with antibacterial solution and drape with sterile towels.
5. Infiltrate 1% lidocaine into the overlying skin.
6. Prepare the ligatures, suture, and catheter. Fill the catheter with saline and leave the syringe attached.
7. Make a small transverse incision in the skin crease overlying the vein.
8. Expose the vein by blunt dissection of the soft tissues under the skin with a hemostat, opening it parallel to the vein. Veins are superficial to the fascia. (The brachial artery is deep to the fascia in the antecubital space.)
9. Pass proximal and distal ligatures around the vein and secure them with hemostats. Do not tie them.
10. Holding the distal ligature on traction, incise the anterior wall of the vein by pinching it up in the smooth forceps and cutting upward with the scalpel to avoid accidentally transecting the vein.
11. Insert the catheter, uncut, so it does not have a sharp leading edge, and pass it 2–3 cm up the vein. Do not advance it beyond the next joint.
12. Aspirate blood. If none is obtained, adjust the position of the catheter. If the patient is in shock, there may be no return of blood, but saline can be infused easily.
13. Tie down the ligatures after also passing the distal one around the catheter to give additional fixation and to permit the vein to recanalize after the catheter is removed.

14. Close the wound with several simple sutures.
15. Apply antibiotic ointment and a sterile dressing to the exit site of the catheter.
16. Tape the dressing and catheter in place before connecting the catheter to intravenous tubing to avoid accidental dislodgment.

C. Complications
1. Accidental **division** of the vein. Avoid by incising with the scalpel only the anterior half, which is held with forceps, not by using scissors.
2. **Perforation** of the vein by the catheter. Avoid by not trimming or tapering the catheter, which gives it a spearlike point.

IV. Central venous catheter insertion.
Either the internal jugular or the subclavian vein may be used. Both are more easily approached from the left side.

A. Indications
1. For monitoring central venous pressure in patients who are hemodynamically unstable or who are receiving large volumes of fluids.
2. For administration of parenteral nutrition when peripheral access is difficult or weight gain is unsatisfactory using peripheral solutions

B. Technique of internal jugular catheterization.
1. Equipment. Central line kit with guide wire, dilator, introducer, and catheter of appropriate size.
2. Position
    a. The patient is placed in the Trendelenburg (head down) position to fill the veins and minimize the danger of air aspiration.
    b. The head is hyperextended by placing a small roll behind the shoulders.
    c. The arms are pulled toward the feet and taped in place.
    d. The face should point straight up.
3. Use an overhead radiant heater for infants to maintain their temperature.
4. Prepare the neck with antibacterial solution and drape with sterile towels
5. Infiltrate 1% lidocaine into the skin medial to the left sternomastoid muscle at the junction of the middle and lower thirds.
6. Standing behind and to the left of the patient, retract the sternomastoid muscle laterally with the gloved left hand until the carotid pulse is felt directly below.
7. Puncture the skin just medial to the fingers of the left hand and advance the needle deep to the fingers, almost parallel to the skin, aiming toward the umbilicus.
8. If blood is not obtained, slowly back the needle out until blood returns. If unsuccessful, repeat the process at a slightly greater angle.
9. When blood is obtained, disconnect the syringe, pass the guide wire into the needle, and advance the wire into the atrium.
10. Pass the dilator over the wire, remove the wire, introduce the catheter, and remove the dilator.
11. Connect the catheter to a syringe, note full and easy aspiration and infusion of blood, and connect to intravenous line.
12. Obtain x-ray to verify that the tip of the catheter is in the atrium. Catheter

may be filled with contrast material if necessary. Adjust position of the catheter.
13. Suture the catheter in place.
14. Apply antibiotic ointment and a sterile dressing.
15. Tape the catheter securely to prevent dislodgment.

C. Technique of insertion of subclavian central venous catheter
1. Equipment and position are the same as for placement of an internal jugular catheter.
2. Prepare the skin of the neck and chest with antibacterial solution and drape with sterile towels.
3. Infiltrate 1% lidocaine into the skin beneath the midpoint of the clavicle.
4. Puncture the skin at the midpoint of the clavicle along the undersurface and advance the needle, aiming it toward the cricoid, applying suction on the syringe.
5. Never change the direction of the needle once it is beneath the clavicle, as this motion may result in a laceration of the vein, artery, or pleura.
6. Once blood is obtained, advance the needle, then remove the syringe and introduce the guide wire.
7. Pass the dilator over the wire, remove the wire, introduce the catheter, and remove the dilator.
8. Verify position and secure catheter in place as described previously under jugular catheter placement.

D. Complications of central venous catheters
1. **Air embolus.** Deep inspiration by the patient after the needle is in the vein and detached can result in aspiration of air into the heart. This mishap can be prevented by placement of the finger over the end of the open needle.
2. **Pneumothorax** can occur if the lung is lacerated (not merely punctured) by misdirection and motion of the needle. Simple puncture of the pleura will not produce a pneumothorax unless the needle is open to the atmosphere.
3. **Hemothorax** can result from laceration of the vein or artery and the pleura.
4. **Hydrothorax** occurs if the catheter is placed into the pleural space—either directly or through the vein wall—and intravenous fluid is infused.
5. **Thromboembolism** may result from atrial thrombi at the end of the catheter.
6. **Catheter sepsis** with bacteremia results from inadequate aseptic precautions during the insertion of the catheter or inadequate care of the entry site thereafter. The incidence of infection increases if the catheter is left in for a long time.

107 Endotracheal Intubation

A. **Indications.** The indication for endotracheal intubation is the inability of the child to ventilate adequately or maintain a patent airway without assistance. Possible causes include:
   1. Airway obstruction
   2. CNS disease, seizures, or trauma depressing respiration
   3. Neuromuscular incoordination or excessive secretions making maintenance of an open airway difficult
   4. Apnea
   5. Cardiac arrest
   6. Severe illness
   7. Labored breathing
   8. Prematurity

B. **Technique**
   1. **Equipment**
      a. A **laryngoscope** of appropriate size. Clinicians other than anesthetists usually find a straight blade easier to use than a curved one.
      b. **Suction** with catheter of proper size attached.
      c. Curved **Magill forceps.**
      d. **Ambu bag,** mask, connectors, tubing, and oxygen for ventilation before and after tube insertion.
      e. A selection of **endotracheal tubes** of appropriate size and length: full-term infant = 3.0 mm; premature infant over 1200 gm = 2.5 mm; infant under 1200 gm = 2.0 mm. In older children, the caliber of the patient's little finger is a reasonable first approximation.
   2. **Position.** Unlike adults, infants and children are more easily intubated in the **flat supine** position, not hyperextended. An assistant holds the shoulders flat against the table and stabilizes the head in the neutral position, preventing side-to-side motion. The operator stands at the head looking toward the patient's feet.
   3. The child is **preoxygenated** by mask ventilation before intubation. Secretions are aspirated.
   4. The **laryngoscope** is held with the left hand and inserted into the right side of the mouth and then to the midline, pushing the tongue out of the way.
   5. A straight **upward pull** against the tongue, taking care not to lever against the upper teeth or gums, is the best way to visualize the larynx.
   6. The tip of the laryngoscope is advanced to the **base** of the epiglottis, not over it as in adults, using upward pressure to reveal the glottis. If visualization is difficult, the assistant should push down the larynx externally.
   7. The **endotracheal tube** is held with the right hand, inserted between the vocal cords, and advanced 2 cm. Magill forceps may be used in guiding the tube. The tube should go in easily. If it is a tight fit, it should be replaced with a smaller tube so the airway is not injured.

8. If the tube is in the airway, the patient cannot phonate and the tube fogs up with each exhalation.
9. The **position** of the tube is checked by auscultation of the chest. If it is correct, satisfactory and equal ventilation of both lungs will be heard.
10. The tube is taped in place securely.
11. Chest x-ray is obtained to verify position of the tube.
12. Prolonged attempts at intubation are very hazardous if the patient is not breathing. Mask ventilation should be interspersed with attempts to intubate in this situation. Oxygen can be supplied to the oropharynx during intubation.

C. **Complications and errors**
1. **Hyperextension** of the head. Although this position is used in adults, it makes intubation more difficult in infants.
2. **Loss of incisor teeth** or laceration of the gums by prying action of the laryngoscope blade. (Lift, do not angulate.)
3. **Overinsertion** of the endotracheal tube with passage into the right mainstem bronchus.
4. **Use of a tube that is too large.** Pressure at the level of the cricoid cartilage causes necrosis, and later, subglottic stricture.

108   Thoracentesis and Tube Thoracostomy

I. Thoracentesis

A. Indications. If **tension pneumothorax** is present, needle aspiration is performed as an emergency lifesaving procedure while preparations are made for insertion of a chest tube. Other indications include:

1. Diagnosis of pleural effusion
2. Treatment of pleural effusion
3. Treatment of pneumothorax

B. Technique

1. **Equipment.** Angiocath vascular catheter, size 20 or 22, with indwelling needle, three-way stopcock, 20- 50-ml syringe, 1% lidocaine local analgesic.

2. **Position**

   a. **Patient**

   (1) Pneumothorax: Supine

   (2) Pleural effusion: sitting

   b. **Needle**

   (1) Pneumothorax: the **second intercostal space** in the midclavicular line.

   (2) **Pleural effusion: midaxillary line** at the level of the nipple for free fluid. If the fluid is sequestered, the needle is inserted where appropriate.

3. **Prepare** the skin with an alcohol wipe or other antibacterial solution, and inject 1% lidocaine into the skin, muscle, and subpleural space. (Omit use of lidocaine in tiny premature infants or if the child is in extremis.)

4. Attach the needle-catheter to a three-way stopcock and syringe.

5. **Puncture** the skin, advance the needle tip over the top of the rib to avoid the intercostal vessels, and puncture the pleura.

6. When air is aspirated, **remove the needle,** reattach the stopcock and syringe to the catheter, and advance the catheter 1–2 cm. Aspirate all of the air by syringe.

7. Remove the needle-catheter once the air or fluid is aspirated. If there is **continuing air leak** or **purulent fluid,** insert **a chest tube.** The vascular catheter is too small for continuous drainage.

C. Complications

1. **Laceration of an intercostal vessel.** Avoid by staying close to the upper surface of the rib during insertion of the needle.

2. Puncture of the **liver** or **spleen** if the puncture site is too low.

3. Laceration of the **lung** with continuing air leak. A chest tube must be inserted. Use of an Angiocath needle-catheter minimizes the risk of lung laceration.

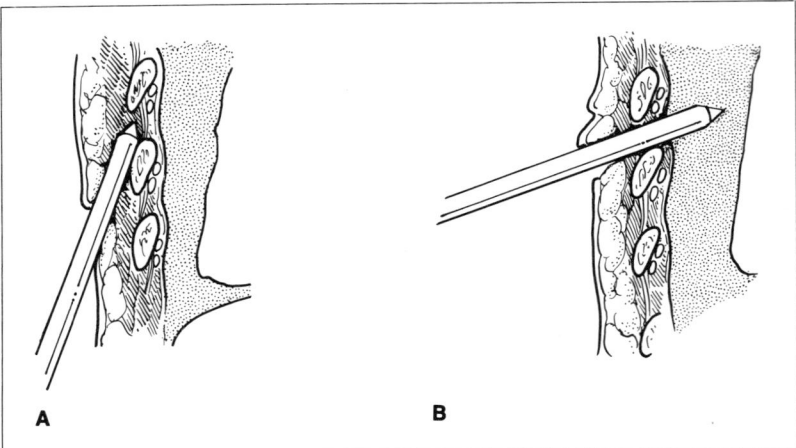

Fig. 108-1. Insertion of chest tube. A. After the trocar is inserted through a small skin incision, it is advanced cephalad one interspace. B. The trocar is then directed perpendicular to the chest wall, entering the pleura along the top edge of the rib to avoid the blood vessels that course along the inferior edge of the rib.

4. **"Dry tap"** when aspirating for fluid. If localization of a loculated pleural effusion is difficult, ultrasound or fluoroscopy can be used to direct the needle accurately.

II. Chest-tube insertion

A. Indications

1. Pneumothorax with continuing air leak
2. Pleural effusion or empyema
3. Traumatic hemothorax or pneumothorax
4. Postoperative chest surgery

B. Technique (Fig. 108-1)

1. **Equipment**
   a. **Thoracostomy set** with hemostats, scissors, scalpel, needle holder, 2-0 sutures, 1% lidocaine.
   b. **Catheter** of appropriate size: 10F for premature infant, 12F for full-term infant, up to 24F for larger child. Large tubes are needed if there is continued bleeding.
2. Position: as for thoracentesis.
3. After **skin preparation** with antibacterial solution, infiltrate lidocaine into the skin at the incision site and into the intercostal space above.
4. Make a **1-cm incision** parallel to the rib in the **midaxillary line at the level of the nipple.**
5. Place a **hemostat** on the tube **2 cm** from the end to prevent overinsertion.
6. **Advance** tube with trocar through skin incision and then cephalad parallel to the surface to make a subcutaneous tunnel up over the **top edge of the rib** above the skin incision.

7. Directing the tube and trocar perpendicular to the chest wall, **puncture the fascia and pleura.** This requires a surprising amount of pressure. A "pop" is felt when the tube enters.

8. **Advance** the tube the full 2 cm while **withdrawing the trocar.** The tube will "fog up" if in the pleural space.

9. **If a trocar is not available,** a hemostat is used to form the subcutaneous tunnel and puncture into the pleural space. (Note: use a "mosquito" hemostat, not a Kelly clamp.) The tube is inserted by grasping the end in the hemostat and directing the clamp and tube into the pleural space.

10. Connect the tube to a **Pleur-evac water seal suction device** with -15 to -20 cm H_2O suction and 2 cm H_2O water seal.

11. **Suture tube in place with heavy (2-0) suture,** tied around the tube with a surgeon's knot that visibly indents the tube. Apply a small gauze dressing and secure it and the tube with **adhesive tape to prevent accidental dislodgment.** Do not rely on the suture to keep the tube in.

12. **Tape the tube connections** securely to prevent accidental disconnection, and tape the tube to the patient's chest or lateral abdomen for extra security.

13. **AP and lateral chest x-rays** are obtained to confirm that the tube is in the proper position and that it has evacuated the air.

C. Complications

1. **Overinsertion or underinsertion of the tube.** Avoid by use of clamp or by premarking the length to be inserted.

2. Placement of the tube in the **subcutaneous** space. Avoid by applying pressure perpendicular to the chest wall at the time of puncture.

3. **Laceration of an intercostal vessel.** Avoid by staying close to the upper surface of the rib during insertion of the tube.

4. **Accidental dislodgment** or disconnection. Avoid by adequate taping of the tube and all connections.

5. **Occlusion** of the tube, which may result from coagulating effusion or clotted blood. Often it can be aspirated or irrigated clear, but sometimes replacement of the tube is necessary.

6. **Leakage** of fluid around the tube. This usually indicates the tube is plugged or not properly positioned.

7. **Subcutaneous emphysema.** This results from air leakage caused by improper positioning, location of a side hole of the tube in the subcutaneous space, inadequate suction, or a plugged tube.

109 Peritoneal Lavage

A. Indications
1. Evaluation of abdominal **trauma**
2. Peritoneal dialysis for **renal failure** or **poisonings**

B. Technique (Fig. 109-1)
1. **Equipment.** Suture set with hemostats, scissors, needle holders, forceps, scalpel, sponges, and 2-0 Vicryl sutures; 1% lidocaine; peritoneal dialysis catheter; lactated Ringer's solution and sterile intravenous tubing.
2. **Position.** Supine.
3. **Empty the bladder** by insertion of a catheter.
4. Prepare the infraumbilical region with antibacterial solution; drape the abdomen; infiltrate lidocaine into the skin, fascia, and peritoneum. (Omit the local anesthetic if patient is unconscious.)
5. Make a midline 2-cm incision just caudal to the umbilicus and extend it to open the peritoneum. Identify the edges of the peritoneum and grasp them with a hemostat on each side.
6. Insert dialysis catheter aiming toward the pelvis on the left or right side.
7. Test catheter for patency and for ease of infusing and aspirating fluid.
8. Suture peritoneum closed tightly around catheter with a pursestring suture of 2-0 Vicryl. Close fascia and skin with similar sutures. Suture the catheter to the skin.
9. Apply a small gauze dressing and secure it and the tube with adhesive tape.
10. **Peritoneal lavage for trauma**
    a. If **blood** is obtained when the catheter is inserted, the diagnosis is established and no lavage is needed.
    b. If blood is not obtained, lactated Ringer's solution is infused, 15 ml/kg, and allowed to drain out.
    c. **Lavage is positive** if the fluid contains:
       (1) Greater than 75,000 RBCs/ml
       (2) Greater than 500 WBCs/ml
       (3) Bile or intestinal contents
    d. The catheter is removed and the peritoneum and fascia are closed with a single running 2-0 Vicryl suture, followed by skin sutures.

C. Complications
1. **Improper placement** of the catheter outside the peritoneal space. The "open" technique described prevents this error.
2. **Failure of infusate to drain.** This is caused by improper catheter position or occlusion with omentum. Repositioning of the catheter is needed. Occasionally, the catheter must be replaced.

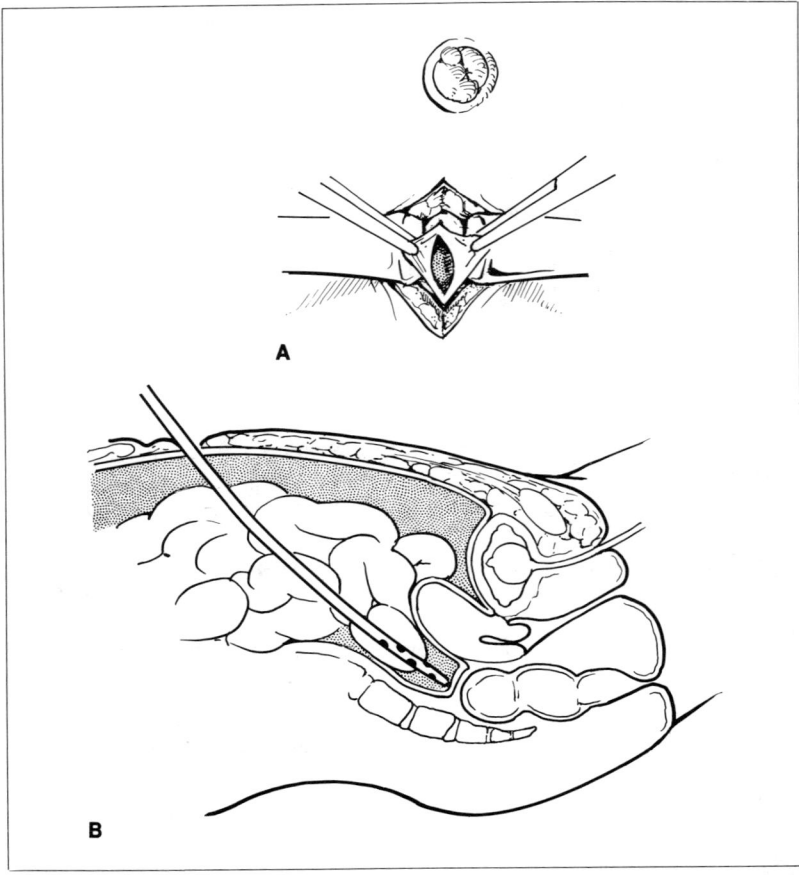

Fig. 109-1. Peritoneal lavage. A. A small incision is made in the midline just inferior to umbilicus. The peritoneum is incised and the edges are grasped with hemostats. B. Position of the lavage catheter in the cul-de-sac.

3. **Bleeding** from catheter trauma to omentum or mesentery. This usually stops spontaneously; it is seldom severe enough to require an operation.
4. **Leakage** of infusate around the catheter. This usually can be corrected by placement of an additional suture or two in the skin or fascia.

110 Bladder Aspiration

A. **Indications.** Percutaneous needle aspiration of the bladder is performed to **obtain a sterile urine specimen** for culture when a urinary tract infection is suspected.
   1. Compared to catheterization via the urethra, bladder aspiration is **less painful,** easier to perform, and less likely to yield a contaminated specimen.
   2. Bladder tap specimens are obtained whenever the child is **unable to cooperate** sufficiently to provide a "clean catch" specimen, i.e., **all infants and most children under the age of 3.** "Bag" specimens should not be used for urine cultures since contamination frequently occurs, making interpretation of a positive culture difficult.
   3. A tap should not be performed if the infant has recently voided.

B. **Technique**
   1. **Equipment.** A size 20–22, 1½-inch needle, attached to a 3- to 10-ml syringe.
   2. **Position.** Supine with legs held by an assistant.
   3. The suprapubic area is prepared with alcohol or other suitable prep solution.
   4. The center of the pubic bone is located by touch, and the needle is introduced through the skin perpendicular to the table, just grazing the superior surface of the pubis.
   5. The plunger of the syringe is pulled back as the needle is introduced in order to aspirate urine as soon as the bladder is entered.
   6. If no urine is obtained after the needle has been introduced to the hub, the needle is slowly withdrawn, maintaining suction.
   7. A second attempt may be made aiming the needle toward the coccyx; if that is unsuccessful, further attempts should be delayed for an hour or two until the bladder fills.
   8. A Band-Aid is applied to the puncture site. Bathing and the use of diapers do not need to be restricted.

C. **Complications.** Bladder tap is a safe procedure with little risk.
   1. Transient, mild hematuria may occur. No treatment is necessary.
   2. Puncture of the rectum will yield stool (and a contaminated culture if not recognized). It is harmless and requires no treatment.

X Appendixes

A Drug Dosages

Resuscitation medications

Drug	Single dose (/per kg)	Route	Comment
Atropine	0.03 mg	IV/IC/IT	
Bicarbonate	1–2 mEq	IV/IC	
Calcium Cl	0.3 ml	IV/IC	
Calcium gluconate	1 ml	IV/IC	
Dobutamine	2–20 μg/min	IV	Infusion
Dopamine	2–20 μg/min	IV	Infusion
Epinephrine	0.1 ml, 1:10,000	IV/IC/IT	
	0.1 μg/min	IV	Infusion
Ephedrine	0.1 mg/min	IV	Infusion
Glucose, 50%	1 ml	IV/IC	
Isoproterenol	1 μg/min	IV	Infusion
Lidocaine	1 mg	IV/IC/IT	
	20–40 μg/min	IV	Infusion
Nitroprusside	1–4 μg/min	IV	Infusion

IC = Intracardiac; IT = Intratracheal.

Antibiotics

Drug	Single dose (/per kg)	Route	Frequency Newborn	Frequency Child	Comment
Amoxicillin	25–100 mg	PO/IM/IV	—	4id	
Ampicillin	25–100 mg	PO/IM/IV	q12h	q6h	
Bactrim	4 mg[a]	PO	—	q12h	q6h for pneumocystis
Carbenicillin	100 mg	IV/IM	q12h	q6h	
Cefazolin	10–20 mg	IM/IV	—	q12h	
Cefoxitin	20–40 mg	IM/IV	q8h	q8h	
Cephalothin	20 mg	IM/IV	q12h	q8h	
Chloramphenicol	25 mg	PO/IM/IV	q24h	q6h	Check blood levels[b]
Clindamycin	5 mg	IM/IV	q8h	q6h	
Erythromycin	5–10 mg	PO/IM/IV	q6h	q6h	
Gentamycin	2.5 mg	IM/IV	q12h	q8h	Check blood levels[c]
Kanamycin	3–5 mg	IM/IV	q12h	q12h	
	100 mg	PO	—	q2h	Preop bowel prep.
Nystatin	100,000 U	PO	q6h	—	
	2% ointment	topic	4id	—	
Oxacillin	25–50 mg	IM/IV	q12h	q6h	
Penicillin	25–50,000 U	PO/IM/IV	q12h	q6h	
Ticarcillin	35–50 mg	IM/IV	q12h	q8h	
Tobramycin	2.5 mg	IM/IV	q12h	q8h	Check blood levels[c]
Vancomycin	15 mg	IM/IV	q12h	q8h	Check blood levels[d]

[a] Dose based on content of trimethoprim.
[b] Peak: 10–20 μg/ml 3 hr after administration.
[c] Peak: 4–8 μg/ml 1 hr after administration.
Trough: <2 μg/ml preceding next dose.
[d] Peak: 25–40 μg/ml 1 hr after administration.
Trough: 12 μg/ml preceding next dose.

Other Commonly Used Drugs

Drug	Single dose (/per kg)	Route	Frequency	Comment
Aldactone	1 mg	PO	q8h	
Aminophylline	5 mg	IV	over 20 min	Repeat prn
	1–1.4 mg/hr	IV	Infusion	TL: 10–20 µg/ml
Aspirin	10–15 mg	PO/PR	q4h	
Benadryl	1 mg	PO/IV	q4–6h	
Bronkosol	0.5 ml/2 ml NS	IN	prn	By nebulizer
Chloral hydrate	50 mg	PO/PR	q4–8h	
Cimetidine	10 mg	PO/IV	q6h	
Decadron	1 mg	IM/IV	q8h	
Demerol	1 mg	IM/IV	q3h	
Diazoxide	5 mg	IV STAT		
Digoxin	40 µg TDD	IV	1/2 STAT	Digitalizing dose
		IV	1/4 at 8h	
		IV	1/4 at 16h	
	5 µg	PO/IM/IV	bid	Maintenance dose
Dilantin	10 mg	IV	loading	
	2.5 mg	PO/IV	bid	TL: 10–20 µg/ml
Diuril	10–15 mg	PO	q12h	
Droperidol	0.1 mg	IM/IV	q8h	
Epinephrine	0.01 ml	SQ	STAT	Bronchodilator
Fentanyl	2–5 µg	IV	q1–2h	Ventilatory assistance
Glucagon	0.025–0.1 mg	SQ/IM/IV	STAT	Repeat q20 min
Heparin	100 U	IV	Bolus	Monitor coagulation
Hydralazine	0.1–0.2 mg	IM/IV	q4–6h	
Insulin	0.1 U/hr	IV	Infusion	
Kayexalate	1 gm	PO	prn	1 gm exchanges
	2 gm	PR	prn	1 mEq K^+ for 2 mEq Na^+
Lasix	1 mg	PO/IM/IV	STAT	
Mannitol	0.24–1.0 gm	IV	Bolus	
Morphine	0.1 mg	IM/IV	q3h	
Narcan	0.01 mg	IV	STAT	Narcotic reversal
Nembutal	2–3 mg	PO/IM/IV	hs	
Pavulon	0.1 mg	IV	q1–2h	Ventilatory assistance
Phenobarbital	10 mg	IV	loading	
	2.5 mg	PO/IV	BID	TL: 20–40 µg/ml
Pitressin	0.005 U/min	IV	Infusion	Max: 0.4 U/min
Prednisone	1 mg	PO	q8h	

Table (Continued)

Drug	Single dose (/per kg)	Route	Frequency	Comment
Pronestyl	2 mg	IV	over 5 min	Repeat q10–30 min
Propranolol	0.01–0.1 mg	IV	STAT	
Prostigmine	0.06 mg	IV	STAT	Atropine first
Racemic epinephrine	0.5 ml/4 ml NS	IN	STAT	Nebulizer
Solucortef	10 mg	IV	q4–6h	
Solumedrol	30 mg	IV	STAT, q2h	Shock dose
Succinylcholine	1–1.5 mg	IV	prn	Ventilatory assistance
Tylenol	10–15 mg	PO/PR	q4h	
Valium	0.1 mg	IV	prn	

TL = therapeutic level; NS = normal saline.

B Normal Laboratory Values

Blood	Premature infant Birth	1 Month	Newborn	Child	Units
HCT	45–65	33–45	45–65	31–43	%
Hb	14–24	11–15	14–24	13–15	gm/dl
WBC	6–32	8–17	9–30	5–10	$\times 1000/mm^3$
Platelets	150–400	150–400	150–400	150–400	$\times 1000/mm^3$
PT	14–22	12–16	13–20	12–14	sec
PTT	35–55	—	30–45	25–35	sec
Fibrinogen	150–300	150–300	150–300	150–300	mg/dl
Na	133–146	133–148	130–160	135–144	mEq/L
K	4.6–6.7	4.5–6.6	5.2–7.7	4.0–5.5	mEq/L
Cl	100–117	100–115	87–114	100–105	mEq/L
HCO_3	14–27	12–26	18–24	18–24	mM/L
Ca	6.1–11.6	8.6–10.5	6–9.9	9–11	mg/L
Mg	—	—	1.5–2.5	1.2–1.8	mEq/L
PO_4	5.4–10.9	5.6–7.9	3.0–8.7	4.0–5.5	mg/dl
Glucose	40–100	60–100	40–100	60–110	mg/dl
BUN	3.1–25.5	2.0–26.5	8–34	4–8	mg/dl
Creatinine	0.8–1.8	0.2–1.0	0.2–0.9	0.5–1.3	mg/dl
Osmolality			270–290	275–295	mOsm/kg
Bilirubin	<1	<2	<1	0.2–0.8	mg/dl
Alk. Phos.	100–150	—	100–150	30–205	IU/L
SGOT	<54	—	<54	5–20	IU/L
SGPT	<29	—	<29	4–25	IU/L
LDH	<84	—	<84	80–165	IU/L
Total Prot.	4.4–6.3	4.1–6.9	4.8–8.5	6.2–8.1	mg/dl
NH_3	14–65	—	14–65	45–80	µg/dl
Amylase	—	—	—	60–160	IU/L
Arterial pH	7.3–7.4	—	7.3–7.4	7.4–7.45	
PaO_2	50–80	—	50–80	60–100	mm Hg
$PaCO_2$	35–45	—	35–45	35–45	mm Hg

C — Trauma Checklists

Trauma Receiving Unit Checklist

Immobilize neck

Remove clothing

Endotracheal intubation if necessary

Perform 60-second examination

Apply ECG leads

Draw blood for CBC, type and crossmatch, amylase

Nasal oxygen

IV

Cutdown

Lateral x-ray of cervical spine

Insert Foley catheter and temperature probe

Insert nasogastric tube

Peritoneal lavage

Arterial line

Dress open wounds

Complete physical examination

Get history

Chest x-ray

Check laboratory results

Calculate Glasgow Coma Score and trauma score

List positive findings

Source: Kiwanis Pediatric Trauma Institute, 1985.

Glasgow Coma Scale

Best response	Stimulus	Score
Eye opening	Spontaneous	4
	To voice	3
	To pain	2
	None	1
Verbal	Oriented	5
	Confused	4
	Inappropriate words	3
	Incomprehensible sounds	2
	None	1
Motor	Obeys command	6
	Localizes pain	5
	Withdraws (pain)	4
	Flexion (pain)	3
	Extension (pain)	2
	None	1
Total		3–15

Trauma score

Scale	Finding	Score
Glasgow Coma Scale	14–15	5
	11–13	4
	8–10	3
	5–7	2
	3–4	1
Respiratory rate	10–24	4
	25–35	3
	>36	2
	1–9	1
	None	0
Respiratory expansion	Normal	1
	Retractive/none	0
Systolic blood pressure	>90 mm Hg	4
	70–89	3
	50–69	2
	0–49	1
	No Pulse	0
Capillary refill	Normal	2
	Delayed	1
	None	0
Total trauma score		1–16

Index

Index

A-V fistula, 231
Abdominal calcifications, 157
Abdominal injuries, 447
Abdominal masses, 127
due to NEC, 159
Abdominal pain, 291
Abscess, perianal, 347
Achalasia, 277
Acidosis
hyperchloremic, 171
troubleshooting, 28
Adrenal insufficiency, 182
Adrenal tumors, 429
Airway obstruction, 89
Alkalosis, troubleshooting, 29
Ambiguous genitalia, 181
adrenal insufficiency in, 182, 182f
Anal disorders, 347
fissure, 347
fistula, 348
stenosis, 171
warts, 348
Anesthesia, 21
Annular pancreas, 141
Anterior ectopic anus, 339, 342f
Anus
disorders of, 347
ectopic, anterior, 339
imperforate, 171, 172f
Apnea
due to GER, 270
troubleshooting, 30
Appendicitis, 317
Apple peel bowel, 149
Ascites, neonatal, 131
Assessment of operative risk, neonatal, 17
Atresia
biliary, 351
esophageal, 109
ileal, 149
rectal, 171
tracheal, 91
vaginal, 188

Battered child, 487
Biliary
ascites, 131
atresia, 351
hypoplasia, 355
Bladder aspiration, 507
Bleeding
GI, neonatal, 133
GI, older child, 299
troubleshooting, 32
Blood volume, 9
Body composition, 9, 100f
Bradycardia, troubleshooting, 34
Branchial cleft cyst, 214

Breast disease, 255
Bronchogenic cyst, 99
cervical, 216
Bronchomalacia, 91
Bronchoscopy, 241
for foreign bodies, 248
Burns, 479

Calcifications
abdominal, 157
scrotal, 157
Cancer, 393
Cardiac arrest, troubleshooting, 35
Cardiac function, neonatal, 12
Caustic ingestion, 279
Central venous catheter insertion, 496
Checklist
neonatal, preoperative, 18
trauma, 515
Chest injuries, 443
Chest tube, insertion of, 501, 502f
Child abuse, 487
Choanal atresia, 90
Cholecystitis, acalculous, 365
Choledochal cyst, 355
Cholelithiasis, 363
Chronic abdominal pain, 291
Chylothorax, 267
Chylous ascites, 131
Circumcision, 389
Cloacal anomalies, 188
Colitis
granulomatous, 325
ulcerative, 329
Colonic polyps, 335
Colostomy, 179
Condyloma acuminatum, perianal, 348
Conjoined twins, 191
Consent, preoperative, 18
Constipation, 339
Costs of care, neonatal, 7
Crohn's disease, 325
Cryptorchidism, 381
Cushing's syndrome, 429
Cutdown
radial artery, 494
venous, 495
Cyanosis, troubleshooting, 37
Cyst
branchial, 214
bronchogenic, 99
cervical, 216
choledochal, 355
dermoid, 214
hypopharyngeal, 90
lung, 99
mesenteric, 349
subglottic, 91
thyroglossal duct, 213

521

Cystic adenomatoid malformation, 99
Cystic fibrosis, 153
Cystic hygroma, 219, 220f

DIC, troubleshooting, 38
Dermoid cyst, 214
Diaphragmatic hernia, 103
Disseminated intravascular coagulation, troubleshooting, 38
Drug dosage, 511
Duhamel procedure, for Hirschsprung's disease, 168
Duodenal
  atresia, 141
  hematoma, 465
  ulcer, 305
Duplications, 311
Dyspnea, 89

ECMO, 107
Edema, troubleshooting, 40
Emergency operations, resuscitation for, 200
Empyema, 263
Encopresis, 340
Endorectal pull-through operation
  for Hirschsprung's disease, 168
  for ulcerative colitis, 332
Endoscopy, 241
Endotracheal intubation, 499
Enterocolitis
  due to Hirschsprung's disease, 165
  granulomatous, 325
  necrotizing, 159
Epiglottis, omega-shaped, 90
Esophageal
  atresia, 109
  varices, 358
Esophagitis, 269
Esophagoscopy, 243
Ethical considerations, 5
Exstrophy of the cloaca, 117

Fever, troubleshooting, 41
Fistula
  A-V, 231
  in-ano, 348
  tracheoesophageal, 109
    due to lye injury, 283
Fluid
  requirements, neonatal, 11
  therapy, child, 203
  therapy, neonatal postop, 23
Foreign bodies, 287
  airway, 247, 248f
Formulas
  components, 77t
  infant, 76t

GI bleeding, neonatal, 133
Gallbladder disease, 363
Gastroesophageal reflux, 269, 271f
Gastrografin enema, 154
Gastrointestinal
  bleeding, 299
  duplications, 311
  function, neonatal, 11

Gastroschisis, 117
Gastrostomy, 175
Gavage feedings, 12
Genetic counselling, 25
Genital injuries, 472
Gestational age
  estimation, 10
  small for, 9
Glasgow Coma Scale, 516
Granuloma, umbilical, 123
Granulomatous enterocolitis, 325

Head injuries, 439
Hemangioma, 231
  laryngeal, 90
  liver, 421
  of salivary gland, 215
  subglottic, 91
Hematoma
  duodenal, 465
Hemolymphangioma, 231
Hepatic
  function, neonatal, 12
  trauma, 455
  tumors, 421
Hepatoblastoma, 422
Hernia
  inguinal, 373
  umbilical, 125
Hirschsprung's disease, 165
  rectal biopsy for, 166
  Swenson's operation for, 168
  total-colon, 168
Hodgkin's disease, 413
Hydrocele, 374f, 379
Hydrometrocolpos, 188
Hymen, imperforate, 187
Hyperbilirubinemia, troubleshooting, 54
Hypercalcemia, troubleshooting, 42
Hyperchloremic acidosis, 171
Hyperglycemia, troubleshooting, 43
Hyperkalemia, troubleshooting, 44
Hypernatremia, troubleshooting, 45
Hyperthyroidism, 228
Hypocalcemia
  neonatal, 13
  troubleshooting, 46
Hypoglycemia, troubleshooting, 48
Hypokalemia, troubleshooting, 50
Hyponatremia, troubleshooting, 51
Hypopharyngeal cyst, 90
Hypothermia, 10
  troubleshooting, 53

Ileal atresia, 149
Ileostomy, 179
Imperforate anus, 171, 172f
Imperforate hymen, 187
Inguinal hernia, 373, 374f
Intersex, 181
Intestinal function, neontal, 11
  injuries, 465
  obstruction, neonatal, 137
  perforation, prenatal, 157
Intravenous fluid requirements, 203

Intubation, endotracheal, 49
Intussusception, 313, 314f

Jaundice, troubleshooting, 54
Jejunoileal atresia, 149
Jitters, troubleshooting, 57

Kernicterus, 54
Kidney
 function, neonatal, 13
 injuries, 475

Laboratory values, 514
Ladd's bands, 145
Laparoscopy, 244
Laryngeal hemangioma, 90
Laryngomalacia, 90
Laryngotracheoesophageal cleft, 91
Lethargy, troubleshooting, 58
Lingual thyroid, 90
Liver
 function, neonatal, 12
 injuries, 455
 tumors, 421
Lobar emphysema, 95
Lung cysts, 99
Lye ingestion, 279, 283f
Lymphadenitis
 cat-scratch, 212
 chronic, 211
 mycobacterial, 212
 suppurative, 211
Lymphadenopathy, cervical, 211
Lymphangioma, 221
 of salivary gland, 215
Lymphedema, 221
Lymphoma, non-Hodgkin's, 417

Macroglossia, 90
Malrotation, 145
Masses
 abdominal, 127
 mediastinal, 257
Meckel's diverticulum, 307, 308f
Meconium ileus, 153
 equivalent, 155
Meconium peritonitis, 157
Mediastinal masses, 257, 259f
Medullary carcinoma of thyroid, 227
Mesenteric cysts, 349
Midgut volvulus, 145
Monitoring, neonatal, postoperative, 23

NEC, 159
Nares, absent, 89
Neck masses, 211, 212f
Necrotizing enterocolitis, 159
Nephroblastoma (Wilms' tumor), 397
Neuroblastoma, 401
Non-Hodgkin's lymphoma, 417, 419f
Nutrition
 neonatal, 73
 total parenteral, 79

Oliguria, troubleshooting, 59
Omega-shaped epiglottis, 90

Omphalitis, 123
Omphalocele, 117
Omphalomesenteric duct, 123
Operation
 care during, neonatal, 21
 neonatal, preparation for, 15
 older child, preparation for, 197
 risk of, assessment in neonate, 17
Opisthotonos, 89
Ovarian tumors, 425

PFC, 107
Pancreas injuries, 459
Pancreatic pseudocyst, 463
Pancreatitis, 367
Papillary carcinoma of the thyroid, 227
Paraphimosis, 389
Parenteral nutrition, 79
Parents
 care of, neonatal, 24
 preoperative consent, 18
Patent urachus, 123
Pectus excavatum, 251
Peptic ulcer, 305
Perforation of intestine
 due to NEC, 159
 prenatal, 157
Perianal abscess, 347
Peritoneal lavage, 505, 506f
Persistent fetal circulation (PFC), 107
Pharyngeal (hypopharyngeal) cyst, 90
Pheochromocytoma, 430
Phimosis, 389
Physiology, neonatal, 9
Pierre Robin syndrome, 90
Pneumatocele, 99
Pneumatosis intestinalis, 159, 161f
Pneumothorax, 93
 traumatic, 444
Polyp
 colonic, 335
 umbilical, 123
Polyposis, 335
Portal hypertension, 357
Portoenterostomy, 354f
 for biliary atresia, 353
Postoperative care
 feeding, 75
 neonatal, 23
 older child, 203
Prematurity, 5, 9
Preoperative check list, neonatal, 18
Preparation for operation, neonate, 15
 older child, 197
Presacral teratoma, 406
Primary peritonitis, 323
Prolapse, rectal, 345
Pseudocyst
 intestinal, 157
 pancreatic, 463
Pull-through operation
 for Hirschsprung's disease, 168, 168f
 for imperforate anus, 173
 for ulcerative colitis, 331, 332f
Pulmonary function, neonatal, 12
Pyloric stenosis, 295, 296f

Radial artery cutdown, 494
Rectal
  atresia, 171
  biopsy for Hirschsprung's disease, 166
  prolapse, 345
Regional enteritis, 325
Renal
  function, neonatal, 13
  injuries, 475
Respiratory
  distress, 85
  distress, troubleshooting, 60
  function, neonatal, 12
Resuscitation
  massive GI bleeding, 301
  neonatal, 16
  preoperative, 200
Retrolental fibroplasia, 13
Retroperitoneal hematoma, 469
Rhabdomyosarcoma, 409
Risk, operative, assessment of in neonate, 17
Ruptured spleen, 451, 452f

Sacrococcygeal teratoma, 405
Salivary gland tumors, 215
Sarcoma botryoides, 410
Scrotal calcifications, 157
Seizures, troubleshooting, 62
Short-gut syndrome, 151
Shunts, portal, 359f
Siamese twins, 191
Small for gestational age (SGA), 9
Soave pull-through operation
  for Hirschsprung's disease, 168
  for ulcerative colitis, 331
Sphincterotomy, for Hirschsprung's disease, 168
Spleen injuries, 451
Splenectomy, 369
Stenosis
  pyloric, 295
  subglottic, 91
  tracheal, 91
Stridor, 89
Subglottic
  cyst, 91
  hemangioma, 91
  stenosis, 91
Surgery, neonatal, 5
Swenson's operation for Hirschsprung's disease, 168
Synechia vulvae, 187

TPN solutions, composition, 80t
Tachycardia, troubleshooting, 65
Temperature
  control during operation, 21
  regulation, 10
Teratoma, 405
  ovarian, 426
  presacral, 406
Testis
  torsion of, 385
  undescended, 381
Thermal neutrality, 10
Thoracentesis, 501

Thoracic trauma, 443
Thyroglossal duct cyst, 213
Thyroid
  lingual, 90
  medullary carcinoma of, 227
  nodules, 227
Thyroiditis, 228
Timing of operations, 17
Torsion of the testis, 385
Torticollis, 223, 224f
Total parenteral nutrition, 79
  composition of solutions for, 80t
Total-colon Hirschsprung's disease, 168
Tracheal
  atresia, 91
  stenosis, 91
Tracheobronchial trauma, 443
Tracheoesophageal fistula, 109
  due to lye injury, 283
Tracheomalacia, 91
Tracheostomy, 235
Transport, neonatal, 15
Trauma
  abdominal, 447
  burns, 479
  checklists, 515
  chest, 443
  child abuse, 487
  general principles, 435
  genital, 472
  head injuries, 439
  intestinal, 465
  kidney, 475
  liver, 455
  pancreas, 459
  retroperitoneal, 469
  score, 517
  spleen, 451
  thoracic, 443
  tracheobronchial, 443
  urinary, 471
Troubleshooting neonatal emergencies, 27–65
Tumors, 393
  adrenal, 429
  liver, 421
  mediastinal, 257
  ovarian, 425
  salivary gland, 215
  Wilms', 397

Ulcer, peptic, 305
Ulcerative colitis, 329, 332f
Umbilical
  anomalies, 123
  artery catheterization, 493
  granuloma, 123
  hernia, 125
  polyp, 123
Undescended testis, 381
Urachus
  cysts, sinuses, 123
  patent, 123
Urinary ascites, 131
Urinary tract injuries, 471
Urogenital sinus, 185

VACTERL syndrome, 109, 171
Vaginal
  anomalies, 187
  atresia, 188
Varices, esophageal, 358
Vascular access, 493
Vascular ring, 91
Ventilation, abnormalities of, 85

Ventilatory assistance, 67
Vitamin requirements, 74t
Vitelline duct, cyst, 123
Vocal cord paralysis, 90
Volvulus, midgut, 145

Water, total body, 9
Wilms' tumor, 397, 398f